BRITISH MILITARY
AND NAVAL MEDICINE,
1600–1830

THE WELLCOME SERIES
IN THE HISTORY OF MEDICINE

Forthcoming:

Control and the Therapeutic Trial:
Rhetoric and Experimentation in Britain, 1918–48

Martin Edwards

'A Cheap, Safe and Natural Medicine':
Religion, Medicine and Culture in John Wesley's Primitive Physic

Deborah Madden

The Wellcome Series in the History of Medicine series editors are
V. Nutton, M. Neve and R. Cooter.
Please send all queries regarding the series to Michael Laycock,
The Wellcome Trust Centre for the History of Medicine at UCL,
183 Euston Road, London NW1 2BE, UK.

BRITISH MILITARY
AND NAVAL MEDICINE,
1600–1830

Edited by Geoffrey L. Hudson

Amsterdam – New York, NY 2007

First published in 2007
by Editions Rodopi B. V., Amsterdam – New York, NY 2007.

Editions Rodopi B.V. © 2007

Design and Typesetting by Michael Laycock,
The Wellcome Trust Centre for the History of Medicine at UCL.
Printed and bound in The Netherlands by Editions Rodopi B. V.,
Amsterdam – New York, NY 2007.

Index by Howard Cooke.

British Library Cataloguing in Publication Data
A catalogue record for this book is available from the British Library
ISBN 978-90-420-2272-0

'British Military and Naval Medicine, 1600–1830 –
Amsterdam – New York, NY:
Rodopi. – ill.
(Clio Medica 81 / ISSN 0045-7183;
The Wellcome Series in the History of Medicine)

Front cover:

'Droll Doings No 29: Shiver my Timbers, Jack.'
© National Maritime Museum. See page 219 for further details.

© Editions Rodopi B. V., Amsterdam – New York, NY 2007
Printed in The Netherlands

All titles in the Clio Medica series (from 1999 onwards) are available to
download from the IngentaConnect website: http://www.ingentaconnect.com

Contents

List of Illustrations

List of Tables

3

Preface

This volume had its origins in a discussion between the editor and the late Professor Roy Porter, the editor's postdoctoral sponsor. They agreed on the need to publish and encourage further work in the field of pre-modern British military and naval medicine. Roy was a generous academic colleague and mentor, and this volume is dedicated to him. He is missed.

I thank the editors of *Clio Medica*, and to Michael Laycock at the Wellcome Trust Centre, for patience and assistance in preparing this work for press. In addition, I thank the external reviewers for their suggestions.

1

Introduction:
British Military and Naval Medicine, 1600–1830

Geoffrey L. Hudson

The introduction reviews the historiography of military and naval medicine for the period, provides an overview of the essays, and concludes that the volume highlights the value of challenging the inherited notion that military medicine was in all respects 'a good thing' for medicine and society. In addition, the essays in this volume tell us more about both how military and naval medicine were components of a wider social, economic, cultural and political framework, and how medicine was part of the process of militarisation.

'Few subjects in the history of medicine have been so poorly served as the relations between medicine and war', wrote Roger Cooter around a decade ago, 'serious research in this field has hardly begun'.[1] This rather sweeping verdict no longer fully applies – thanks in part to his own important studies, both empirical and critical;[2] and most scholars would accept that certain fields of the history of military medicine are now yielding a good harvest, especially in the modern period.[3]

How far that brighter picture applies to the subject of seventeenth- and eighteenth-century British military and naval medicine is perhaps more moot, with only a few recent exceptions. Official histories, and other works similarly rather traditional in their approaches, have been compiled and published during the last fifty years. These tend to focus on the pioneers of military and naval medicine and surgery, the development of career and administrative structures, as well as institutions. Most prominent among them include the indispensable first three volumes of *Medicine and the Navy* by J.J. Keevil (Vol. 1, 1200–1649, Vol. 2, 1649–1714) and C. Lloyd and J.L.S. Coulter (Vol. III, 1714–1815). For military medicine, the first volume of N. Cantlie's *A History of the Army Medical Department* is similarly a foundation work for those interested in developments in the nature of administration, medical personnel, and treatments in the period.[4] Certain sources have been made more easily available, with perhaps the most useful volume for students being C. Lloyd's *The Health of Seamen,* which includes well-chosen selections from the works of James Lind, Gilbert Blane, and Thomas Trotter.[5]

Despite a new interest in the history of war itself, and certain innovative general military and naval histories – N.A.M. Rodger's *The Wooden World: An Anatomy of the Georgian Navy* springs to mind[6] – there have been few published monographs or path-breaking works of synthesis for Britain. This scholarly *lacuna* is reflected, for example, in Lindsay Granshaw's chapter on 'The Rise of the Modern Hospital in Britain' (1992) which does not even mention the enormous military and naval hospitals that developed in Britain during this period, let alone discuss their influence on medicine and society.[7] This scholarly gap in the literature is also apparent in history course offerings.

More recently, a contributor to this volume, Eric Gruber von Arni, has published a monograph entitled *Hospital Care and the British Standing Army, 1660–1714* (2006)[8] which investigates the nature of medicine and nursing in hospitals for soldiers using a wide variety of sources during an important developmental period. In addition, Laurence Brockliss, John Cardwell and Michael Moss have recently published *Nelson's Surgeon: William Beatty, Naval Medicine, and the Battle of Trafalgar* (2005).[9] Here, the authors draw on the work of Lloyd and Coulter, as well as an ongoing prosopographical study of nine hundred army and naval surgeons, to analyse the nature of the naval medical service (education, training, work) in the late-eighteenth and early-nineteenth centuries. They also explore the role of naval medicine, including preventative medicine, in the Napoleonic Wars, but more work clearly needs to be done.

The relative paucity of British work in this area is in marked contrast to work on the Continent. This is reflected in Ole Peter Grell's chapter on 'War, Medicine and the Military Revolution' in Peter Elmer's recent textbook for the Open University entitled *The Healing Arts: Health, Disease and Society in Europe, 1500–1800* (2004), where Grell relies on contributions to the literature from scholars such as Geoffrey Parker.[10] In *The Four Horsemen of the Apocalypse: Religion, War, Famine and Death in Reformation Europe* (2000), Grell, with co-author Andrew Cunningham, discusses war and medicine within the overall context of an argument for the pervasiveness of a belief in the apocalypse, *circa* 1490–1648. In particular they argue that:

> [E]arly modern warfare with its extensive use of guns and gunpowder caused suffering and injuries on an unprecedented and horrific scale, which was more often not beyond any relief. As such it also affected the views and attitudes of the leading thinkers and theologians of the day.[11]

War and medicine lost their apocalyptic connotations with the 1648 Peace of Westphalia and the end of the wars of religion. Grell and Cunningham provide an interesting example of how military medicine can be incorporated into wider social, intellectual, and political frameworks.

Arguably the most prominent book on which Grell relies is *The Medical World of Early Modern France* (1997) by Laurence Brockliss and Colin Jones.[12] A truly impressive synthesis of their own work and that of other French historians, this book deals with important and illuminating aspects of the relationship between war, medicine, and society, among many other topics. They argue that, contrary to the arguments made by Erwin Ackerknecht and Michel Foucault, medicine was transformed well before 1789, and that military medicine was part of that evolution:

> The armed forces proved a testing ground for the content of medical and surgical training. Thus although historians conventionally date the 'birth of the clinic' from the 1790s, many of the elements of the approaches associated with that development – teaching practice, an emphasis on bedside medicine, the routine practice of autopsies, and a concern with medical statistics – had all been found in Ancien Régime military hospitals.[13]

In addition, they maintain that naval and military health services also served as laboratories for experimenting with preventative and environmental medicine. They also point specifically to the Hôtel des Invalides for disabled ex-servicemen, established in 1670, as the pioneer of the medicalised hospital,[14] and it is no accident that three of the papers in this volume focus to a greater or lesser extent on the British Royal Hospitals for ex-servicemen at Greenwich and Chelsea, established in the late-seventeenth century.

There are good, or at least plausible, reasons for the relative lack of attention to military and naval medicine for Britain in this period. For one thing, the Hanoverian British Army was not organised on such a connected and centralised footing as its counterparts in other parts of Europe, notably France, Prussia, and Austria. In terms of institutions, there is not the equivalent bureaucracy, nor is there the same continuity, cohesion and clarity in the archives. The occasionally hand-to-mouth nature of the British Army enterprise, together with its atomisation and localism, make research into various aspects of it more arduous.

Research and its dissemination are also rendered more difficult by one peculiar and unfortunate circumstance. The most important reformer of military medicine in Georgian Britain was arguably Sir John Pringle, a President of the Royal Society and Physician General to the Army. The Scottish physician kept extensive and well-organised records of his thinking and his endeavours. On his death he bequeathed them to the Royal College of Physicians of Edinburgh, on condition that they should never be published. The College continues to uphold the conditions of that bequest, allowing consultation but not publication; and the sad, if unavoidable, result is that Pringle's key role in reforming and transforming British medicine remains – and is likely to remain – less than perfectly understood.[15]

A third reason may be cited. Eighteenth-century British military medicine has always worn the mark of comedy – *black* comedy. In this case, cultural tradition has perhaps inhibited research. With regard to medicine at large, Georgian Britain has been popularly and jocularly characterised as an 'age of agony', full of ignorant apothecaries, proud physicians, sporting extravagant wigs and gold-tipped canes, and – worst of all – butcher-like surgeons, sadistically indulging in excruciating bleedings, blisterings and amputations.[16] This is the epithet which has been applied almost universally to medicine on the battlefield, in camps and on board ship.

One reason for this is that pain, medical cruelty and ineffectuality were so habitually exploited in Georgian fiction for comic or sentimental effect. Take Tobias Smollett's first novel, *Roderick Random*. In 1740, poverty led the young Scottish surgeon to seek employment as second surgeon's mate on board *HMS Chichester*, about to be sent to reinforce Vernon in the West Indies during the War of Jenkin's Ear.

Smollett was soon to project his experiences onto his hero, Roderick Random. To obtain a warrant as surgeon's mate, Random is advised to go to Surgeons' Hall. There, he is summoned by a beadle before a table of grim-faced examiners who inquire after his qualifications and quiz him: 'If during an engagement at sea, a man should be brought to you with his head shot off, how would you behave?' The examination ends with a demand for a five shillings fee.[17]

Random is subsequently dragged onto *HMS Thunder*, whose Captain, Oakum, has a simple philosophy: 'Harkee, sir, I'll have no sick people on board, by God!' Shown down to the surgeon's mess, a square about six feet wide, surrounded with medicine chests and a canvas screen, a shock awaits him: 'I was much less surprised that people should die on board, than that any sick person should recover'.[18]

A sick parade follows, dominated by Oakum's denial. So when the subservient surgeon, Mackshane, examines the first fever-stricken patient, he protests the man is perfectly fit 'and the captain delivered him over to the boatswain's mate, with orders that he should receive a round dozen at the gangway immediately for counterfeiting himself sick'. Truth? Or just a good yarn? Throughout his career, Smollett seemingly rejoiced in exposing the shortcomings of military and other sorts of medicine, evidently understanding very well the psychology of black humour.[19]

Smollett's military doctors are worse than the disease. In another classic fictional portrayal of war-inflicted wounds, it is not the medical attendants who can take much credit for the cure. Laurence Sterne tells us in *Tristram Shandy* of his character, who had been wounded in the groin at the seige of Namur:

> Whoever has read Hippocrates, or Dr James Mackenzie, and has considered well the effects which the passions and affections of the mind have upon the digestion... may easily conceive what sharp paroxysms and exacerbations of his wound my uncle Toby must have undergone...[20]

As a man of feeling, 'My uncle Toby could not philosophize upon it; – 'twas enough he felt it was so'; and such feelings led to a remarkable self-cure:

> He was one morning lying upon his back in his bed, the anguish and nature of the wound upon his groin suffering him to lie in no other position, when a thought came into his head, that if he could purchase such a thing, and have it pasted down upon a board, as a large map of the fortifications of the town and citadel of Namur, with its environs, it might be a means of giving him ease.

> [...] When my uncle Toby got his map of Namur, he began immediately to apply himself to the study of it; for nothing being of more importance to him that his recovery, and his recovery depending, as you have read, upon the passion and affections of his mind, it behoved him to take the nicest care to make himself master of his subject.

> With the aid of Gobesius's military architecture and pyroballogy, translated from the Flemish, ...my uncle Toby was able to cross the Maes and Sambre; make diversions as far as Vauban's line, the abbey of Salsines, &c. and give his visitors as distinct a history of each of their attacks, as of that of the gate of St Nicolas, where he had the honour to receive his wound.

The old soldier, it will be noted, grew obsessed with historical research.

> [M]y uncle began to break in upon the daily regularity of a clean shirt, – to dismiss his barber unshaven, – and to allow his surgeon scarce time sufficient to dress his wound.... When, lo! – all of a sudden... he began to sigh heavily for his recovery.[21]

Finally, Toby comes up with the true solution, or cure, which is a full-scale model of the seige, erected at the cost of the ruination of his bowling green. The wound heals, a true self-cure.

The story of Uncle Toby and the healing of his wound might be said to reflect one of the themes which have come to the fore in the new, and mainly social, history of medicine in Britain during the long eighteenth century which grew up during the 1980s and '90s: the agency of the sick person in orchestrating his or her own therapy.[22] Alongside this – the 'patients' view' – various other threads and themes have been formulated and followed. There have been attempts by historians of military medicine to get away from Whiggish, heroic and teleological histories, and a new insistence can be heard upon avoiding anachronism in interpretations of the meanings of terms – 'antiseptic' for instance. A number of historians have attempted to apply the insights and categories of Foucauldian inquiry – notions of disciplinarity, the 'gaze', or the pre-modern hospital. A distinguished example of such reinterpretations is Christopher Lawrence's 'Disciplining Disease: Scurvy, the Navy, and Imperial Expansion, 1750–1825'.[23] In that article, Lawrence, without at all debunking the importance of James Lind, shows the importance of a true grasp of the story of scurvy, of recovering the historical meanings of terms easily misunderstood through conflation with today's usages (for instance, 'putrefaction'), and of reconstructing earlier notions of medical institutions. While drawing on Foucault, Lawrence, like Jones, also challenges the Foucauldian chronological emphasis on rapid 'medicalisation' in the late-eighteenth and early-nineteenth century Paris clinic.[24] Lawrence highlights the significance of earlier developments in British naval medicine, including the gradual evolution of ideas and practices, such as the medical discipline of anonymous populations onboard ship, the rise of preventative medicine, routine observation, as well as regularised examination and punishment. Naval medicine influenced, and was influenced by, these changes – in forums such as the Royal Society – and was affected by wider social processes, such as the development of class-consciousness.

Lawrence is part of another important move in historical scholarship since the mid-1970s: the urge to break down the walls sequestrating the history of British military medicine. Peter Mathias and, later, Hal Cook and others[25] have argued that developments in military and naval medicine had a great impact on the nature of civilian medical care. Peter Mathias examines medicine, the armed forces, and public health in the late-eighteenth century. He notes that the military spent a large component of public and national monies, and that ever-greater numbers of physicians and surgeons were employed in the naval and military medical services. These services had unique institutional conditions – an authoritarian community – and purposes – military effectiveness via manpower management – that enabled military medics to apply Baconian scientific practices. Mass observation and experimentation led men like John Pringle, Thomas Trotter and Gilbert

Blane to promote within the services and in society more generally the value of preventative medicine – cleanliness, ventilation, clean water, as well as good nutrition and clothing. Mathias argues that these ideas had an impact on hospital practice and public health over time, especially by the mid-nineteenth century: to study the work of eighteenth-century military medicine 'is to stand in the hills observing streams from which great rivers were eventually sustained'.[26]

Hal Cook in his essay 'Practical Medicine and the British Armed Forces after the "Glorious Revolution"' is concerned with the impact of military medicine on medicine itself. He argues that military medicine had an emphasis on identifying diseases as entities and developing corresponding – and quick – medical and surgical cures for the masses in the forces. This was in contrast to traditional learned medicine that sought to emphasise physic and the individual and his or her own particular disease. In the military, it was simply not possible nor desirable to apply humoral therapeutics for each and every serviceman, based as it was on intimate knowledge of the patient and the course of his own disease. Cook argues that military medicine over several decades legitimised medical empiricism and the development of standardised diagnosis and treatment. It did so via reform of military medical institutions, with the move to take on board the clinical ideas of Thomas Sydenham – the clinical emphasis on observation, note-taking, and the identification of disease from symptoms. In doing so, Cook argues, military medicine not only trained new doctors – creating many career opportunities – but more crucially 'inculcated in them certain medical values'.[27]

If the history of eighteenth-century British military medicine is not yet fully ablaze, there are sparks of life. Many of the themes developed by Mathias, Cook, and Lawrence influence the questions explored by the contributors to this volume. A number focus, to a lesser or greater degree, on the effect of military medicine on wider developments: architecture, nursing, the medical profession, therapeutics, and domestic hospitals. Several contributors concentrate on the ways in which military medicine allowed for experimentation on, and observation of, subjects, and the impact of this development on medicine in the period.

The essays in this volume have been divided up along broad thematic and chronological lines: military and naval medicine in an imperial context (James D. Alsop, 1600–1800; Paul E. Kopperman, 1753–88; Mark Harrison, 1750–1830); military and naval hospital nursing and medicine in Britain (Eric Gruber von Arni, 1642–60; Philip R. Mills, *c.*1714–1800); naval medicine (Patricia Kathleen Crimmin, 1700–1800; Margarette Lincoln, 1750–1815); as well as military and naval medicine, the state and

13

society (Christine Stevenson, long-eighteenth century; Geoffrey L. Hudson, early-eighteenth century).

Military and naval medicine in an imperial context

With the growth of an Empire came the development of military medical services in a new context.[28] Three contributors address this theme explicitly. J.D. Alsop discusses 'Warfare and the Creation of British Imperial Medicine, 1600–1800', reviewing the literature of British naval and imperial medicine. He observes that very little was published before 1680 and that the key growth in the literature was concomitant with the wars of the late-seventeenth and early-eighteenth centuries, when the Navy started to maintain a regular fleet overseas. The growth of the literature thereafter followed major imperial wars and was focused on the needs of state in war; white, young males – servicemen – were the subjects of attention – with women invisible. Prescriptions for cures were universal, empirical, and economical, and the need to experiment on servicemen to develop remedies was recommended. There was a Hippocratic emphasis on the environment (the dangers of hot climate) and a perceived need to regulate and educate servicemen; their hygiene, diet, sexual activities and drinking proclivities.

Paul E. Kopperman examines 'The British Army in North America and the West Indies, 1755–83' drawing on a database of over eight hundred medical officers, regimental returns, lists of drugs used, and contemporary correspondence and publications. He provides an analytical overview of the operational structure, personnel, hospital and regimental systems of army medical practice in these colonies. Health and medical practice varied depending upon location (Canada/Caribbean), season (campaigning/ garrison duty), and time of year. For effective medicine, what was crucial was co-operation between medical and general officers. Practice was influenced by Pringle – avoidance of swamps, preference for open airy conditions – and medics were active in arguing for the benefits of prevention (cheaper, improved fighting effectiveness). Preventative treatments employed included proper rest, food and exercise, hygiene and sanitation campaigns. Scurvy treatments included fresh greens and spruce beer. Experimentation was cautiously employed. Kopperman also sees army practitioners being at the forefront of a move towards moderate therapeutics, including a move away from bleeding and expulsive drugs by medical officers in the West Indies.

Mark Harrison examines the treatment of fevers and the emergence of tropical therapeutics in British India, 1750–1830. He provides an overview of the size – considerable – and structure of the East India Company's medical establishment. It was noted for innovation and experimentation, tested economical mass remedies and in so doing objectified its patients (post-mortem examination were common). Harrison comments that the service's control of its patients was important and that much of this activity prefigured the birth of the clinical–anatomical medicine of Paris of the 1790s.

He also argues that the sheer size of the East India Company's medical services enabled it to develop different ideas and treatment than those current in Britain. A unique disease environment created a distinctive medical culture: tropical medicine. Harrison focuses in particular on the treatment of fever – for which there was a high incidence – and hospital records from Calcutta. The climate was blamed for fever, with medics influenced by Pringle's notion of the effect of adverse atmospheric conditions on the body. In India the particular focus was on malfunction of the liver, with hot weather making it over active, stimulating the creation of too much bile. The dominant treatment was purgation via mercury – in the period 1790–1830 – with bloodletting frowned upon. This treatment also spread to the West Indies. Harrison stresses that the dominance of this method was due to the ability of senior military officers to impose their views on their juniors. Military medicine was therefore not simply innovative, experimental empiricism; it was also dogmatic and conformist, with senior officers able to control the drugs and therapies employed.

Military and naval hospital nursing and medicine in Britain

Eric Gruber von Arni examines military nursing of servicemen and ex-servicemen during the mid-seventeenth century. The chronological focus is significant, given that very little work has been done on nursing, let alone military nursing, in England prior to the nineteenth century. In his essay Gruber von Arni uses Commonwealth Exchequer papers from the Long Parliament's Committee for Sick and Wounded Soldiers to examine nursing in the State's Ely House and Savoy hospitals. Gruber von Arni sets the context by examining the numbers treated, the nature of contemporary military treatment by surgeons and physicians, and the extant evidence for medical and nursing practice at these hospitals, including the provision of bedding, heat, treatment, food, and activities for the patients. His conclusion is that the quality was far superior to that assumed by many historians, and he encourages further research.

Philip R. Mills focuses on the treatment of hernias at the Greenwich Hospital in the mid-eighteenth century, in his chapter on experimentation and innovation within British military medicine. Hernias were prevalent among servicemen, drawn as they were from among the poor and malnourished. In service, they often lacked proper food and exercise, and often drank too much and moved too little. Contemporary medical practice accepted that the rupture could not be cured, and a palliative approach was taken – rest, trusses, better diet. For the military, this was unacceptable:

wastage rates due to ruptures were high, and seasoned servicemen were a valuable commodity. Certain military patrons were prepared, therefore, to support experiments conducted by medical entrepreneurs prepared to offer cures rather than simply chronic care. Mills uses two excellent examples to illustrate that experimentation was a very contentious activity, reliant on the whims of patronage and war-time budgets. Although military hospitals provided a good place to engage in such experimentation – with patients subject to discipline unlike in civilian practice – it was contested hotly by other military medics, who were ultimately successful in ending the experiments. Experimentation was possible within the military framework, but was not necessarily efficacious and could be successfully contested.

Naval medicine

Patricia Kathleen Crimmin questions whether British naval health improved over the course of the eighteenth century, based on her ongoing study of the Sick and Hurt Board – the Navy's administration body responsible for Navy hospitals, medical care and food. Over the course of the century the Board created the national military hospitals of Haslar and Portsmouth – moving away from a reliance on private houses and inns – and responded to complaints about improper medical care. In addition, it sought to discover cures for common ailments such as ruptures, scurvy, and the flux, and did so by encouraging experimentation and the development of cheap universal cures. It also strove to provide healthy ventilation, clothing, cleanliness, as well as adequate and appropriate food – for example, development of portable soup. Overall, Crimmin argues that prevention rather than the development of cures was very much the focus.

Crimmin also argues that Mathias placed too much emphasis on the authoritarian nature of the Royal Navy in the eighteenth century. She maintains that each ship was ruled differently by its own officers – there was remarkably little central direction – especially early in the century. It was only in the late-eighteenth century when this changed – with increased authoritarian central control and discipline. With that change the various measures that the Board advocated were increasingly implemented, and health improved.

Margarette Lincoln focuses on the interrelationship between naval medicine and broader society in 'The Medical Profession and Representations of the Navy, 1750–1815'. Lincoln discusses medical representations of the Navy in the late-eighteenth century, utilising medical publications and the popular *Gentleman's Magazine* and *The Times*, and reveals that naval medicine was a matter of keen debate, as it was perceived as important for the country. She also argues that publications were used to promote the status of Navy surgeons. Navy servicemen were represented in

16

contradictory ways: as a tool of Empire, heroes worthy of care for their service to their country (hospitals, pensions) and as a source of contagion and ill discipline in need of paternal attention from officers and medics. There was perceived to be a role for physicians and surgeons in improving the naval medical service, via observation and prevention, and an increasing emphasis on statistics that reveal an increasingly caring and effective Navy.

Military and naval medicine, the state and society

Christine Stevenson's book on early British hospital architecture is a good example of breaking down the walls separating medicine from society; she stresses the similarities and continuities between the civilian and the military.[29] In her essay in this volume, Stevenson critically reviews military and naval architectural history, focusing largely on late-seventeenth and eighteenth centuries, placing the experience within the wider European and North American context. The hospitals examined include those for the sick and wounded in the Empire and later at home (Minorca, Jamaica, Gibraltar, Haslar, Plymouth), and those built for long-term chronic cases (Kilmainham in Dublin, Greenwich and Chelsea). She includes consideration of how matters of state affected architecture, arguing that a concrete manifestation of the military revolution included the growth of royal control over armed forces. Her main focus is very much on how medical theory affected architecture, and in particular on how John Pringle – and subsequently his disciples – in the context of the fever epidemics of 1739–40, synthesised and promoted earlier ideas about how environment – camp, ship, hospital, and gaol – created fever, and the necessity of promoting circulation of air, and, in a later edition of his work, separation of patients.

John Brewer and Linda Colley have echoed Mathias, arguing that historians would be wise to focus on the military aspects of the eighteenth-century British state. This argument has been picked up by scholars, such as Joanna Innes, who point to the domestic face of the military–fiscal state, including provision for sick and disabled ex-servicemen.[30]

Geoffrey L. Hudson takes a look at the domestic face when he examines the minutes of the council, which administered discipline at the Royal Greenwich Hospital for ex-sailors. In doing so, he analyses the nature of care in the early-eighteenth century, including the ways in which chronically disabled patients experienced the hospital. Traditionally, historians have argued that Greenwich was architecturally magnificent, providing both excellent care and a happy environment for its patients – in contrast to the seventeenth-century county system for ex-servicemen which preceded it. An examination of the extent of provision in the county system, and Greenwich's inner life challenges this assumption. Many more were provided for in the seventeenth century than has been assumed by scholars. In addition, Greenwich was a 'reverse' institution, one in which the ex-servicemen were closely regulated and treated like unruly visitors, with only the officers and medics given free movement and obvious influence. Initially, the inner life of the Hospital owed much to almshouse and shipboard models. Increasingly, however, medical considerations became influential, and a new type of institution took shape. Physicians and surgeons were actively involved in its governance, intervening to change the nature of punishment, promoting ventilation and dietary changes, and agitating, successfully, for the creation of a separate infirmary. In addition, a medical monopoly was imposed, and military medics took the opportunity to experiment and observe continuous subjects. Hudson includes consideration of the ways patients negotiated the terms of their incarceration. The men did negotiate their position in the institution with some limited success, both as individuals and in combination. Overall, however, Hudson concludes that central provision in the Royal Hospital was problematic for disabled ex-servicemen, and that, as with Colin Jones' analysis of the French situation, hospitals for disabled veterans were police operations first and foremost. Greater discipline and bureaucratic control of ex-serviceman were also visited on serving men, both when they were well and when they were sick. The state had an increased interest in controlling its men, as well as conserving them.[31]

Conclusion

With the move to standing armies and navies in this period came permanent military medical establishments and a corresponding shift from the management of disease in individuals to groups. Prevention, discipline, and surveillance brought results and career opportunities for physicians and surgeons. These developments had an impact on medicine and society, and were in turn influenced by them. The essays in this volume explore these and related developments and point to opportunities for further research. More work on military nursing and other health care providers is needed, for example. The focus on the long eighteenth century, while positive, must be balanced by more work on earlier periods. The so-called monopoly of military medicine and the authoritarian structures within the military were complex. At times, they were successfully contested. At other times, they imposed changes that cannot be characterised as improvements. Overall, this volume, following on from the ideas of Roger Cooter and others, highlights the value of challenging the inherited notion that military medicine was in all respects 'a good thing' for medicine and society.[32] Furthermore, medicine and war were, indeed, components of a wider social, economic, cultural, and political framework. Medicine was part of the process of militarisation. Continued research is needed and will tell us more about the history of the development of institutions, medical practice, the relationship between medicine and society, and much more besides.

Notes

1. R. Cooter, 'War and Modern Medicine', in W.F. Bynum and R. Porter (eds), *Companion Encyclopedia of the History of Medicine* (London: Routledge, 1993), 1536–73: 1536.

2. R. Cooter, *Surgery and Society in Peace and War: Orthopaedics and the Organization of Modern Medicine, 1880–1948* (Basingstoke: Macmillan Press, 1993); see also, R. Cooter, 'Medicine and the Goodness of War', *Canadian Bulletin of Medical History*, 12 (1990), 637–47; R. Cooter, 'Of War and Epidemics: Unnatural Couplings, Problematic Conceptions', *Social History of Medicine*, 16, 2 (2003), 283–302.

3. This is especially the case for the modern period. See R. Cooter, M. Harrison and S. Sturdy, *War, Medicine and Modernity* (London: Sutton, 1998) and the review article by M. Harrision, 'The Medicalization of War: The Militarization of Medicine', *Social History of Medicine*, 9, 2 (1996), 267–76. For another overview see M. Harrison, 'Medicine and the Management of Modern Warfare', *History of Science*, 34 (1996), 379–410. An instance of a particularly strong field is that of histories of shell-shock: see for instance P. Leese, *Shell Shock: Traumatic Neurosis and the British Soldiers of the First World War* (London: Palgrave Macmillan, 2002) and P. Barham, *Forgotten Lunatics of the Great War* (New Haven: Yale University Press, 2004).

4. J.J. Keevil, *Medicine and the Navy, 1200-1900: Vol. 1, 1200–1649* (Edinburgh: Livingstone, 1957); J.J. Keevil, *Medicine and the Navy, 1200–1900, Vol. II, 1649–1714* (Edinburgh: Livingstone, 1958); C. Lloyd and J.L.S. Coulter, *Medicine and the Navy 1200-1900: Vol. III: 1714-1815* (Edinburgh: Livingstone, 1961); N. Cantlie, *A History of the Army Medical Department*, 2 vols (Edinburgh: Churchill Livingstone, 1974). See also, F.H. Garrison, *Notes on the History of Military Medicine* (Washington: Association of Military Surgeons, 1922); R.C. Engelman and R.J.T. Joy, *Two Hundred Years of Military Medicine* (Fort Detrick: US Army Medical Department, 1975); 'The Medical Service' in C.G. Cruickshank, *Elizabeth's Army*, 2nd ed. (Oxford: Oxford University Press, 1966), 174–88; S. Selwyn, 'Sir John Pringle: Hospital Reformer, Moral Philosopher and Pioneer of Antiseptics', *Medical History*, 10, 3 (1966), 266–74; R.L. Blanco, 'Henry Marshall (1775–1851) and the Health of the British Army', *Medical History*, 14, 3 (1970), 260–76; R.L. Blanco, 'The Soldier's Friend: Sir Jeremiah Fitzpatrick, Inspector of Health for Land Forces' *Medical History*, 20, 4 (1976), 402–21; J. Watt, 'Some Forgotten Contributions of Naval Surgeons', *Journal of the Royal Society of Medicine*, 78, 9 (1985), 753–62. Some more

recent examples: G.C. Cook, 'Influence of Diarrhoeal Disease on Military and Naval Campaigns', *Journal of the Royal Society of Medicine*, 94, 2 (2001), 95–7; H. Ellis, 'John Hunter's Teachings on Gunshot Wounds', *Journal of the Royal Society of Medicine*, 94, 1 (2001), 43–5; M.H. Kaufman, *Surgeons at War: Medical Arrangements for the Treatment of the Sick and Wounded in the British Army during the Late Eighteenth and Nineteenth Centuries* (Westwood, CT: Greenwood, 2001). A recent survey in this tradition, but less well done and on occasion unreliable: R.A. Gabriel and K.S. Metz, *A History of Military Medicine, Vol. 2: From the Renaissance through Modern Times* (New York: Greenwood Press, 1992). Popular, recent, heroic and teleological treatments: D.I. Harvie, *Limeys: The True Story of One Man's War against Ignorance, the Establishment, and the Deadly Scurvy* (Phoenix Mill, UK: Sutton, 2002) and S.R. Bown, *Scurvy: How a Surgeon, a Mariner and a Gentleman Solved the Greatest Medical Mystery of the Age of Sail* (Toronto: Thomas Allen, 2003).

5. C. Lloyd (ed.), *The Health of Seamen, Selections from the Works of Dr James Lind, Sir Gilbert Blane and Dr Thomas Trotter* (London: Navy Records Society, 1965). More recently excerpts from a number of naval surgeon's medical journals were published in B. Lavery (ed.), *Shipboard Life and Organization, 1731–1815* (Aldershot: Ashgate, 1998).

6. N.A.M. Rodger, *The Wooden World: An Anatomy of the Georgian Navy* (London: Collins, 1986).

7. L. Granshaw, 'The Rise of the Modern Hospital in Britain', in A. Wear (ed), *Medicine in Society: Historical Essays* (Cambridge: Cambridge University Press, 1992), 197–218.

8. E. Gruber von Arni, *Hospital Care and the British Standing Army, 1660–1714* (Aldershot: Ashgate, 2006).

9. L. Brockliss, J. Cardwell and M. Moss, *Nelson's Surgeon: William Beatty, Naval Medicine, and the Battle of Trafalgar* (Oxford: Oxford University Press, 2005).

10. O. P. Grell, 'War, Medicine and the Military Revolution,' in P. Elmer (ed.), *The Healing Arts: Health, Disease and Society in Europe, 1500–1800* (Manchester: Manchester University Press, 2004), 257–83; Grell greatly draws on G. Parker, *The Army of Flanders and the Spanish Road 1567–1659*, 2nd edn (Cambridge: Cambridge University Press, 2004, 1st edn 1974).

11. A. Cunningham and O.P. Grell, *The Four Horsemen of the Apocalypse: Religion, War, Famine and Death in Reformation Europe* (Cambridge: Cambridge University Press, 2000), 136–7.

12. L. Brockliss and C. Jones, *The Medical World of Early Modern France* (Oxford: Oxford University Press, 1997).

13. *Ibid.*, 692. See also E.H. Ackerknecht, *Medicine at the Paris Hospital, 1794–1848* (Baltimore: Johns Hopkins, 1967); M. Foucault, A. Sheridan

trans., *The Birth of the Clinic: An Archaeology of Medical Perception* (London: Tavistock, 1973); and C. Jones, 'The Construction of the Hospital Patient in Early Modern France' in N. Finzsch and R. Jutte (eds), *Institutions of Confinement: Hospitals, Asylums, and Prisons in Western Europe and North America, 1500–1950* (Cambridge: Cambridge University Press, 1996), 55–74.

14. *Ibid.*, 689–90.
15. See J. Pringle, *Observations on the Nature and Cure of Hospital and Jayl-Fevers* (London, 1750), and *Observations on the Diseases of the Army*, 4th edn (London, 1764).
16. G. Williams, *The Age of Agony: The Art of Healing c.1700–1800* (London: Constable, 1975); significantly, Williams headed his book about the nineteenth century, *The Age of Miracles: Medicine and Surgery in the Nineteenth Century* (London: Constable, 1981).
17. T. Smollett, *Roderick Random*, David Blewitt (ed.), (Harmondsworth: Penguin, 1995 [1748]), 92.
18. *Ibid.*, 154, 143.
19. *Ibid.*, 161; A. Douglas, *Uneasy Sensations: Smollett and the Body* (Chicago: University of Chicago Press, 1995); G.S. Rousseau, *Tobias Smollett: Essays of Two Decades* (Edinburgh: Edinburgh University Press, 1982); J.F. Sena, 'Smollett's Matthew Bramble and the Tradition of the Physician–Satirist', *Papers on Language and Literature*, xi (1975), 380–96.
20. L. Sterne, *The Life and Opinions of Tristram Shandy*, Graham Petrie (ed.) (Harmondsworth: Penguin, 1967), 90f.; D. Furst, 'Sterne and Physick: Images of Health and Disease in *Tristram Shandy*' (PhD Diss., Columbia University, 1974); R. Porter, 'Against the Spleen', in V. Grosvenor Myer (ed.), *Laurence Sterne: Riddles and Mysteries* (London and New York: Vision, 1984), 84–99; L. Landa, 'The Shandean Homunculus: The Background of Sterne's "Little Gentleman"', in C. Camden (ed.) *Restoration and Eighteenth-Century Literature: Essays in Honour of Alan Dugald McKillop* (Chicago: Chicago University Press, 1963), 49–68; J. Stedmond, *The Comic Art of Laurence Sterne* (Toronto: Toronto University Press, 1967). It should be remembered that Sterne himself was a soldier's son: O.P. James, *The Relation of Tristram Shandy to the Life of Sterne* (The Hague: Mouton, 1966).
21. Sterne, *ibid.*, 111.
22. L. McCray Beier, 'In Sickness and in Health: A Seventeenth Century Family Experience', in R. Porter (ed.), *Patients and Practitioners* (Cambridge: Cambridge University Press, 1985), 101–28; L. McCray Beier, *Sufferers and Healers: The Experience of Illness in Seventeenth-Century England* (London: Routledge & Kegan Paul, 1987); R. Porter (ed.), *Patients and Practitioners: Lay Perceptions of Medicine in Pre-Industrial Society* (Cambridge: Cambridge University Press, 1985), 283–314; R. Porter and D. Porter, *In Sickness and in*

Health: The British Experience 1650–1850 (London: Fourth Estate, 1988); D. Porter and R. Porter, *Patient's Progress: Doctors and Doctoring in Eighteenth-Century England* (Cambridge: Polity Press, 1989).

23. C. Lawrence, 'Disciplining Disease: Scurvy, the Navy, and Imperial Expansion, 1750–1825', in D.P. Miller and P.H. Reill (eds), *Visions of Empire: Voyages, Botany, and Representations of Nature* (Cambridge: Cambridge University Press, 1996), 80–106.

24. For the Paris clinic thesis see, in addition to Ackerknecht and Foucault, *op. cit.* (note 12), T. Gelfand, *Professionalizing Modern Medicine: Paris Surgeons and Medical Science and Institutions in the Eighteenth Century* (Westport: Greenwood, 1980), and more recently, C. Hannaway and A. La Berge, *Constructing Paris Medicine* (Amsterdam: Rodopi, 1998).

25. See also J. Riley, *The Eighteenth Century Campaign to Avoid Diseases* (Basingstoke: Macmillan, 1987).

26. P. Mathias, 'Swords and Ploughshares: The Armed Forces, Medicine and Public Health in the Late Eighteenth Century' in J.M. Winder (ed.), *War and Economic Development: Essays in Memory of David Joslin* (Cambridge: Cambridge University Press, 1975), 73–90: 88.

27. H. Cook, 'Practical Medicine and the British Armed Forces after the "Glorious Revolution"', *Medical History*, 34 (1990), 1–26: 16.

28. See M. Harrison, '"The Tender Frame of Man": Disease, Climate, and Racial Difference in India and West Indies, 1760–1860', *Bulletin of the History of Medicine*, 70 (1996), 68–93; M. Worboys, 'Germs, Malaria and the Invention of Mansonian Tropical Medicine: From "Diseases in the Tropics" to "Tropical Diseases"', in D. Arnold (ed.), *Warm Climates and Western Medicine: The Emergence of Tropical Medicine* (Amsterdam: Rodopi 1996), 181–207.

29. C. Stevenson, *Medicine and Magnificence: British Hospital and Asylum Architecture 1660–1815* (New Haven and London: Yale University Press, 2000). For the French parallel, see Brockliss and Jones, *op. cit.* (note 13).

30. J. Brewer, *The Sinews of Power: War, Money and the English State, 1688–1783* (New York: Knopf, 1989); L. Colley, *Britons: Forging the Nation, 1707–1837* (London: Pimlico, 1994); J. Innes, 'The Domestic Face of the Military–Fiscal State: Government and Society in Eighteenth-Century Britain' in L. Stone (ed.), *An Imperial State at War: Britain from 1689 to 1815* (London: Routledge, 1994), 96–127.

31. C. Jones, *The Charitable Imperative: Hospitals and Nursing in Ancien Régime and Revolutionary France* (London: Routledge, 1989), 217–19.

32. Cooter, *op. cit.* (note 1).

2

Warfare and the Creation of British Imperial Medicine, 1600–1800

J.D. Alsop

The literature of British maritime and imperial medicine is reviewed here, noting that the key growth in the area coincided with the wars of the late-seventeenth and early-eighteenth centuries when the navy started to maintain a regular fleet overseas. Thereafter, the literature followed major imperial wars and focused on the needs of the state in war, and male servicemen. Medical prescriptions for cure were universal, empirical, and economical; experimenting on servicemen to develop cures was a necessity. The emphasis was on control of the human environment and regulation of the men.

Introduction

The period from 1600 to 1800 witnessed growth in the numbers, and natures, of British peoples exposed to the varied health risks associated with economic and military expansion. Hundreds of thousands of Britons came to work at sea or to reside overseas: men, women, and children, indentured, free and coerced. They were joined by even larger numbers of slave and indigenous populations. In the process, hitherto largely separate disease environments came into direct contact. Recent analysis has demonstrated that prior to the mid-nineteenth century, oceanic travel lowered average life expectancy, while residence beyond the shores of Europe often entailed serious risks to life and health.[1] Any sampling of published autobiographical accounts of overseas travel in the seventeenth and eighteenth centuries will reveal significant contemporary anxiety.[2] The majority of Britons who travelled, worked, or resided overseas in this period were civilians. Nevertheless, the medical literature of the first British Empire was overwhelmingly martial in its conception and content. The requirements of war exerted a profound influence upon the literature of British naval and imperial medicine prior to 1800. Military and naval authors dominate the genre. These authors wrote from a perspective acquired in state service, and they published their work as an aid to, and a preparation for, war. The result was that the formal discourse of a growing body of specialist medical literature within an age of empire possessed fundamental characteristics: it was white, elitist, masculine, and state-centred.

Development prior to 1680

The most notable statement to be made about British naval and imperial medicine prior to the 1680s is that it scarcely existed in print. There were numerous practitioners – sea surgeons, army surgeons and physicians, and colonial 'doctors' – but strikingly little publication. This is in direct contrast to the period from 1690 to 1800, when a rich, mature, increasingly specialised, literature came into existence.[3] Why? Certainly the decades at the centre of the transition, circa 1675–1740, witnessed the establishment of a large, vibrant, 'British Atlantic' world of extensive trade, increased governance, and expanding migration.[4] These developments did not create the need for a specialist literature; that had existed since the 1550s.[5] However, they undoubtedly enhanced the societal recognition of this lacuna, and perhaps provided commercial incentives for publication. Nonetheless, as will be seen, the emergence of a maritime and imperial literature after 1690 was too rapid and concentrated to be explained solely, or primarily, as a product of gradual economic expansion. Rather, the pivotal event was the onset of sustained European and colonial warfare from 1689 through to the conclusion of the Revolutionary and Napoleonic Wars in 1815. This context indelibly marked the character of the medicine of overseas expansion.

Before the 1680s only two publications arose which can be labelled, retrospectively, as belonging to the genre of British imperial medicine. From the outset, the needs of war were front and centre. In 1598, one G.W. authored *The Cures of the Diseased, in Remote Regions: Preventing Mortalitie, Incident in Forraine Attempts, of the English Nation.*[6] This was an attempt, the writer stated, to prevent a recurrence of the horrendous death and misery of the Cadiz expedition of 1596. The author, a former sea surgeon, provided the first account in English of hot climate diseases, knowledge acquired while a prisoner-of-war in Spain but also based – in part – upon his own experience at sea. Although a short treatise of only twenty-one pages, G.W.'s work addressed the causation and treatment of two of the principal afflictions of overseas expansion: scurvy and fevers. The description of the causes of scurvy began what would prove to be an enduring emphasis upon the dangers of putrefied meat, contaminated drink, mouldy flour, wet apparel, and slothful habits of body. This publication was relevant to both commercial and military expansion abroad, but the context for its creation, and its stated purpose, was service to the state in time of war. The Anglo-Spanish War of 1585–1604 was the very first where England's armed forces engaged an enemy extensively at sea, and in sub-tropical and tropical locations. The *Cures of the Diseased*, for all its limitations, was therefore timely.

The second publication was more authoritative and enduring. This was John Woodall's *The Surgions Mate* (London, 1617), a comprehensive treatise on 'the most frequent diseases at Sea', which acquired lasting fame as the first in English to recommend citrus juice in the prevention and treatment of scurvy.[7] The context for Woodall's publication was distinctive, and this initially set it apart from the martial character of the genre overall. Woodall, subsequently master of the Barber–Surgeons' Company of London (1633), had already risen to a position of local prominence when, in 1613, he became the first Surgeon–General of the English East India Company. Published, 'chiefly for the benefit of young Sea–Surgeons, imployed in the East-India Companies affaires', the treatise discharged one obligation of Woodall's office.[8] In this initial period of high-risk voyages, the Company depended heavily upon apprenticed labour to provide the commercial agents, junior ships' officers, and surgeons in Asia. Lengthy voyages with high morbidity rates and sustained mortality created obvious problems in the recruitment and retention of seamen, and limited commercial success.[9] Woodall's task, therefore, was to provide a textual aid for the 'many young Surgions, (who by reason of their youth and lacke of practise have not attained to that perfection of knowledge, that were requisite).'[10] Thus, a particular and quite specific need led to the publication of a text of general utility.

It is interesting, however, to observe the alteration in the positioning of *The Surgions Mate* as it came to be reprinted. The expanded second edition of 1639 and the third, final, edition of 1655 each displayed prominently a new title: *The Surgions Mate. or Military & Domestique Surgery*. References to both sea surgeons and to the East India Company were dropped from the title pages, and the original motivation for publication – the effective management of personnel resources and morale in a new high-risk area of overseas commerce – was obscured by the supplementary information on military medicine and the plague. Although invariably studied by scholars in the context of imperial medicine, *The Surgions Mate* from the outset had always been a multi-purpose text. It was a compendium of diverse surgical information drawn from the author's Company service, private practice, and wide reading. Mariners did not require advice on the treatment of scrofula, salves for the inflammation of female breasts, or medicine to ease pain for women in menstruation and childbirth.[11] Woodall had created in 1617 the first published treatise in England to address at length some of the health problems inherent in overseas expansion, but he had also taken a new multi-faceted general surgical text and positioned it for a particular need and market. By 1639 the Company had an established, fairly circumscribed, position in the East, with experienced crews and known health risks. At the same time, the Bishops' Wars had brought military surgery to the forefront of public attention. Already, in 1626, Woodall had been appointed supervisor of medical chests in the Army and Navy for the Anglo-Spanish War, and in 1628 he exploited the opportunity of war with France to publish *Woodalls Viaticum: The Pathway to the Surgions Chest. For Younger Surgeons Now Employed at the Siege of Rochelle.*[12] The second edition of *The Surgions Mate* came to be used in the British Isles during the civil wars of the 1640s, while the third edition was published in 1655 at the outbreak of the Anglo-Spanish War, and in the very year of the conquest of Jamaica.

This repositioning of the only prominent early Stuart text directly relevant to overseas expansion is important. It reveals that from the outset, British imperial medical advice would be developed within the context of military medicine, occasionally as relatively minor features of texts of more general applicability. Woodall, moreover, would prove to be typical of several of the most illustrious eighteenth-century authors within this genre in respect to his relative lack of first-hand experience: his early service was in the English army on the continent of Europe; he possessed no direct experience of extra-European health challenges; indeed, it cannot be established that he was ever employed at sea.[13] It is not surprising, therefore, that he and many of the authors who followed in his footsteps would produce encyclopaedic works arising out of their past experiences and aimed at the largest market, or the greatest public utility. The changes to *The Surgions Mate*, and the complete lack of any competition from, or development by, Woodall's contemporaries, strongly suggests that there did not exist in early Stuart Britain a market for, or sustained professional interest in, the developing themes of imperial medicine. The neglect is obvious. Spanish and Portuguese publications remained un-translated, and largely uncommented upon in the medical literature.[14] There was no English equivalent to Jacobus Bontius's *De Medicina Indorum* of 1642, and this treatise initially received scant attention within the British Isles.[15] Johann Rudolph Glauber's *Consolatio Navigantium* of 1657 provided the first extended study of maritime illness, but this remained un-translated and references in print were sparse before the turn of the century.[16] It was left to an Italian academic, Bernardino Ramazzini, to produce, in 1700, the first occupation-specific study of the diseases of mariners. Although this was speedily translated and published in London in 1705 as *A Treatise of the Diseases of Tradesmen*, it is telling that only the second edition of Ramazzini's text (1713) contained his full analysis of seamen and this remained un-translated until 1746.[17]

The reasons for this relative neglect are difficult to comprehend. Certainly, the educated English public was aware that a century and more of exploration, commerce, and initial settlement had created lasting health concerns for the English, Welsh, Scots, and Irish who ventured overseas in increasing numbers. The pages of Richard Hakluyt's *Principall Navigations* and Samuel Purchas's *Purchas His Pilgrimes* contained startling eye-witness accounts of death and suffering from strange, terrifying diseases.[18] The risk to health was a recurring theme within the seventeenth-century literature on overseas expansion.[19] Nor can the almost total absence of a professional literature prior to 1690 be explained by the presence of effective apprenticeship for sea surgeons in the Navy and merchant marine, which would have negated the necessity for printed texts. In spite of regular complaints about the abilities of its practitioners, the apprenticeship system remained unaltered prior to the naval reforms of the nineteenth century.[20] Moreover, most oceanic commercial vessels did not retain surgeons and we are left to ask: why did this not give rise to the type of self-help medical manuals which flourished only much later, from the end of the eighteenth century?[21] Although many of the Tudor and Stuart sea surgeons were men of modest competency, on the periphery of professional medicine, there were some of ability. John Conny, for example, a sea surgeon of the 1650s who rose to be twice mayor of Rochester, compiled extensive manuscript case records of his maritime practice, as sound as many of those which later found their way into print.[22] The noted naval surgeon of the Restoration, James Yonge (1647–1721), authored treatises on head wounds and amputation but published virtually nothing during his lifetime on his recognised specialty of maritime medicine.[23] Finally, by way of illustration, there is the case of Richard Boulton. A pupil of Richard Wiseman (1620–76) Sergeant–Surgeon to Charles II, Boulton served in the Restoration navy, but chose to capitalise on this experience through publication only long after the fact, in 1699.[24] Wiseman himself, although possessing first-hand knowledge of tropical illnesses, published almost exclusively on the treatment of wounds.[25] Well might Dr William Cockburn, physician to the Blue Squadron of the Royal Navy, state in 1706:

> The Methods of former Sea-Physicians in the curing of Distempers are no more to be discover'd then the Furrows a Ship makes in the Sea, neither of them leaving the least footsteps for the direction of them who come after.[26]

This wholesale failure to create a literature on maritime health during the Restoration period has been commented upon, but never explained.[27] The answer is that the contemporary emphasis upon the particular nature of the sea battles of the Second and Third Dutch Wars directed medical attention towards the treatment of wounds and away from maritime health in general.

Maritime medicine

Only after 1689 did attention shift towards a broader concern for naval health. That development arose in the context of an extended period of naval warfare, frequently pursued in distant locales. The wars of 1689–97 and 1702–13, for example, were the first in which the Royal Navy maintained regular fleets in the Mediterranean and West Indies, and the first in which the Admiralty practised the unhealthy system of year-long impressed service.[28] Health problems multiplied at the same time as the manpower needs of the Navy increased exponentially.[29] The result was the rise of a state concern for, and a published literature on, the 'manning problem' of the Royal Navy.[30] It was in this context that there arose a professional medical literature on maritime medicine, which over the course of the succeeding decades evolved into a more generally applicable imperial medicine. It is readily apparent that it was the needs of the state, rather than those of the private sector – the merchant marine and the colonising movements – which led to this development. There was little incentive for the creation of an imperial medical literature so long as the principal sufferers were common sailors and labourers in an era of extended population increase, when many marginal young males found the sea to be the occupation of last resort.[31] Professional medicine did not direct its attention to these issues until after the state placed a premium upon healthy skilled labour, first the able seaman, and later in the eighteenth century, the trained soldier.

Apart from a flurry of publications in the 1680s on methods to purify sea water, there was no advance on Woodall's *Surgions Mate* until John Moyle published his *Abstractum Cirurgiae Marinae* in 1686.[32] Moyle speedily capitalised upon new-found interest by expanding this initial treatise into *Chirurgus Marinus, Or, the Sea Chirurgion, being Instructions to Junior Chirurgie Practitioners Who Design to Serve in This Imploy.* First published in 1693, this text of over three hundred pages was already in its fourth edition by the outbreak of the War of the Spanish Succession in 1702. Moyle, an experienced naval surgeon on second- and fourth-rate ships of the line, provided the first systematic study of maritime medicine derived from personal practice and observation. Although Moyle had served on board merchantmen on voyages to the Mediterranean and West Indies, *Chirurgus Marinus* was focused upon the health risks of war. He devoted lengthy sections to wounds because, he stated, even experienced sea surgeons possessed little acquaintance with these as a consequence of the long period of peace between 1674 and 1689.[33] The appraisals of internal and external ailments covered all afflictions experienced by seafarers. Only rarely did he deviate from his theme, as in his comments on the treatment of worms in children.[34] There were, however, important omissions in relation to imperial medicine. Although Moyle observed that fevers were more common and epidemical to the 'Southward', his analysis was limited to camp fever (typhus) and intermittent fever (malaria).[35]

Moyle was soon joined by other enterprising authors and publishers. Some of the literature of the 1689–1713 period repackaged earlier civilian writings for the new priority of war. This, for example, was true of a 1691 reprint of a plague tract by the late esteemed Dr Thomas Willis, *A Plain and Easie Method for... the Plague, Or Any Contagious Distemper in City, Camp, Fleet, etc.... Written in the Year 1666*.[36] Richard Boulton in his *System of Rational Surgery*, likewise stressed the relevance of earlier practice in the Dutch Wars.[37] Other writers drew upon current surgical practice in the wartime navy, notably Thomas Bates, the naval surgeon who published in 1708, *An Enchiridion of Fevers Incident to Sea-Men, (during the Summer) in the Mediterranean*, and James Christie, the master surgeon of a hospital ship in service in the Mediterranean, who authored *An Abstract of Some Years Observations Concerning such General and Unperceived Occasions of Sickliness in Fleets and Ships of War* (1709).[38] These latter two works were the first publications to focus upon specific, singular health issues in imperial medicine (respectively, fevers, and disorderly living and diet); eventually there would be many successors, although only after the onset of war, once again, in 1739. The Mediterranean was clearly the medical 'frontier' of this era, and the theatre of operations which held the attention of both the government and the general public.[39] Bates wrote for the marketplace. However, Christie's short but insightful tract was a product of an older tradition: he turned to print only after a virtually identical manuscript text submitted to the Admiralty went unheeded, and the publication itself was intended solely for the use of government officials.[40]

The principal competitor to Moyle, however, was a sea-going physician, not a fellow surgeon. After the innovative step was taken in 1691 of appointing one physician to each English naval fleet in active service, a Leyden-educated Scot, William Cockburn (1669–1739), was one of the first appointees, in 1694. He speedily exploited his knowledge of disease and injury acquired in the Navy during the Nine Years' War to produce in 1696–7 a two-volume study of maritime health, subsequently reworked and retitled in 1706 (and republished in 1736) as a standard work, *Sea Diseases*.[41] Cockburn was a son of Sir William Cockburn, Baronet, a Fellow of the Royal Society (elected 1697) and the physician to Greenwich Hospital, 1731–9; he was well placed and well respected.[42] The sixty-three case histories of illnesses in the fleet during 1695–6 which formed the core of Cockburn's analysis were biased towards the socially prominent and were representative neither of the range of patients nor the practice of wartime maritime medicine. Nonetheless, Cockburn speedily gained the respect of the naval establishment. In 1694, he exploited his developing reputation by having the Admiralty conduct a sea trial of his anti-dysentery remedy, and then utilised the limited endorsement from the Navy to advertise the medicine to the general public via a series of self-promoting publications.[43] As late as 1757, those claiming to hold the secret of this electuary were still trading on Cockburn's Europe-wide reputation.[44]

The era of Moyle and Cockburn was one of rapid state expansion combined with a fixation for economies of scale.[45] British military medicine in the wars of 1689 to 1713 consciously attempted to establish universally applicable, empirical remedies which would return the men to service as quickly, efficiently, and cheaply as possible.[46] Cockburn succeeded not least because he identified himself with this perspective. The Navy was the largest employer of seamen, and its health problems were viewed as being the most intractable of any found in maritime experience.[47] Little wonder, then, that naval science constituted the most common path in the eighteenth century to acknowledged expertise in maritime and imperial medicine. As soon as this perspective was fixed in public consciousness, it was exploited. The title pages of the general surgical works by Richard Boulton (1699) and James Handley (1705) each proudly proclaimed the previous naval service, and thus presumed surgical competence, of the respective authors.[48] When John Moyle published his *Experienced Chirurgion* in 1703 for the benefit of young surgeons who practised on land, he was identified as one of Her Majesty's 'Ancient Sea Surgeons'.[49] These were but the first texts in a century-long trend whereby naval practice was deemed to provide outstanding surgical expertise.[50] As we have seen, most of this early generation of maritime writers enjoyed long experience at sea, but this period saw, as well, the development of another eighteenth-century phenomenon: the exploitation of publication for career advantage by relative novices. Thomas Bates was perhaps the earliest to seize upon the new-found pre-occupation with naval health for advancement. When he published his *Enchiridion of Fevers* in 1708 he was only a junior naval surgeon. He had entered the Navy as a surgeon's third mate on *HMS Chichester* in April 1701, having served a five-year apprenticeship under his own father, a Newcastle surgeon. Described as a 'young man', diligent and sober, he nevertheless rose slowly before being appointed surgeon of a fifth-rate ship of the line in August 1705 on active service in the Mediterranean theatre. Following his emergence as an author, he took up the practice of physic in London and eventually gained admission to the Royal Society in 1719.[51]

Not all who followed the route to preferment were as well known or socially prominent as Cockburn, a physician who dined with admirals and had Jonathan Swift as a patient. John Atkins (1685–1757), for example, was a sea surgeon who began a long employment in the Navy as a junior surgeon's mate in 1701, qualified as surgeon of a second-rate ship of the line only in 1718 and served until 1723.[52] He self-consciously parleyed his expertise into *The Navy-Surgeon: Or, a Practical System of Surgery* of 1734, with subsequent editions in 1737 and 1742. Atkins pointedly observed that, 'for the common and general Parts of Surgery... I know no better School to improve in, than the NAVY, especially in Time of War, Accidents are frequent, and the Industrious illustrate Practice by their Cures'.[53] Atkins seized upon his fortuitous naval service on the equatorial coast of Africa on *HMS Swallow* in 1721–2 to include an appendix, prominently displayed on the title page of his work as 'Physical Observations on the Heat, Moisture, and Density of the Air on the Coast of Guiney; the Colour of the Natives, the Sicknesses which they and the Europeans trading thither are subject to; with a method of Cure'.[54] *The Navy-Surgeon* was the first British maritime publication based principally upon experiences acquired in extra-European service. Although Atkins's racial theories are now considered innovative,[55] the author was not well placed for preferment and his naval career was particularly halting. After 1723, he entered private practice in Plaistow, Essex.

Expertise and empire

The comment by Atkins that war produced the best school in which to advance professional expertise was frequently echoed in the eighteenth century. Gideon Harvey, the noted royal physician to Charles II, considered it commonplace as early as 1683 that surgeons would learn their trade through 'practice in Armies, or Fleets at Sea'.[56] James Lind (1716–94), the celebrated and most widely read of all eighteenth-century writers on imperial medicine throughout Europe and America, commented blandly in 1768: 'There is a large field for medical observations during a very sickly season in the West Indies, when thousands of Europeans are sent thither at once, in case of a war in that part of the world.'[57] Lind's famed scurvy trials on board *HMS Salisbury* in 1747 were merely the best known of numerous experiments conducted upon Britain's servicemen.[58] A philosophy and practice of experimentation which began with Cockburn's anti-dysentery remedy in the 1690s progressed through a multitude of natural restoratives to the exploration of the medical benefits of electricity, nitric acid, and other chemicals at the close of the eighteenth century.[59] The unprecedented health challenges at sea and overseas were favoured targets of those actions, and trials were conducted at appropriate times upon sailors, soldiers, prisoners-of-war and incapacitated allied servicemen alike. Individual illustrations abound: the surgeon of *HMS Magnificent* in 1782 experimented with tobacco smoke forced into the nostrils of a seaman as a cure for tetanus; in the 1790s the internal use of mercury was introduced into the British Army

31

and Navy as a cure for yellow fever.[60] Many afflictions were the objects of experimentation, but the most extensive and best documented actions were directed at the 'scourge' of servicemen in every theatre of operations: venereal disease.[61] Experimentation was not restricted to the controlled population-at-risk of servicemen, of course. Plantation owners, and their hired medical practitioners, experimented upon slaves:[62] James Lind, surgeon of the East India Company, in 1762 allowed malaria to run its course on 'a black boy' in Bengal to observe its symptoms,[63] and there exists the intriguing account of how one Surgeon Vage in Senegal during 1759 conducted a trial of the efficacy of bleeding in tropical fevers upon (unidentified) unwitting white subjects. Vage already was 'surprised' at the inability of his patients to recover following the removal of eight to ten ounces of blood when he conducted a trial by evacuating six ounces of blood from one subject only in each of two sets of twinned patients. Vage concluded that bloodletting doubled the time of recovery, and rendered the sick 'always comatose and stupid'.[64]

Servicemen, though, remained the principal subjects of experimentation, for they were at the same time coerced, plentiful, and the intended beneficiaries of any improvements. Indeed, from at least the 1750s, there existed an expectation on the part of innovators that new, speculative, remedies for unresolved disease problems deserved to be accorded experimental trial at sea on ships' companies. John Travis argued in 1757 when promoting his cure for scurvy:

> [S]urely, in a case of such vast importance, at this dangerous crisis of public affairs [in the war with France], it merits at least an impartial trial in a large ship: for a proposal, which promises a benefit so extensive, and invaluable, should stand, or fall, by the test of truth, and experience only[65]

State personnel were also among the most adventurous on the medical fringes of the empire: Henry Warren of Barbados noted that when the island's medical practitioners declined to conduct autopsies during an outbreak of yellow fever in the 1730s due to fear of infection and the intolerable stench, a naval surgeon, 'an ingenious Young Gentleman', was the only one to accept the challenge by dissecting the body of a deceased crewman.[66] Early practitioners of overseas medicine were frequently involved, formally or informally, in experimentation, for they worked in relative seclusion from the medical elites, amidst morbidity or mortality crises, where the focus was upon the effective recovery of the military unit, not the survival of the individual serviceman. As J.B. Sheppard, a Royal Navy surgeon and member of the Royal College of Surgeons of London, later commented in reference to the yellow fever epidemic of 1793 in the

West Indies: 'credulity generally keeps pace with apprehension.'[67] Within the professional culture of the British Army and Navy overseas during the second half of the eighteenth century, there was an expectation of experimentation and no effective restriction.

British maritime medicine, therefore, developed within boundaries set by medical authorities who placed the requirements of the state front and centre. The focus established in the wars of 1689 to 1713 remained unaltered through to 1815. Publications continued to be derived almost exclusively from experience gained in state service, and they tended to bunch in periods of warfare: 1739–48, 1756–63, 1776–83, 1793–1815. The principal topics selected for study – scurvy, fresh water, tropical fevers, dysentery, venereal disease – were relevant to all seafarers but they were the pressing concerns of central government between 1689 and 1815. It is noteworthy that there was no parallel profusion of publications on army medicine prior to the mid-eighteenth century. The first general treatises were John Pringle's highly influential *Observations on the Diseases of the Army in Camp and Garrison* (1752), and Donald Monro's *An Account of the Diseases which were Most Frequent in the British Military Hospitals in Germany* (1764).[68] This relative neglect was frequently commented upon at the time.[69] State and public attention initially focused upon the manning problem of the Navy. Medicine followed suit. Military medicine was, to quote from John Hennen's experience of his early career in the Georgian army, 'the lowest step of professional drudgery and degradation', and initially it was largely divorced from the themes of imperial health and healing.[70] With the notable exception of George Cleghorn's *Observations on the Epidemical Diseases of Minorca from the Year 1744 to 1749* (London, 1751), the first detailed studies drawn from imperial service appeared only after 1776.[71] Even then, the army practitioners who published in the final decades of the eighteenth century sometimes deferred to the more developed maritime literature on health and illness overseas.[72] The opinions of the authors of the standard texts on military medicine, especially Pringle and Monro, were, however, widely disseminated within the imperial literature. The authoritative lessons on the maintenance of health during the heat of a European summer were perceived to be directly applicable to the health problems of servicemen in tropical climates.

From maritime to imperial

Maritime medicine had developed inexorably into a broader imperial medicine by the mid-eighteenth century. Naval writers came increasingly to offer advice relevant to places overseas, not simply on sea travel itself. This was first apparent in Bates's *Enchiridion of Fevers* and Atkins's *Naval Surgeon*. These authors commented extensively upon the health risks, and remedies, for the Mediterranean, and Equatorial Africa and the West Indies, respectively. This was a general development which followed upon the revival of the Hippocratic emphasis upon the environment, and the increasing concern in eighteenth-century treatises for hot climate fevers. Now identified principally as yellow fever and malaria, these fevers were customarily understood within the context of the doctrines of climatology.[73] In the well-regarded treatises of Dr James Lind, naval surgeon during the War of the Austrian Succession, and founding physician of the Royal Navy's Hasler Hospital, considerations of maritime health were dominated by the micro-climates of the ports and shorelines of Africa, Asia, and the Americas.[74] Not surprising, therefore, naval writers became responsible for some of the most prominent analyses of the hot climate diseases encountered within the expanding British empire, and these views were summarised in standard geographical reference texts.[75]

Parallel to an increasingly rich naval medicine, there arose a 'hot climate' medical literature which was readily incorporated into the prevailing themes of maritime health. This was the location-specific literature which frequently relied upon climatology to comprehend disease occurrence as a consequence of locale, weather, and season. The first publication in this genre was *A Discourse on the State of Health in the Island of Jamaica*, published by Thomas Trapham in 1679.[76] Development was initially haphazard and ephemeral, limited to short descriptions of distant locales.[77] Even Sir Hans Sloane, dispatched to Jamaica early in his career in 1687, as physician to the Governor, limited his appraisal of the connection between environment and disease within his celebrated *Natural History* to several paragraphs of superficial observation, followed by a selection of unadorned, partly undigested, case records drawn from his practice.[78] As Sloane stated, it was accepted wisdom that the diseases of imperial possessions, 'were all very different from what they are in Europe', but there was a noticeable lack of published description and professional advice.[79] The latter circumstance remained essentially unaltered prior to the 1740s and the absorption of this sub-genre into the mainstream of imperial medicine. Authorities came to differ on whether the disease environment at colonial locations was distinctive, and the literature reflected the contemporary contestation between contagion and anti-contagion theories. However, the most notable development was the method through which the medical topography of individual, dispersed locations on the globe became part of the unified literature of British imperial medicine.

The earliest publications in the medical topography of empire were unrelated to the requirement of military and naval medicine. The first, uncritical, public commentary arose within the boosterism of the colonial expansion movements of the seventeenth and early-eighteenth centuries.

The attempt to engage in scientific study began with Trapham. Although several of the early writers, Sloane included, held government posts, their experience lay primarily in private practice and their concerns were with the health of colonial populations, including immigrants and transient labour. This initially provided a perspective which was rarely found within the previously examined maritime literature. For example, it was Henry Warren, in his *Treatise Concerning the Malignant Fever of Barbados*, who asserted that the value of his observations during the years 1734–8 lay in the future avoidance of large-scale attrition within the merchant marine: he estimated that within the six years ending in May 1739, the British Crown had lost in the sugar colonies of the West Indies 20,000 useful subjects to yellow fever, the greatest part of whom were merchant seamen.[80] Nevertheless, Warren's *Treatise* was situated on the cusp of change: although his interest lay in the economical vitality of Barbados, it is doubtful whether the tract would have been published in 1741 had it not been for the extensive public interest and state concern which arose out of the War of Jenkin's Ear and the disastrous mortality of Admiral Vernon's expedition to the Caribbean.[81]

From 1740, the publications in the medical topography of empire reflected the needs of state and, in particular, the priorities of war. At first, the authors felt obligated to justify the general utility of their particular practices. Cleghorn prefaced his *Observations on Epidemical Diseases of Minorca* with the observation that his treatise was restricted to:

> '[T]is true, an Account of the Diseases only, of a small, remote Part of the British Dominions; but of a Part in which Numbers of his Majesty's Subjects... are often brought together, both in Time of Peace and War: And as the Qualities of the Air, and the Course of the Seasons in Minorca correspond nearly with those in several other Parts of the World; to which our Fleets frequently repair, it is probable the Diseases may likewise be similar. Would all who practice Physick in our Factories and Colonies abroad embrace the Opportunity their Situation affords, to make proper Obervations on the Sick, and communicate them to the Public, we should soon have a more exact and ample History of Diseases... and no small benefit to their Country.[82]

In contrast, John Tennent capitalised in 1741 on the current concern for the mortality of 'Northern Foreigners' in the West Indian campaigns to assert confidently that he possessed knowledge derived from his experience in Virginia, 'on which depend, in a great measure, the lives of Admirals, Generals, Officers, and Thousands of brave Men, engaged in obtaining Justice to their Country, and defending its Honour'.[83] However, by 1766, Dr Charles Bisset included in his *Medical Essays* over one hundred pages of observation derived from his military service in Jamaica during the 1740s without the need for either justification or hyperbole.[84] By then, reliance upon location-specific observation and treatment was commonplace, and incorporated into the developing literature on health in the tropics.[85] Publication was monopolised by military practitioners who, as in the case of Dr John Bell, late surgeon to the Fifth Regiment of Foot, wrote for 'the attention equally of the statesman and the physician',[86] but who, in effect, devoted more attention to attracting the attention of the state to their favoured remedies.

The national interest

Professional expertise was portrayed from the 1690s through to 1815 within a context of hard-won, generally useful, experience either acquired in state service or of notable benefit to the nation in its wars. Appeals to the national interest were frequently invoked in this context. The oft-published civilian writer on medical topics, Stephen Hales, dedicated his *Instructions for Such as Undertake Long Voyages at Sea* of 1739 to the Commissioners of the Admiralty with the observation that those in charge of the 'most numerous and Powerful Fleet in the World' had particular use for a work intended chiefly for seafaring persons.[87] John Moyle published *Chirurgus Marinus*, he stated, for the good of every one of the Queen's seamen, soldiers, and other subjects who would henceforth be wounded or diseased at sea.[88] Nothing less than 'the Public Welfare' was at issue, wrote the physician John Tennent in 1742, in describing his remedy for the thousands of needless deaths in the late campaigns.[89] Shortly thereafter, Dr John Huxham called upon the state to adopt his favoured (and expensive) method for the eradication of scurvy, by way of a comparison with the fabled Roman soldier of old:

> [I]f that glorious prudent People thought the life of a Roman Soldier so valuable, and were at such Expence to preserve it; why should not we have as much Regard to that of a British Sailor, who is altogether as brave and as useful to the Commonwealth?[90]

The state was entreated repeatedly to concern itself with the welfare of the individual serviceman, for he 'always must be of importance to Britain, while she wishes to maintain her possessions either in the Eastern or Western World.'[91] The improvement of imperial medicine, therefore, was both a public duty and a valuable gift, provided by the qualified expert to the 'faithful guardian of the state' as a means of preserving the royal naval and military forces in health and vigour.[92] Dutiful servants of the public, of course, recognised the value of economy, and they invariably couched their proposals in the language of thrift and value for money.[93]

The imperial medicine which emerged within this context of war, state service, and professional expertise possessed particular characteristics. To observe that it was state-centred is an understatement. The literature was overwhelmingly focused upon the requirements of the state, conceptualised within a fairly narrow understanding of war and defence, with scant attention devoted prior to 1800 to the broader themes of imperial commerce, immigration, or population vitality. The tone of the literature was white. The premises of environmentalism asserted that Europeans who traversed climatic zones, from temperate to semi-tropical or tropical, were at greatest risk and thus, in need of particular, experienced, protection.[94] Transported Africans, on the other hand, moved merely from one hot, moist climate to another, and could be expected to adapt with relative ease. Africans do appear in the medical literature of overseas expansion, but they do so infrequently and as foils for the perceptively far more difficult experiences of Europeans.[95] The superior health record of transplanted Africans in respect to tropical fevers was held to provide definitive proof of the 'seasoning' provided by exposure to climate. The closest link between the developing literature on imperial medicine and slavery lay in the fact that a professional expertise focused upon economic prevention or treatment for a large servile population of servicemen at risk, and could readily be translated into parallel, watered-down advice for plantation slavery.[96] Moreover, the economics of slavery provided a marketable expertise for those who could claim some first-hand knowledge of the epidemiology of the peoples of sub-Saharan Africa. Enterprising naval surgeons were among the first to exploit this opportunity, prior to the rise of a literature on plantation medicine.[97]

Imperial medicine was focused upon the European body, but this was a peculiar body: gendered male, identified as a young adult, characterised as temperamentally childlike and in need of firm guidance. All these characteristics arose as a consequence of the fixation upon the lessons and requirements of war and state service. Prior to 1800, references to women within the literature were rare. Within a genre which depended upon extensive reproduction of, and commentary on, individual medical case histories, women were almost invisible; the professional practices of authors who acquired their expertise primarily in the services or long-distance commerce were dominated by the experiences and health needs of young males.[98] The ostensible object of the discourse is the European body, but the advice is all focused, silently, upon the youthful male. For women, we learn merely that they were less prone to sea-sickness, and less likely to contract or to die from yellow fever, but more inclined to be hysterical in the tropics.[99] As with the more numerous references to Africans, women appear as counter examples in an effort to understand better the male experience.[100] The same is true of the aged, who truly are invisible in the text.[101] Essential, rudimentary advice for children – child doses for prescriptions (which are always implicitly set for adults) – appear extremely infrequently prior to 1800. Instead, the emphasis was firmly upon the youthful, male, European body. This was a sensible focus if the object of the literature was to provide practical advice in maintaining service personal healthy and effective throughout the empire; this most certainly was the stated intent of the genre overall. It was not the nature of the empire. As important in establishing this preoccupation, however, was the unstated bias which permeated all texts, even those such as Lind's *Diseases Incidental to Europeans*, which purported to provide universally applicable medical knowledge for health overseas. Most writers on imperial health prior to 1800 arose from within the services. Those who did not, in turning to the standard authorities, almost invariably acquired a similar perspective and bias. There existed no counter perspective, no identification of the limitations. Instead, the call was for more, superior, and quantitative knowledge derived from the armed services.[102] The essential message, therefore, was a depiction of the common experience of all Europeans confronted by all hot, humid climates, even though the medical expertise was very largely dependent upon observing and treating young males under arms in very specific locales.

Finally, an important sub-text within the literature of British imperial medicine is the theme of the control and regulation of the body. The desire to regulate the bodies of the poor, the slaves, and the servicemen became a pre-occupation of the medical, political and commercial elites of eighteenth-century Britain and its empire. An imperial medicine grounded in the care of servicemen, not surprisingly, emphasised the importance of enforced hygiene, control of diet and prevention of excess and licence. From an early period, sailors were conceived of by their superiors as improvident, childlike, and indifferent to their long-term health.[103] The moral improvement literature of the eighteenth century further encouraged these attitudes.[104] The stated judgements of standard authorities on the responsibility for ill health within the empire were frequently starkly judgmental. James Christie referred to the 'childish Indiscretion' of naval seamen as a principal cause of their morbidity.[105] Dr Richard Brocklesby, physician to the British Army, fellow of the College of Physicians, and Fellow of the Royal Society, was particularly pointed in his critique: common soldiers 'are in general foul feeders' prone to 'filth', who possess 'squalid' bodies.[106] Atkins attributed 'the Filth and Nastiness bred from such a Number [of a ship's crew], by Neglect and Idleness', as the principal cause of epidemic and contagious distempers within the Royal Navy overseas.[107] Condemnations of licentious, alcoholic, and disorderly conduct were commonplace in this era. Writers on imperial medicine were at pains to demonstrate that such behaviour was particularly destructive in tropical climes.[108] Hilliar confidently attributed the mortality of Europeans on the Gold Coast to 'their ill Diet, and ill Government';[109] this general interpretation was repeated across the empire.[110] Servicemen, of necessity, engaged in abnormally strenuous exercise, were forced to encamp in hazardous locations, and were required to participate in 'wood and water' parties at inopportune times.[111] Nonetheless, the literature emphasised the frailty of the human condition: 'We are under the necessity of observing', stated Dr Rollo, 'that many in the Army despise every rule, and, without discretion, expose themselves, in the most unnecessary manner, to causes they are perfectly conscious give rise to disease.'[112] Servicemen were simply 'ungovernable in their Actions, Debauchery and Appetites'.[113] The solution was obvious: imperial authorities must regulate, sanitise, and (if possible) educate.

Conclusion

By the second half of the eighteenth century writers on the themes of imperial medicine were cognisant that they wrote within a particular genre, with cross citations, the conscious labelling of identical medical problems, and the like. However, overlap with, and borrowings from, other areas of medical investigation, both domestic and foreign, were routine. The empire encompassed diverse populations, geographies and climates, including many where the lessons of domestic physic and surgery were immediately applicable.[114] The medical concerns of empire were far too multifaceted for there to have arisen a specific, narrowly construed tropical medicine.[115] An emphasis within the military publications upon generic advice relevant to all servicemen prevented fine distinctions, and experience garnered in the British Isles, Europe, and overseas was sometimes run together in a seamless manner.[116] Moreover, the authors, especially upon the conclusion of wars, were at pains to emphasise the general utility of their expertise: in 1763, James Lind confidently proclaimed that the hard-won knowledge of typhus and typhoid fever acquired among servicemen in the West Indies, Nova Scotia, and Minorca was readily applicable to British male and female boarding schools.[117] Such linkages, though, were generally by way of casual allusion rather than specific demonstration.

This knowledge acquired in war, published at least in part as a preparative for war, and based upon the experiences and care of young adult males, found its way into the general medical textbooks and the specific advice literature for the merchant marine, passengers, and colonists, as for example in Thomas Masterman Winterbottom's (1765–1859) *Medical Directions for the Use of Navigators and Settlers in Hot Climates* (London, 1803) and the highly popular *Sailor's Physician* by the American naval surgeon and physician, Usher Parsons (1788–1868).[118] Not surprisingly, therefore, the writers on imperial medicine on the eve of the great population movements of the early-nineteenth century tended to offer guidance portrayed as applicable to all persons – all Europeans – with extremely little advice specifically for the elderly or mature, children, or women. This narrowness only began to disappear in the writings of Winterbottom and Parsons,[119] a trend encouraged by the publication in the late-eighteenth century of broadly conceived works on the state of health and medicine in specific political jurisdictions overseas, beginning with the former American colonies.[120]

In the present state of knowledge, it is difficult to evaluate the consequences of a published literature on British imperial medicine prior to 1800 which possessed the characteristics described in this study. On the one hand, the requirements of the state in war and defence led to the creation of a complex, voluminous literature on health and illness within an expanding empire. On the other hand, this genre was governed by a narrow conception of the requirements of the state and an uncritical assumption on the part of the authors that their particular experience possessed general applicability. An imperial medical expertise grounded in military medicine, so susceptible to morbidity and mortality crises, implicitly emphasised the health problems of the empire. Moreover, if one believed, as did John Bell, that the cause of yellow fever mortality was alcoholism,[121] then what consequences did this carry for epidemiology? Medical practitioners in the port cities and tide-water regions of the empire – the geographical areas covered by this literature – treated a wide variety of patients, most of whom did not resemble, and were not in conditions identical to, early modern servicemen. Did it matter that prior to the late-eighteenth century there was a significant disjunction between published medical advice and the clientele of private practitioners within the empire? These are fruitful areas for further investigation in comprehending the significance of a British imperial medicine which was predominately state centred, elitist, white, and masculine in its conception and execution.

Notes

1. L. Cohn, 'Maritime Morbidity in the Eighteenth and Nineteenth Centuries: A Survey', *International Journal of Maritime History*, i (1989), 159–91; R. Haines, R. Shlomowitz and L. Brennan, 'Maritime Morbidity Revisited', *International Journal of Maritime History*, viii (1996), 133–72; J.R. McNeill, 'The Ecological Basis of Warfare in the Caribbean, 1700–1804', in M. Ultee (ed.), *Adapting to Conditions: War and Society in the Eighteenth Century* (Alabama: University of Alabama Press, 1986), 26–42; P.D. Curtin, *Death by Migration: Europe's Encounter with the Tropical World in the Nineteenth Century* (Cambridge: Cambridge University Press, 1989); P.D. Curtin, *Disease and Imperialism before the Nineteenth Century*

(Minneapolis: University of Minneapolis Press, 1990), 1–14; K.F. Kiple and K.C. Ornelas, 'Race, War and Tropical Medicine in the Eighteenth-Century Caribbean', in D. Arnold (ed), *Warm Climates and Western Medicine: The Emergence of Tropical Medicine, 1500–1900* (Amsterdam: Rodopi, 1996), 65–79. The author gratefully acknowledges the assistance provided for this investigation by the Associated Medical Services, Toronto, the College of Physicians of Philadelphia, the John Carter Brown Library, and the Osler Library, McGill University.

2. K.O. Kupperman, 'Fear of Hot Climates in the Anglo-American Colonial Experience', *William and Mary Quarterly*, 3rd ser., xli (1984), 213–40. Examples include: *A History of the Voyages and Travels of Captain Nathaniel Uring* (London, 1726), 8, 11–13, 20; *A Journal of the Life, Travels and Labours of Love, in the Work of the Ministry of... Thomas Wilson* (Dublin, 1728), 27, 39; W. Seward, *Journal of a Voyage from Savannah to Philadelphia, and from Philadelphia to England, MDCCXL* (London, 1740), 1, 3, 42, 53; *A Journal of the Life of Thomas Story* (Newcastle upon Tyne, 1747), 434, 444, 454–6; *An Account of the Life and Travels in the Work of the Ministry of John Fothergill* (London, 1753), 38, 51; *An Account of the Life, Travels, and Christian Experience in the Work of the Ministry of Samuel Bownas* (2nd edn, London, 1761), 107, 136–8, 168–71; W. Spavens, *The Seamen's Narrative: Containing an Account of a Great Variety of such Incidents as the Author Met with in the Sea Service* (Louth, 1796), 5, 9, 17–18, 22, 33.

3. T.R. Adams and D.W. Waters (eds), *English Maritime Books Printed Before 1801* (Providence, R.I.: John Carter Brown Library, 1995), 317–30; J.J. Keevil, *Medicine and the Navy, 1649–1714* (Edinburgh and London: Livingstone, 1958), 298–306; C. Lloyd and J.L.S. Coulter, *Medicine and the Navy, 1714–1815* (Edinburgh and London: Livingstone, 1961), 381–91.

4. I.K. Steele, *The English Atlantic, 1675–1740* (Oxford: Oxford University Press, 1986).

5. J.D. Alsop, 'Sea Surgeons, Health and England's Maritime Expansion: the West African Trade, 1553–1660', *Mariner's Mirror*, lxxvi (1990), 215–21; P.E.H. Hair and J.D. Alsop, *English Seamen and Traders in Guinea, 1553–1565* (Lewiston, N.Y.: Mellen, 1992).

6. G. Wateson, *The Cures of the Diseased in Forrein Attempts of the English Nation. London, 1598*, C. Singer (ed.), (Oxford: Oxford University Press. 1915).

7. J. Woodall, *The Surgions Mate* (1617), facsimile edn. with introduction and appendix by J. Kirkup, (Bath: Kingsmead, 1978), 185–5.

8. *Ibid.*, title page and 'Epistle Dedicatorie' fo. 2v.

9. W.N. Sainsbury (ed.), *Calendar of State Papers, Colonial Series East Indies, China and Japan, 1513–1616* (London: Longman, 1862), *passim; idem., Calendar of State Papers, Colonial Series, East Indies, China and Japan,*

1617–1621 (London: H.M.S.O., 1870), *passim*; K.J. Carpenter, *The History of Scurvy and Vitamin C* (Cambridge: Cambridge University Press, 1986), 18–22.

10. Woodall, *op. cit.* (note 7), fo. 3.

11. *Ibid.*, 80, 117–20.

12. *Ibid.*, xv. This text was republished in 1639 for use by the royalist army and the subtitle was altered to: 'Chirurgical Instructions for the younger sort of Surgeon, imployed in the Service of his Majestie, or for the Common Wealth upon any occasion whatsoever'.

13. Woodall, *op. cit.* (note 7), xii–xvi; J.J. Keevil, *Medicine and the Navy, 1200–1649* (Edinburgh and London: Livingstone, 1957), 177, 220–26.

14. F. Guerra, *Historia de la Materia Medica Hispanoamericana y Filipina en la Epoca Colonial* (Madrid, 1973). Of those who published before 1617, Woodall referred only to the writing of Nicolas Monardes.

15. Keevil, *op. cit.* (note 13), 153.

16. J.R. Glauber, *Consolatio Navigantium* (Amsterdam, 1657). A French translation, *La Consolation des Navigants*, appeared in Paris in 1659. For early Dutch medical interest in maritime disease, see also J. Harskamp (ed.), *Dissertatio Medica Inauguralis... Leyden Medical Dissertations in the British Library 1593–1746: Catalogue of a Sloane-inspired Collection* (London: Wellcome Trust, 1997).

17. The Latin edition of 1700 was translated and published as: B. Ramazzini, *A Treatise of the Diseases of Tradesmen, Shewing the Various Influences of Particular Trade Upon the State of Health* (London, 1705). Mariners received modest attention in this first edition, considered alongside fishermen (181–4). Only in the second Latin edition of 1713 did Ramazzini include a longer, separate, chapter on sailors and rovers. B. Ramazzini, *Diseases of Workers*, W.C. Wright (trans), (New York: Hafner, 1964), vii, 459–69.

18. R. Hakluyt, *The Principall Navigations Voiages and Discoveries of the English Nation [1589]*, D.B. Quinn and A. Quinn (eds), 2 vols, (Cambridge: Cambridge University Press, 1965); R. Hakluyt, *The Principal Navigations, Voyages, Traffiques and Discoveries of the English Nation* [1598–1600], J. Masefield (ed.), 8 vols (London: J.M. Dent, 1907); S. Purchas, *Hakluytus Posthumus Or Purchas His Pilgrmes*, 4 vols (London, 1625).

19. Kupperman, *op. cit.* (note 2), 213–40.

20. C. Lloyd and J.L.S. Coulter, *Medicine and the Navy, 1815–1900* (Edinburgh and London: Livingstone, 1963), 11–32.

21. E. Gordon, 'Sailors' Physicians: Medical Guides for Merchant Ships and Whalers, 1774–1864', *Journal of the History of Medicine and Allied Sciences*, xlviii (1993), 139–56.

22. *Dictionary of National Biography*, sub. Robert Conny [father of John]; British Library, additional ms. 2779. It is relevant to observe that while household

medical 'receipt' books were frequently copied within lay and professional circles, and exist for early modern England in some abundance, this was not true for maritime practice. There is no known instance of medical receipts, such as those by Conny, being used at sea by other practitioners. The absence of a published literature, therefore, cannot be explained by reference to a manuscript tradition.

23. F.N.L. Poynter (ed.), *The Journal of James Yonge (1647–1721): Plymouth Surgeon* (London: Longmans, 1963); Keevil, *op. cit.* (note 3), 81–2, 108, 149, 154–7.

24. R. Boulton, *A System of Rational and Practical Surgery*, 2nd edn, enlarged (London, 1733).

25. R. Wiseman, *A Treatise of Wounds* (London, 1672); *idem, Severall Chirurgical Treatises* (London, 1676); *Dictionary of National Biography*, sub. R. Wiseman.

26. W. Cockburn, *Sea Diseases: Or a Treatise of Their Nature, Causes, and Cure,* 2nd edn (London, 1706), 3.

27. Keevil, *Medicine and the Navy, 1649–1714, op. cit.* (note 3), 43.

28. J.P. Ehrman, *The Navy in the War of William III, 1689–1697* (Cambridge: Cambridge University Press, 1953); S.F. Gradish, 'The Establishment of British Seapower in the Mediterranean, 1689–1713', *Canadian Journal of History,* x (1975), 1–16; J.H. Owen, *War at Sea Under Queen Anne, 1702–1708* (Cambridge: Cambridge University Press, 1938); R.D. Merriman (ed.), *Queen Anne's Navy: Documents Concerning the Administration of the Navy of Queen Anne, 1702–1714* (London, Navy Records Society, 1961).

29. M. Duffy, 'The Foundations of British Naval Power', in M. Duffy (ed.), *The Military Revolution and the State, 1500–1800* (Exeter: University of Exeter, 1980), 67–72.

30. N.A.M. Rodger, *The Wooden World: An Anatomy of the Georgian Navy* (London: Fontana, 1988), 145–82; Adams and Waters, *op. cit.* (note 3), 419–53.

31. E.A. Wrigley and R. S. Schofield, *The Population History of England, 1541–1871: A Reconstruction* (Cambridge, Mass: Harvard University Press, 1981), 220 and *passim*; R. Davis, *The Rise of the English Shipping Industry in the Seventeenth and Eighteenth Centuries* (Newton Abbot: David and Charles, 1962), 114–16. For contemporary recognition of this fact, see H. Warren, *A Treatise Concerning the Malignant Fever in Barbados, and the Neighbouring Islands: With an Account of the Seasons There, from the Year 1734 to 1738* (London, 1741), 19–20, 73.

32. Adams and Waters, *op. cit.* (note 3), 317–8.

33. J. Moyle, *Chirurgus Marinus: Or, the Sea-Chirurgion. Being Instructions to Junior Chirurgie Practitioners, Who Design to Serve at Sea in This Imploy*, 4th edn (London, 1702), A3v-4r, 35–6; Keevil, *op. cit.* (note 3), 157–59.

34. Moyle, *ibid.,* 318.

35. *Ibid.,* 2, 226–38.

36. This work was edited by Willis's former amanuensis, J. Hemming; it appeared again in the following year, with the same title, in T. Willis, *The London Practice of Physick* (London, 1692).

37. Boulton, *op. cit.* (note 24), *passim.*

38. A second, corrected, edition of Bates's treatise was printed in London in 1709.

39. J.D. Alsop, 'Sickness in the British Mediterranean Fleet: The *Tiger's* Journal of 1706', *War and Society,* xi (1993), 57–76.

40. J. Christie, *An Abstract of Some Years Observations Concerning such General and Unperceived Occasions of Sickliness in Fleets and Ships of War,* unpaginated dedication; *idem.,* 'Such Occasions of Sicklyness in Flects, and Ships of War', in British Library, add. ms. 9331, fols. 158r-168v.

41. W. Cockburn, *An Account of the Nature, Causes, Symptoms and Cure of the Distempers that are Incident to Seafaring People* (London, 1696); *idem., A Continuation of the Account of the Nature, Causes, Symptoms and Cure of the Distempers that are Incident to Seafaring People* (London, 1697); *idem., op. cit.* (note 26).

42. Keevil, *op. cit.* (note 3), 286–96.

43. W. Cockburn, *Sea Diseases: Or a Treatise of Their Nature, Causes, and Cure,* 3rd edn (London, 1736), A3v-4v, 216–18; *idem., Profluvia Ventris: Or the Nature and Causes of Looseness Plainly Discovered* (London, 1701); *idem., An Account of the Nature, Causes, Symptoms and Cure of Looseness,* 2nd edn (London, 1710); *idem., The Nature and Cure of Fluxes* (London, 1724).

44. H. Boeshier De La Touche, *Some Observations of the Power and Efficacy of a Medicine Against Looseness, Bloody Fluxes, etc. By the late William Cockburn,* 2nd edn (London, 1757).

45. J. Brewer, *The Sinews of Power: War, Money and the English State, 1688–1783* (New York: Knopf, 1989). For evidence of long-running emphasis upon economy, see the correspondence of the Lords of the Admiralty to the Commissions for Sick and Wounded Seamen between 1702 and 1728, National Maritime Museum, Greenwich, ADM/E/1–6.

46. H.J. Cook, 'Practical Medicine and the British Armed Forces after the Glorious Revolution', *Medical History,* xxxiv (1990), 1–26; J.D. Alsop, 'Royal Navy Morbidity in Early Eighteenth-Century Virginia', in D. Meyers and
M. Perreault (eds), *Colonial Chesapeake: New Perspectives* (Nanham: Lexington, 2006), 141–77.

47. For example: J. Christie, 17 April 1704, British Library, Add. Ms. 5439, fol. 108; J. Burchett, *Memoirs of Transactions at Sea During the War with France: Beginning in 1688 and Ending in 1697* (London, 1703), A1–A2; William

Hodges, *Humble Proposals for the Relief, Encouragment, Security and Happiness of the Loyal, Couragious Seamen of England* (London, 1695), 5, 22, 30.

48. Boulton, *op. cit.* (note 24); J. Handley, *Colloquia Chirurgica; Or, the Whole Art of Surgery Epitomized and Made Easy... By One of Her Majesty's Surgeons for Many Years Employed in Her Navy* (London, 1705).

49. J. Moyle, *The Experienced Chirugion* (London, 1703).

50. Later examples include: R. Robertson, *An Essay on Fevers* (London, 1790), 3.

51. Barber–Surgeons' Company of London certificates, naval warrants, and letters of recommendation for Thomas Bates, Public Record Office, ADM 106/2953, part I.

52. Public Record Office, ADM 106/2952.

53. J. Atkins, *The Navy-Surgeon* (London, 1734), x.

54. See also, J. Atkins, *A Voyage to Guinea, Brasil, and the West Indies: In His Majesty's Ships the Swallow and Weymouth... Describing the Colour, Diet, Languages, Habits, Manners, Customs, and Religions of the Respective Natives and Inhabitants* (London, 1735; 2nd edn 1737), 149–80.

55. N. Saakwa-Mante, 'Western Medicine and Racial Constructions: Surgeon John Atkins' Theory of Polygenism and Sleep Distemper in the 1730s', in W. Ernst and B. Harris (eds), *Race, Science and Medicine, 1700–1960* (London and New York, Routledge, 1999), 27–57.

56. G. Harvey, *The Conclave of Physicians* (London, 1683), 40.

57. J. Lind, *An Essay on Diseases Incidental to Europeans in Hot Climates* (London, 1768), 121.

58. K.J. Carpenter, *The History of Scurvy and Vitamin C*, 2nd edn (Cambridge: Cambridge University Press, 1988), 52–4.

59. P. Mathias, 'Swords and Ploughshares: The Armed Forces, Medicine, and Public Health in the Late Eighteenth Century', in J.M. Winter (ed.) *War and Economic Development* (Cambridge: Cambridge University Press, 1975), 76–87. Examples include: J. Badenoch, 'Observations in the Use of Wort, in the Cure of Scurvy at Sea', *Medical Observations and Inquiries*, v (London, 1776), 61–72; J. C. Smyth, *An Account of the Experiment Made at the Desire of the Lords Commissioners of the Admiralty on Board the Union Hospital Ship, to Determine the Effects of the Nitrous Acid in Destroying Contagion* (London, 1796); *Some Letters upon the Application of the Nitric Acid, to Medicine: From the Bombay Courier* (Bombay, 1797), 9–10, 32.

60. T. Duncan, 'Case of Tetanus Cured by Injections of Tobacco Smoke', *New England Journal of Medicine and Surgery*, v (1816), 195–202; J.B. Sheppard, 'On the Mercurial Treatment of Yellow Fever', *ibid.*, vii (1818), 247–58.

61. For example, W. Fordyce, 'An Attempt to Discover the Virtues of the Sarsaparilla Root in the Venereal Disease', *Medical Observations and Inquiries*, vol. i (2nd edn, London, 1758), 149–83; A. Gordon 'The Cure of the Lues

Venerea by the Mercurius Corrosivus Sublimatus', *ibid.*, 365–87; R. Miller, 'Some Further Observations upon the Use of Corrosive Sublimate', *ibid.*, vol. ii (London, 1762), 70–87; *Some Letters* (note 59), 26–29.

62. R.B. Sheridan, *Doctors and Slaves: A Medical and Demographic History of Slavery in the British West Indies, 1680–1834* (Cambridge: Cambridge University Press, 1985), *passim.*

63. J. Lind, *A Treatise on the Putrid and Remitting Marsh Fever, Which Raged at Bengal in the Year 1762* (Edinburgh, 1776), 46.

64. 'An Extract of a Letter from Mr. Vage, dated at Senegal, Oct. 15 1759', *Medical Observations and Inquiries, op. cit.* (note 61), ii, 269–72.

65. 'A Letter from Mr. John Travis...[on] One Principal Cause of the Sea Scurvy', *ibid.*, ii, 16.

66. Warren, *op. cit.* (note 31), 67.

67. Sheppard, *op. cit.* (note 60), 251.

68. S.J. Rogal, *Medicine in Great Britain from the Restoration to the Nineteenth Century, 1660–1800: An Annotated Bibliography* (New York: Greenwood, 1992), 211–14.

69. For example, see J. Bell, *An Inquiry into the Causes Which Produce, and the Means of Preventing Diseases Among British Officers, Soldiers, And Others in the West Indies* (London, 1791), vii, 122–3; R. Brocklesby, *Oeconomical and Medical Observations, in Two Parts. From the Year 1758 to the Year 1763, Inclusive, Tending to the Improvement of Military Hospitals and the Cure of Camp Diseases, Incident to Soldiers* (London, 1764), 44–9.

70. J. Hennen, *Principles of Military Surgery* (London, 1829), 2; H.A.L. Howell, 'The Story of the Army Surgeon and the Care of the Sick and Wounded in the British Army, from 1715 to 1748', *Journal of the Army Medical Corps*, xxii (1914), 320–34, 455–71; P.E. Kopperman, 'Medical Services in the British Army, 1742–1783', *Journal of the History of Medicine and Allied Sciences*, xxxiv (1979), 428–55.

71. Rogal, *op. cit.* (note 68), 211–14, 227–9.

72. J. Rollo, *Observations on the Diseases which Appeared in the Army on St Lucia*, 2nd edn (London, 1781), x; J. Anderson, *A Few Facts and Observations on the Yellow Fever of the West Indies* (Edinburgh, 1798), 34. It is worthy of note that Cleghorn dedicated the second edition of his treatise to the surgeons of the Royal Navy, in 1751, in the belief that they, not his army companions, would find his work on malaria of most benefit: George Cleghorn, *Observations on the Epidemical Diseases in Minorca, from the Year 1744 to 1749*, 2nd edn (London, 1752), iii–xii.

73. C. Hannaway, 'Environment and Miasmatics', in W. Bynum and R. Porter (eds), *Companion Encyclopedia of the History of Medicine*, 2 vols (Cambridge: Cambridge University Press, 1993).

74. Lind, *op. cit.* (note 57).

75. Lloyd and Coulter, *op. cit.* (note 3), *passim*; W. Northcote, *The Marine Practice of Physic and Surgery, Including that of Hot Countries* (London, 1770); G. Blane, *Observations on Diseases Incident to Seamen* (Edinburgh, 1785); R. Robertson, *Observations on Fevers and Other Diseases which Occur on Voyages to Africa and the West Indies* (London, 1792); T. Trotter, *Medicina Nautica: An Essay on the Diseases of Seamen*, 3 vols (London, 1797–1800); T. Salmon, *A New Geographical and Historical Grammar* (Edinburgh, 1767), 479, 485, 508, 518, 521, 542, 545, 567, 570, 579, 586. The *Grammar* was in its 12th edition by 1772.

76. T. Trapham, *A Discourse on the State of Health in the Island of Jamaica* (London, 1679); G. Miller, 'Airs, Waters, and Places in History', *Journal of the History of Medicine and Allied Sciences*, xvii (1962), 129–40.

77. Examples include: 'A Letter from Mr. John Clayton, Rector of Croston at Wakefield in Yorkshire, to the Royal Society, May 12, 1688, giving an Account of Several Observations in Virginia, and His Voyage Thither, More Particularly Concerning the Air', *Philosophical Transactions*, xvii (1694–95), 781–95, 941–8, xviii, 121–35; J. Cunningham, 'Observations on Weather in a Voyage to China, 1700', *Philosophical Transactions*, xxiv (1704), 1639–48; J. Cunningham, 'A Register of Wind and Weather... at Chusan', *idem.*, xxiv (1704), 1648–98. An excellent early first-hand analysis of medical topography for portions of West Africa is contained in the letters by J. Hilliar of 1688: William Denham (ed.), *Miscellanea Curiosa*, 3 vols, 3rd edn (London, 1727), III, 356–80.

78. H. Sloane, *A Voyage to the Islands Madera, Barbados, Nieves, S. Christophers and Jamaica, with the Natural History of the... Last of Those Islands; to which is prefix'd an Introduction, Wherein is an Account of the Inhabitants, Air, Waters, Diseases, Trade, etc. of that Place*, 2 vols (London, 1707 and 1725), I, xxx–xxxiii, xc–cliv. See also: W.D. Churchill, 'Bodily Differences? Gender, Race, and Class in Hans Sloane's Jamaican Medical Practice, 1687–1688', *Journal of the History of Medicine and Allied Sciences*, 60 (2005), 391–444.

79. Sloane, *ibid.*, I, xc.

80. Warren, *op. cit.* (note 31), 19–20, 73, and *passim*.

81. For the medical context, see: D. Crewe, *Yellow Jack and the Worm: British Naval Administration in the West Indies, 1739–1748* (Liverpool: Liverpool University Press, 1993).

82. Cleghorn, *op. cit.* (note 72), iv–v.

83. J. Tennent, *A Reprieve From Death: In Two Physical Chapters* (London, 1741), iv–v, 3.

84. C. Bisset, *Medical Essays* (Newcastle upon Tyne, 1766), *passim*.

85. B. Mosely, *Observations on the Dysentery of the West Indies* (London, 1781); T. Dancer, *A Brief History of the Late Expedition Against Fort San Juan, so far as it relates to the Diseases of the Troops* (Kingston, Jamaica, 1781); J. Hunter,

Observations on the Diseases of the Army in Jamaica (London, 1788);
R. Jackson, *A Treatise on the Fevers of Jamaica, with Some Observations on the Intermitting Fever of America* (London, 1791).

86. Bell, *op. cit.* (note 69), vii.
87. S. Hales, *Philosophical Experiments: Containing Useful, and Necessary Instructions for Such as Undertake Long Voyages at Sea* (London, 1739), i–ii. See also *idem.*, *A Description of Ventilators: Whereby Great Quantities of Fresh Air May with Ease be Conveyed into Mines, Gaols, Hospitals, Work-Houses and Ships, in Exchange for Their Noxious Air* (London, 1743), i–iv.
88. Moyle, *op. cit.* (note 33), A3–4.
89. J. Tennent, *Physical Inquiries* (London, 1742), unpaginated dedication.
90. J. Huxham, 'A Method for Preserving the Health of Seamen in Long Cruises and Voyages', in his *Essay on Fevers* (London, 1750), 264.
91. Bell, *op. cit.* (note 69), ix, xiv.
92. J. Millar, *Observations on the Management of the Prevailing Diseases in Great Britain, Particularly in the Army and Navy* (London, 1783), iv.
93. Cockburn, *Profluvia Ventris, op. cit.* (note 43), preface, n.p.; Bell, *op. cit.* (note 69), 3–4, 124–32; J. Pringle, *Observations on the Diseases of the Army*, B. Rush (ed.), (Philadelphia, 1810), xxxv; D. Monro, *An Account of the Diseases which were More Frequent in the British Military Hospitals in Germany, from January 1761 to the Return of the Troops to England in March 1763: To which is Added, an Essay on the Means of Preserving the Health of Soldiers, and Conducting Military Hospitals* (London, 1764), 312.
94. Trapham, *op. cit.* (note 76), 20, 50, 140–2; Bisset, *op. cit.* (note 84), 19, 37–8; F. Fuller, *Medicina Gymnastica*, 2nd edn (London, 1705), 223, 228; R. Towne, *A Treatise of the Diseases Most Frequent in the West-Indies* (London, 1726), 1–2, 7, 9–10; J. Williams, *An Essay on the Bilious or Yellow Fever of Jamaica*, Charles Blicke (ed.), (London, 1772), *passim*; J.P. Purry, *A Method for Determining the Best Climate of the Earth* (London, 1744), 22.
95. Denham, *op. cit.* (note 77), III, 361–2; Towne, *op. cit.* (note 94), 100, 114, 183–8, 189; Lind, *op. cit.* (note 57), 120, 134–5, 141; Atkins, *op. cit.* (note 53) 17–20, appendix, 17; W. Northcote, *The Anatomy of the Human Body* (London, 1772), x–xi, 12; P. Browne, *The Civil and Natural History of Jamaica* (London, 1789), 25; V. Seaman, *An Account of the Epidemic Yellow Fever, as it appeared in the City of New York in the Year 1795* (New York, 1796), 6, 12, 20; T. Aubury, *The Sea-Surgeon, or the Guinea Man's Vade Mecum* (London, 1729), *passim*. See also Kiple and Ornelas *op. cit.* (note 1), 71–5.
96. Slave and plantation medicine is examined in Sheridan, *op. cit.* (note 62), 42–71, 98–126, 292–342.
97. Atkins, *op. cit.* (note 53), appendix, 17–28.
98. For the dominance of youthful males see, for example: J.P. Wade, *Select*

Evidence of the Successful Method of Treating Fever and Dysentery in Bengal (London, 1791), *passim*; R. Robertson, *Observations on the Jail, Hospital and Ship Fever*, new edn (London, 1789), *passim*; Bisset (note 84), 47–65; J. Clark, *Observations on the Diseases in Long Voyages to Hot Countries* (London, 1773), *passim*. For case histories of women, see W. Churchill, *op. cit.* (note 78), 391–444.

99. M. Adanson, *A Voyage to Senegal, the Isle of Goree, and the River Gambia* (London, 1759), 217–18 (observation inserted by the anonymous English translator); Tennent, *op. cit.* (note 89), 34; Tennent, *op. cit.* (note 83), 14; Lind, *op. cit.* (note 57), 59, 102–3,117, 126; Williams, *op.cit.* (note 95), 15, 65; Trapham, *op. cit.* (note 76), 13, 101; Sloane, *op. cit.* (note 78), I, xxxi; Towne (note 94), 115–8, 163, 169.

100. W. Hillary, *Observations on the Changes to the Air, and the Cocomitant Epidemical Diseases on the Island of Barbados*, B. Rush (ed.) (Philadelphia, 1811), vi; Clark, *op. cit.* (note 98), 41–2.

101. Wade, *op. cit.* (note 98), 166 and *passim*.

102. Rollo, *op. cit.* (note 72), 135; Robertson, *op. cit.* (note 75), 1, 49; Clark, *op. cit.* (note 98), viii; C. Lloyd (ed.), *The Health of Seamen* (London: Naval Records Society, 1965), 136, 217.

103. C. Fury, *Tides in the Affairs of Men: The Social History of Elizabethan Seamen, 1580–160* (Westport: Greenwood, 2002), 162–4, 198–201.

104. J. Woodward, *The Seaman's Monitor; Or, Advice to Sea-faring Men, with Reference to Their Behaviour Before, In, and After Their Voyage,* 7th edn (London, 1767), 32, 39; J. Hanway, *The Seaman's Faithful Companion* (London, 1763), 20, 28, 33, 37; D. Morrice, *The Young Midshipman's Instructor* (London, 1801), 2, 3, 5–7.

105. Christie, *Abstract, op. cit.* (note 40), 6.

106. Brocklesby, *op. cit.* (note 69), 207, 217, 229.

107. Atkins, *op. cit.* (note 53), appendix, 4.

108. Hales, *Philosophical Experiments* (note 87), 17–20; Hillary, *op. cit.* (note 100), vi.

109. Denham, *op. cit.* (note 77), III, 361–2.

110. Monro, *op. cit.* (note 93), 332–4; Brockesby, *op. cit.* (note 69), 112–3; Sloane, *op. cit.* (note 78), I, xxxi; Robertson, *Fevers* (note 50), 87–8, 100–2, 107, 234–7; Atkins, *op. cit.* (note 54), 234; Tennent, *Reprieve* (note 83), 8, 11; Williams, *op. cit.* (note 94), 20–1; T.M. Winterbottom, *Medical Directions for the Use of Navigators and Settlers in Hot Climates* (London, 1803), 7, 9, 11–13, 23; G. Freiherr Van Swieten, *The Diseases Incident to Armies... To which are Added the Nature and Treatment of Gun-shot Wounds... Likewise, Some Brief Directions, to be Observed by Sea Surgeons in Engagements. Also, Preventative of the Scurvy at Sea.... Published for the Use of Military, and Naval Surgeons in America* (Philadelphia, 1776); J. Jones, *Plain*

Concise Practical Remarks, on the Treatment of Wounds and Fractures, to which is Added, an Appendix, on Camp and Military Hospitals; Principally Designed, for the Use of Young Military and Naval Surgeons in North America (Philadelphia, 1776); Anon., 'Remarks upon Bilious Fevers and Innoculation, being an Extract from a letter by Dr Rush, of Philadelphia', *Medical Observations and Inquiries*, 5 (London, 1776), 33. See also, Lind, *op. cit.* (note 57), 113, 129; Towne, *op. cit.* (note 94), 11–12, 19–20, 128.

111. Williams, *op. cit.* (note 95), 5; Rollo, *op. cit.* (note 72), 146–7; Anderson, *op. cit.* (note 72), 42; Lind, *op. cit.* (note 57), 132–6; Clark, *op. cit.* (note 98), 67–8.

112. Rollo, *op. cit.* (note 72), 144, and see 150, 152.

113. Atkins *op. cit.* (note 53), appendix, 7–8. See also Bell, *op. cit.* (note 69), 9.

114. For example: Jones, *op. cit.* (note 110), *passim*; Winterbottom, *op. cit.* (note 110), 71–3, 83, 86–7, 93–107, 110–7; Towne, *op. cit.* (note 94), 17, 19, 29–30, 119, 158; Bisset, *op. cit.* (note 84), 37–41, 46.

115. M. Worboys, 'The Emergence of Tropical Medicine: A Study in the Establishment of a Scientific Specialty', in G. Lemaime, *et al.* (eds), *Perspectives on the Emergence of Scientific Disciplines* (Mouton, The Hague and Paris: Aldine, 1976), 78–80; M. Worboys, 'Germs, Malaria and the Invention of Mansonian Tropical Medicine: From "Diseases in the Tropics" to "Tropical Diseases"', in Arnold, *op. cit.* (note 1), 181–207: 182–6 ; D. Arnold, 'Introduction: Tropical Medicine before Manson', in *idem.*, 1–19: 6–13.

116. For example: Millar, *op. cit.* (note 92), *passim*.

117. J. Lind, *Two Papers on Fevers and Infections* (London, 1763), 105.

118. Winterbottom, *op. cit.* (note 110), 5–6, 10–13, 16–18, 59, 66–7; U. Parsons, *Sailor's Physician, Containing Medical Advice for Seamen and Other Persons at Sea, on the Treatment of Diseases, also on the Preservation of Health in Sickly Climates,* 2nd edn (Providence, Rhode Island, 1824), 139, 146, 150–62 and *passim*. Subsequent editions up to 1877 employed the title *Physician for Ships*.

119. Winterbottom, *op. cit.* (note 110), 20; Parsons, *op. cit.* (note 118), 180 and *passim*.

120. W. Curry, *An Historical Account of the Climates and Diseases of the United States of America* (Philadelphia, 1792); D. Ramsay, *A Sketch of the Soil, Climate, Weather, and Diseases of South-Carolina* (Charleston, 1796).

121. Bell, *op. cit.* (note 69), 1, 6–9, 121–3.

3

The British Army in North America and the West Indies, 1755–83: A Medical Perspective

Paul E. Kopperman

This chapter provides an analytical overview of the operational structure, hospital and regimental systems of military medical practice of the British Army in North Amercia and the West Indies, 1755–83, using a database of medical officers, regimental returns, lists of drugs used, correspondence and publications. Practice varied depending on location, season, and time of year, but cooperation between medical and general officers was crucial. Pringle's emphasis on environment influenced practice, with medics advocating preventative treatments. Army practitioners were among medical officers in the West Indies, at the forefront of moderate therapeutics.

One of the advantages of studying medical history in the military context is that the historian can make use of data that are in many respects fuller than would be available on contemporary practice in the civilian sphere. This essay will focus on British Army practice in North America and the West Indies, 1755–83. In the course of it, I intend to make use of databases that I have created in association with a book project. One database contains information on 858 men who served as medical officers in America or the Indies at some point during the period in question. A second consists of regimental returns; a third, of casualties and overall mortality; a fourth, of lists of drugs distributed for the use of the army abroad, 1703–97. There is also a wealth of evidence available in contemporary correspondence, diaries, and publications. The data taken *in toto* are sufficiently strong to allow a fair assessment of the medical services that were available to the British soldier in the eighteenth century. Contemporary medicine was limited in its ability to prevent and cure disease and was characterised by premises that have been shown to be mistaken. It appears, however, that on the whole the medical services performed well and beneficially.

The organisation of medical services

The British Army was present in North America regularly after 1664, but prior to 1755 this was usually in the form of detachments and independent companies. Several regiments were stationed in the West Indies during Queen Anne's War, and afterwards the 38th Foot remained in Antigua, while independent companies were stationed in Jamaica and Bermuda. Large numbers of British regulars participated in the Walker expedition of 1711 and the Vernon expedition of 1741/2. Three regiments relieved the Americans at Louisbourg in 1746, then remained in Canada. Besides a military presence, the army brought a medical presence. As of July 1750, the garrison hospital at Halifax was quite large, including even a midwife.[1] But while army units were stationed in the New World, it does not appear that prior to 1755 the high command or the government back in Britain were sensitive to the health issues peculiar to service there.

During the eighteenth century, army medical services operated on five levels. Outlines of medical policy were set at the War Office, though the consent of the king and of other departments of government might be required. The Secretary-at-War issued directives for the services, but almost always did so on the advice of key medical personnel. Prior to 1756, his main advisors were the Surgeon-General and, of somewhat less importance, the Physician-General. Under this system, central direction was rather weak and medical services in theatres of war tended to be dominated by hospital physicians, Sir John Pringle, the pre-eminent medical figure during the War of the Austrian Succession, being a case in point. In 1756, however, Lord Barrington, the Secretary-at-War, possibly acting at the behest of the Duke of Cumberland, created the position of Inspector of Regimental Infirmaries and gave it to Robert Adair. Unlike the Physician-General and the Surgeon-General, the inspector was a full-time official, with an office at Horse Guards. Nevertheless, Adair made the office as much as it made him. By 1758, his authority was fully established, and between that time and his death in 1790 he dominated medical policy; his advice being frequently sought and almost automatically accepted by a series of Secretaries-at-War. Personal charm helped him establish his influence, as did his marriage into the Keppel family, but he was also able, and he dealt with a vast range of issues.[2]

Serving men in the field were four categories of staff.[3] Each regiment or battalion had a surgeon on its establishment. Foot regiments, though generally not cavalry or dragoons, also employed a mate, and several regiments that served in America 1758–60 had two mates.[4] Medical personnel were on establishments for most major garrisons. Hospitals were often created in Britain to accompany expeditions going abroad.

In theatres of war, the general hospital was the most important medical institution, for both administration and treatment. The term 'hospital' referred to an institution, its facilities, and officers alike. Hospital physicians and surgeons were the elite of army medical personnel. Other hospital staff included apothecaries and surgeons' mates – also, prior to 1763, apothecary's mates. If the staff included a matron, she was listed among the officers.[5]

The hospital in North America was created in the autumn of 1754, initially for service on the projected expedition under Major-General Edward Braddock. The choices of personnel reflect care. James Napier, the director, had served as a hospital surgeon on the Continent during the preceding war. Another surgeon had previously served on an expedition to Brittany in 1746. With only three exceptions, the balance of the staff, including Charlotte Browne, the matron, were veterans of American service, all having tended the troops at Louisbourg during the British occupation of 1746–9.[6] A list of necessities for the hospital, prepared in late 1754, included 800 flock beds and bolsters.[7] Given that Braddock's army primarily consisted of just two regiments, these were large numbers, and may suggest that the planners anticipated a buildup. On the other hand, there was a marked omission in the hospital as first set out. It included no physician, and none was to be designated until Richard Huck, commissioned a surgeon in March 1756, was appointed physician in August 1757, probably at the instance of Lord Loudoun, his mentor and the Commander-in-Chief in North America.

From the time it landed in America, the hospital was mobile. Although some medical staff stayed at Fort Cumberland, most, including Napier, followed Braddock, and were present at the Battle of the Monongahela, which on 9 July 1755 concluded the campaign in disaster. After the battle and subsequent retreat, Napier recommended breaking up the hospital. On 22 July, he wrote to Henry Fox, Secretary of State for the Southern Department,

> As the Forces acting on this Continent are in several Divisions, at some hundreds of Miles distance from one another, an Hospital can be of Use but to few... therefor [*sic*] submit it to your Consideration whether the Service would not be full as well answer'd, if not better... by having no Establishment for an Hospital, and allowing two or three additional Mates to each Regiment.[8]

In that letter and others, however, he also laid out an alternate plan for reform. If the hospital was to be maintained, he argued, it would be necessary to increase the staff and to confirm his authority over the other surgeons. It was this set of suggestions that was ultimately accepted. At some point in 1756 the War Office issued instructions for the hospital officers, with the aim of regularising management. The directive established the chief surgeon and the physicians as the 'Principal Officers' and directed the apothecaries and mates to heed their orders. Not only did this document set out the governing structure of the hospital for the balance of the war, but it was reaffirmed during the War of Independence.[9] Finally, in April 1757, Loudoun appointed Napier to Chief Surgeon, providing him with clear authority over all personnel in the hospital.[10]

Although the number of hospital officers increased during the course of the French and Indian War, growth was roughly commensurate with that of the army. Reduced in 1764, the hospital was revived in 1775 and, after Napier declined to serve again as head, it fell increasingly under the control of a physician, John Mervin Nooth, whose predominance was confirmed when in April 1779 he was appointed Superintendent General. Under Nooth, the size of staff proliferated, causing Adair to advise him in March 1782, 'Your List of Mates is exceedingly large, & I must recommend it to you to have Attention to keep it within Bounds.'[11]

The issue of size was tied to that of expense, an obsession at the War Office. Keeping a tight rein on the size of staff during wartime, reducing the hospital during peacetime, and generally relying as much as possible on regimental and garrison personnel – these were standard policies.[12] Furthermore, no matter how well run, the hospital was regularly compared negatively to the regimental infirmary in military medical literature. There were complaints that troops who were hospitalised for lengthy periods became depressed, lethargic, and unsoldierly. The hospital was thought by many to be wasteful and unnecessarily expensive. Writers asserted that soldiers died needlessly, in transit to hospital. But the overriding criticism was that the hospital actually encouraged disease, by confining many contagious patients in central facilities. That the hospital was seriously flawed was regarded by critics as beyond dispute. Adair himself saw the matter this way. In a letter that he wrote in 1779 he observed, 'The advantages attending regimental, in preference to General Hospitals, are... obvious to Practitioners.'[13]

Education and credentials of army medical officers

In one important respect, however, the hospital was seen as markedly superior to the infirmary: the quality of personnel. The physicians and surgeons of the hospital were generally considered the elite of the medical services in the field, being better educated, more experienced, and generally more competent than were regimental or garrison medical officers. In May 1781, Barrington wrote to Sir Henry Clinton, the Commander-in-Chief in North America:

I have had frequent conversations with Mr Adair upon the propriety of filling up Vacancies in the General Hospital with Regimentall Surgeons: and I find it to have ever been his Opinion (as it is also that of Dr Nooth) that the charge is of too serious a nature to be entrusted to the Surgeons of Regiment, who have very rarely had opportunities of acquiring sufficient skill to perform the great Operations of Surgery, or sufficient Judgement to decide upon the necessity of performing them.[14]

Hospital mates, too, were regarded far more favourably than were their regimental counterparts. It was standard policy for the War Office to recommend that regimental surgeons be drawn from the ranks of hospital mates, rather than regimental mates. Since surgeoncies were usually bought and sold, however, and since the regimental mates were on the scene and were known to the colonels, they were usually able to succeed retiring surgeons if they wished to and had the purchase price.[15]

During the eighteenth century, no separate medical school or programme existed in Britain for training army medical officers.[16] Future medical officers were trained or educated in a civilian environment, often by men who had themselves known no other and could relate little to what practising medicine in the military might entail.[17] Furthermore, most officers left the army to enter private practice while still young. Nevertheless, military medicine was a distinct field of practice. It required a range of surgical and medical competence that was greater than in the civilian world, and medical personnel on duty abroad often faced diseases almost unknown in Britain. Military medicine was, indeed, a speciality that precluded the sort of specialisation that was then becoming more popular in civilian practice. The irony is reflected in a notation by Thompson Forster, a hospital surgeon during the American War of Independence. In October 1776, he served on a hospital ship that supported the army before and after the Battle of White Plains. In his diary, he noted, 'Upon all Expeditions of this sort we act in the threefold capacities of Physician, Surgeon and Apothecary; Physicians or Apothecaries are never detached, but remain in Garrison, I have frequently had more Physical cases than Surgical, which was the case here.'[18]

Throughout the century, and especially toward its close, there were frequent complaints that the army was being failed by the educational system. Robert Jackson, whose four decades of army service began in the War of Independence, suggested reforms in education, the founding of a school to train medical officers, and an upgrade of standards for promotion.[19] John Bell proposed the establishment of a 'School of Naval and Military Surgery' and even detailed a curriculum for the institution.[20] Among critics of regimental personnel, none was more vociferous than Robert Hamilton, who, as a former medical officer, wrote from personal knowledge but with the passion and perhaps tendency to exaggerate of a reformer. While noting that there were regimental surgeons who had completed a strong programme of medical education before entering the service, he added,

> [I]t is a truth too well known to be denied, that many more have, and do daily find their way into it thro' interest and mis-applied recommendation, whose opportunities of qualifying themselves to undertake so important an office, have been almost none, or, at best, extremely limited.[21]

Acknowledging that the problem could not immediately be corrected, he instead addressed his work to medical officers who were 'Young and inexperienced in the profession in which they are engaged, and without that foundation to build on, which it behooved them to possess.'[22] Bell complained:

> A young man for example in no affluent circumstances struggles for one or two years to obtain the most ordinary points of knowledge; or without knowledge, he learns by rote to answer the common questions. He undergoes a slight examination, is allowed a diploma, and goes along with troops to the most sickly climates on the most dangerous service. He is at first, indeed, received only as a mate, but by gradation he becomes a surgeon.[23]

Other observers were more willing to accept the educational shortcomings of medical officers, especially if they were young and showed a desire to improve. There was a traditional sense that quality improved through experience.

Most of the men who served as army medical officers were indeed young when they entered the service, and this was especially so of the regimental surgeons' mates. For the 115 mates whose year of birth and month of warrant can be determined, the average age at appointment was 20.8. Only eighteen were over twenty-five when appointed, while nineteen were eighteen or younger, the youngest being sixteen. These were young men, but not children. Given the average timetable of those entering practice, it can be said that most of them would have had the time to serve out an apprenticeship, and many to have had more extensive training. The new mates were probably at least on a par with young men entering private practice in the civilian world. In May 1756, John Stevenson, a Scottish physician, wrote to Loudoun:

> William McMyne who goes Surgeons Mate [of the 42ⁿᵈ] to America is my acquaintance. He has not only seen what a Scots Infirmary afords, and been

in an apothecarys Shops, & study'd surgery and anatomy, but attended all of the medical colleges here, with application.[24]

Regimental surgeons tended to be somewhat older at the time of appointment. The thirty-four men in my data base who attained a surgeoncy without first having served as mate had an average age of 24.2 on the date of commission, and there was one case of a 16-year-old being appointed. Many, and probably most men in this category, had practiced in the civilian world before seeking commissions. In some cases, at least, their practice had been unsuccessful. In January 1757, Thomas Oswald wrote Loudoun from Philadelphia, seeking a surgeoncy in the Royal Americans for his friend, Lauchlan McLean. Asserting that McLean 'had a very fine Education first at Dublin and then at Edinburgh,' he added that he had failed to establish a practice in America, but only because the Americans were too 'Connected with what they call physicians.'[25] Most regimental surgeons were men who had entered the army as mates, and they were typically older than those who moved directly to surgeoncies. The seventy surgeons who had first served as regimental mates averaged 29.2 when commissioned, and the fifty who had been hospital mates when appointed averaged thirty-one years old.

Only a dozen medical officers held MDs at the time they entered army service, and three of these were Loyalists who served the British during the War of Independence. The remainder were hospital or expeditionary physicians, and indeed the MD was generally a prerequisite for such appointments.[26] An additional sixty-two officers went on to receive MDs during, or more typically after, their period of service. Most men in this category gained their degrees at St Andrews or Aberdeen, universities that did not have medical programs but nevertheless granted the MD on the basis of an oral examination and certificates of competence. Contemporaries roundly denounced the practice, and there appears indeed to have been abuse.[27]

Usually some inquiry was made into the credentials of would-be medical officers. Prior to 1745, it was the function of the Surgeon-General to consider the qualifications of regimental surgeons. When the Company of Surgeons was chartered in 1745, it gained a monopoly on examining candidates. In fact, however, many surgeons' mates and some surgeons were not examined at all, and a few were examined not in London but in Edinburgh or Dublin.[28] The Army, unlike the Navy, did not require that applicants for all surgical posts be examined, but individual appointments were made contingent on passing. Most regimental surgeons and mates who served in America did so only after having first been tested, and surgeons who did not submit a certificate confirming that they had passed were often required to do so, or face being superseded.[29] Virtually all hospital surgeons received their appointments only after passing an examination by the board in London. The company sometimes examined hospital mates, but it was more common for them to be reviewed by a hospital board or by senior personnel. On 8 October 1776, Charles (later Sir Charles) Blagden, physician to the hospital in North America, noted in his diary that he and a second physician had examined two mates and that 'they appeared duly qualified'.[30]

The prospect of review by company examiners may have discouraged some men from even making an attempt to proceed, but the examination itself was notoriously inadequate. The questions asked were easy and standard, and a number of writers complained that examiners were too lenient in assessing the responses. Bell claimed that candidates prepared themselves for the examination by memorising lists of common questions and answers. Even those who did poorly, he asserted, usually got through:

> Often I have heard the president of a board of examiners address a young
> man in the following terms: 'You seem, Sir, to be exceedingly ignorant in
> many very important matters, but you are young and may improve, we have
> granted you a diploma with this expectation; and we lay our injunctions
> upon you to be diligent.'[31]

John Ring, a member of the company but a critic of its leadership, asserted that leniency grew from greed, since examinees who passed paid a fee.[32] Even some successful candidates expressed disdain for the process. In 1796, Thomas Robertson recorded in his diary his impressions on being examined so that he could be certified a naval surgeon:

> The first examination (by the surgeons) I found teasing and inadequate to
> ascertain ability. The physician's examination superficial. Four of us went for
> the same time for that purpose; all, out of compliment and from its being
> customary, purchased his books.[33]

In wartime, the numbers of candidates being examined increased, and this resulted in examinations that were still more hurried, cursory, and superficial. On 7 March 1776, no fewer than seventy-four candidates for various appointments and diplomas were reviewed. All passed.[34]

Although some men may have been poorly trained and educated prior to their entry into service, the Army afforded them an unexcelled opportunity to improve. John Buchanan, who served as surgeon to the Blues, 1733–45, recalled his interaction with other medical officers during a tour on the Continent during the War of the Austrian Succession.

> We have a weekly Club where all are welcome to come, the chief Subject of
> conversation relates to our own business; it being a standing rule with us,

that if any thing remarkable happen'd during the last weeks practice, it's to be made publick for the good of the Society; by this means we know the practice of the whole army during the Campn, [and] in winter quarters that of the Garrison, where we have an opportunity of attending the hospital. All talk freely, nor can I perceive any reservedness or fondness for Secret medecines, or a private method of practice; some are regular bred Physicians.[35]

The network of medical men provided an excellent opportunity for young practitioners to learn. So did the ready availability of bodies to dissect. But not everyone took advantage. Mates, both regimental and hospital, had a reputation for indifference to duty. In 1770, Richard Hope, surgeon to the 52nd Foot, reported from Quebec:

I have no one to give me the least assistance, my Mate (who ought to attend all cases, report the disorders to me, and make up the medicines) is so fine a gentleman, so much above his business, and such a man of gallantry, that I don't see his face once in a month.[36]

There were some checks on the impact that poorly educated medical men could have on the soldiery. On the regimental level, the more difficult medical and surgical cases were normally handled by the surgeon, rather than by his mate. Men who were seriously ill or who required major surgery ideally went not to the regimental infirmary but to the hospital, where the surgeons and physicians, the elite of the medical services, were in charge. When the Army was concentrated and did not face a health crisis, these safeguards were probably observed in most cases. If, however, the regimental surgeon was absent or incapacitated or if his regiment was divided, the mate often had charge of difficult cases. Furthermore, in the face of a battle or epidemic, any medical officer might have to handle serious wounds or diseases on his own.

The military circumstance

The relative health or illness of the Army depended more on circumstances than on the quality of medical personnel. To provide a yardstick for analysis, we might first consider the 1/84th – prior to March 1779, the 'Royal Highland Emigrants' – a battalion unique in having left an unbroken string of ninety-four monthly returns. The 1/84th suffered some spikes of illness, but the monthly percentage of men returned as sick averaged only 11.1. The annual mortality rate was 3.1.[37] The men who composed this battalion were relatively old, being in large part discharged veterans who returned to service in 1775, when the Americans invaded Canada. Aside from age, however, all of the health factors for the battalion were positive. By September 1776, when the set of returns begins, the 1/84th had already passed through its most active phase. For the balance of its existence, it did garrison duty, mainly in Quebec and Montreal. Life may have been dull, but it was seldom unhealthful. As Thomas Anburey, a Loyalist volunteer in Lieutenant-General John Burgoyne's army, observed, 'The air of Canada is reckoned the most salubrious and healthy of any in the world.'[38] Army units that served in Canada for extended periods and were largely sedentary typically maintained a level of health roughly on the order of that enjoyed by the 1/84th.

The same was true of regiments serving in New England and in the middle colonies of British North America. It is not surprising that 1770 should have been a healthy year for the British troops in North America, with a sickness rate of only about 5.7 per cent and annual mortality of only 2.3 per cent.[39] Most of the troops were engaged in garrison activity in Boston and New York. Duty was seldom fatiguing, and the stress level was low. The men generally enjoyed good accommodation, and they were well supplied. Soldiers who became sickly were discharged or recommended to Chelsea. This was a model peacetime circumstance, with almost every variable encouraging health. But any of the variables could change quickly, in which case the level of illness and the mortality rate was almost certain to rise.

By way of contrast to the Army of 1770, we might note the force that Sir William Howe commanded in 1777. It began the year in New York, recuperating from the campaign of 1776 – this, despite the fact that it had emerged victorious from every significant engagement. The Army spent most of 1777 in and around New York before moving on toward Philadelphia that autumn, an effort also marked by major battles, each of them a victory, and by ultimate achievement of the objective. This was an army that averaged 14.2 per cent sick monthly and suffered 11.3 per cent mortality for the year. Its healthiest months, and those with lowest mortality, were July–October, despite the fact that contemporary wisdom considered late-summer to early-autumn to be the period most dangerous to an army. The reason for this incongruity is that although the Army suffered several outbreaks of illness, its poor health numbers were primarily driven by the violence and fatigue of war, rather than by disease.

Eighteenth-century medical men and officers saw a close connection between disease and fatigue, and while military duty was often fatiguing, the French and Indian War, which included many campaigns in the interior, was exceptionally arduous. The march on Montreal in 1760 marked a fitting climax to campaigns in the north. On 17 August, Huck wrote to Loudoun:

> The Fatigue and Labour the Troops have had is inconceivable. Men and Officers all Day almost in the Water dragging the Batteaus with Provision

over the Shoals and Rifts.... No Campaign has hitherto been attended with the Fatigue which this Army has already undergone.[40]

Huck added that if the Army were defeated at Montreal, it would be impossible for it to get back.

Even for men in stationary circumstances, living conditions might be so poor as to threaten health. When Colonel Henry Bouquet and his battalion, the 1/60th, arrived in Charleston on 18 June 1757, they could find no accommodation and were forced to encamp at a racecourse, which during the summer that followed, was often inundated. In late July, Bouquet applied to the Governor for accommodation, but was provided only with four 'bad empty houses', where soldiers were obliged to lie on the floor.[41] Only after repeated remonstrations did the Province provide quartering in public houses, and then only for 160 men, the rest remaining in the empty houses. By October, Bouquet was reporting, 'We have Lost a good Number of Men by Death and Desertion, owing in part to the bad Accommodations given us.'[42] The Assembly voted funds to build a barracks, but not to furnish it immediately, putting that consideration off until the next session. This led Bouquet to berate the Governor and to complain to Loudoun:

> Till now I had expected that the Troops having been Sent here at the request of the Governor, they would be taken care of, but it Seems that People in this Province are apt to believe that any thing is well enough for officers and Soldiers.[43]

Meanwhile, the sickness continued. On 22 October, Bouquet informed Richard Peters, the Secretary of Pennsylvania, 'Our men die very fast'.[44] To make matters worse, the Assembly provided very little firewood.[45] It finally voted funds for furniture, but construction of the barracks went slowly, and until late-winter most of the men remained in the decrepit houses that had been allotted to them earlier. Only on 19 February 1758, did they occupy their new barracks.[46]

It goes without saying that a battle could within hours change a healthy army into one that desperately needed medical aid, but often a series of small engagements was as damaging as a major battle. Furthermore, assuming that the casualty figures were not wholly one-sided, as they were at Paoli, the identity of the victor was less important than which army could more quickly make good its losses. During the War of Independence the Continental Army drew on greater manpower resources than could the British, and this played a major role in its victory in a war that saw Americans lose most major battles and suffer far heavier casualties.

Medical services were severely strained by battle. In the wake of large-scale engagements, wounded soldiers often went untended for many hours.

As might be expected, the problem was especially severe if the army was forced into a quick retreat after the action. Such was the case in the hours after Braddock's army retreated. Although some wounded officers, including Braddock, received prompt treatment, it appears that most of the rank-and-file had to fend for themselves. Years later, George Washington recalled the first hours of retreat:

> The shocking Scenes which presented themselves in this Nights March are not to be described. The dead, the dying, the groans, lamentations, and crys along the Road of the wounded for help... were enough to pierce a heart of adamant.[47]

It was not until 13 July (the day of Braddock's death), after the main force had reached the camp of Colonel Thomas Dunbar, that troops first received dressings on their wounds, and by then these were filled with maggots.[48]

Braddock's defeat was problematical not only because of the precipitous retreat, but because the battle itself was unexpected. The British were often surprised by attacks during both wars, and this had significance for the medical services. It was common for the hospital base to be some miles behind the army, and in case of a sudden attack it was seldom in a position to offer immediate assistance. On 13 July 1777, six days after Burgoyne's army had been surprised and mauled at Skenesborough, John Macnamara Hayes, a surgeon in the hospital, wrote of his recent experiences. He had arrived at Skenesborough on the 8th, after riding twenty-five miles through the wilderness. What he had encountered there he communicated to a friend in England.

> Most of [the wounded] are in sheds made of Boughs, which are no defence from rain, now wch unfortunately set in these three or four days past almost constantly.... I never experienced more uneasiness at seeing the Wounded Suffer, nor do I wish ever to be in so disagreeable a Situation again. Had I the Common Necessaries for their relief, I shd. not Complain, but without them, how great must Man's feelings be; – My hands embrued in Blood, My face as dirty & my beard as long as a Capuetien fryar with every thing filthy on me is my prest. Situation, nor can I help it, as my things are 25 Miles off.[49]

It was risky to site medical facilities close to an action. In the wake of the Battle of Harlem Heights, Forster established a facility in three nearby houses, only to be driven out, amid derisive laughter from his own camp, when American artillery opened up on it. He reported in his diary, 'The whole blame of this rested upon my Shoulders.'[50]

Armies spread disease, and this was one reason why communities seldom welcomed them. In a letter written in June 1757, Bouquet reported that his battalion had recently arrived in Charleston. Smallpox was spreading among the troops, he noted, and 'The people are so afraid of this Distemper that I was doubtful if they wou'd let us come in Town.'[51] Of course, the army circumstance also encouraged the spread of disease among the troops. Forces that were in transit regularly picked up and spread epidemics. Such was the case in the most devastating epidemic that struck the British Army in the New World between 1755 and 1783: the visitation of yellow fever that virtually destroyed the force that had been sent out under the Earl of Albemarle to seize Havana. The epidemic appears to have begun in Martinique, which the British had seized during the winter of 1761/2. Albemarle arrived in April 1762 to merge some of the troops there with the force that he had brought from Europe, and he informed Sir Jeffery Amherst, the Commander-in-Chief in North America, 'upon my arrival I found the Troops very Sickly, many dead, & the Sick list increasing dayly'.[52] The taking of Havana was not without cost, for five-to-six hundred men were killed or wounded.[53] Overwhelmingly, however, the men suffered from illness. A weekly return dating from 16 August, just after the city was taken, showed 4,205 men fit for duty; 5238, fully 55.5 per cent, sick; and 196 dead in the past week alone.[54] Worse was to come. A return of 11 October noted 886 fit, 5,713 – 86.6 per cent – sick, and 306 dead in the past week. The 22nd Foot had not a single man fit for duty, and the 46th, which had been in Cuba for only about eight weeks, had just seven men fit, 339 sick.[55] In a letter written to Amherst on 6 October, Albemarle reported, 'we have buried above *3000* Since the Capitulation.'[56] By the time the British evacuated Cuba in 1763, the mortality associated with the enterprise probably exceeded 5,000, more than had died in North America during the entire course of the war.

Just as battles might overwhelm the medical services, so might epidemics. The numbers of medical officers were adequate for an army in good health and were geared to this situation, largely for the sake of economy. In the reality of New World service, however, shortages of staff were common. Not only were there the crises provoked by epidemics and battles, but troops were often scattered, with the result that some detachments lacked medical care. The problem was greatest during the 1760s, and it was exacerbated by the reduction of the hospital in 1764, for prior to this time, and after the hospital was re-established in 1775, it was possible to detach mates to do duty in remote garrisons or to tend regiments that lacked one or both medical officers. In a health crisis, commanding officers might augment the nursing corps by recruiting more soldiers' wives or might seek the assistance of civilian practitioners in the vicinity.

Nevertheless, the quality of medical care that troops could expect declined markedly during crises, and such situations were not at all unusual.

The role of the officers in combating illness

The military circumstance was sufficiently dangerous, arduous, and unhealthy to suggest that it is not surprising that so many men died in the service but that – aside from those who were sent to the Indies – a considerable majority survived. That such was the case was in large part due to co-operation between medical officers and officers of the line. In confronting disease and in regulating the medical aspect of army life, line officers, especially those in command, played an important part and generally a positive one. Historians have dealt little with their role, but contemporaries familiar with army life recognised it and some sought to cement a partnership between line and medical officers. Several writers on military medicine directed their works to the officers, among them Richard Brocklesby, who in introducing his highly influential *Oeconomical and Medical Observations*, noted that the scheme that he proposed to improve medical services and health in the army would be addressed 'to the Colonels in the army, or to such other commanding Officers of battalions, and their regimental surgeons, on whom principally it will at all times depend.'[57] There is strong evidence that many officers read medical works and were influenced by them. In assessing the impact of Pringle's *Diseases of the Army*, a writer asserted:

> By the instructions received from this book, General [Robert] Melville... was enabled, while governor of the Neutral Islands, to be singularly useful. By taking care to have his men always lodged in large, open, and airy apartments, and by never letting his forces remain long enough in swampy places, to be injured by the noxious air of such places, the general was the happy instrument of saving the lives of seven hundred soldiers.[58]

A sense of humanity might prompt officers to work to preserve their men. If not, there was the common knowledge that it was militarily advantageous. John Bell, who served in the Indies as surgeon to the 94th Foot, wrote:

> The preservation... of any number of lives must be of important benefit to the state; for if five hundred men either die, or are so far weakened by disease as to be unfit for actual service, that number must be replaced, at a great expence to the nation. But independent of the expence occasioned by the death of a soldier on foreign service, it ought to be considered that success in every military operation must, in a great measure, depend on the health and vigour of the troops.[59]

Policies directed toward maintaining the troops comprehended a number of categories, and not all focused on those who might be expected to endure combat. Old or sickly soldiers were often given light duty. An order given in Halifax in July 1777 specified, 'Any man who can shave and is old and Infirm will be appointed to the Infirmary.'[60] It was common to assign invalids to garrison duty. The army usually included an invalid regiment, and in 1779 the Royal Garrison Battalion was established in America and promptly sent to guard Bermuda.

During the late-1750s and the 1760s a rotation system was used in America to balance the burden of frontier duty. In October 1759, Amherst advised Gage, 'As Abercromby's Regiment has been two Winters Quartered in what they call the best Quarters, that Regiment must now take the Advanced Posts.'[61] There was considerable effort to limit fatigue on the march. Braddock's march was highly fatiguing, particularly for the men whose job it was to cut a road through the forest, and the general observed the practice of 'halting days' – days when troops on the march remained in camp. The army moved so slowly that on 16 June Braddock decided to leave much of his baggage and manpower behind and press on quickly. Nevertheless, he allowed two further halting days.[62]

Officers took precautions to try to maintain their men in the face of epidemics. In the autumn of 1766, disease raged at Mobile. Responding, Colonel William Taylor divided his regiment and distributed detachments around West Florida.[63] In an attempt to avoid the sickness that often afflicted new troops when they embarked in Florida during the sickly season, on at least one occasion Gage ordered that recruits for the 21st and 31st Foot spend the summer in New York before joining their regiments.[64] A common duty for junior officers was to watch over convalescents. In July 1780 ,Lieutenant-Colonel Richard Boycott of the 91st Foot ordered, 'An Officer of a Company is to See that the Convalescents keep themselves properly Clean, & for the future the Orderly Officer is to turn them out of their hutts Every Evening at 5 oClock, & march them about till Retreat beating if the Weather will Permit.'[65] In the 19th Foot, a standing order issued in September 1769 prescribed that men being released from hospital be commended to the particular attention of the captain of their company, 'which Offr. will see him before he lows him to Mount Guard & not to Put him on Duty untill he thinks him Able to undergo the Fatigue.'[66]

Hospitalised soldiers were routinely provided with food that was deemed to be of higher quality or more nutritious than would be found in standard rations. In the wake of Bunker Hill, Howe ordered that wine and oatmeal be served to patients when the surgeons of their regiments deemed it desirable.[67] Special attention was always given to supplying the sick. On 20 August 1775, Hope noted in a letter that a ship carrying sheep, cattle, and pigs had recently landed. Soon, he reported, the men would have fresh provisions, 'and the sick and wounded (who are first to be considered) will be refreshed.'[68]

Medical opinion saw exercise as being extremely important. Jackson recommended that upon awakening, soldiers wash in cold water, then exercise for two hours before breakfast.[69] Whether inspired by such advice or simply adhering to common practice, many officers exercised their troops rigourously. On 23 September 1778, Earl William Cathcart, colonel to the British Legion, informed Clinton, 'All the Troops under my Command are now, thank God, fit for any Service,' and added that he had that morning marched them seven miles, fully encumbered.[70]

William Rowley, who served as a medical officer in the West Indies during the Seven Years' War, stressed, 'Above all things, where there is a large army, cleanliness not only in dress, but in all other respects should be strongly inculcated, and even insisted on.'[71] Several other writers likewise emphasised the importance of cleanliness and personal hygiene, including regular bathing and good grooming.[72] Numerous orders reflect the tendency of officers to promote personal hygiene. For example, at Fort Stanwix, in 1759, Major James Clephane ordered his men to have 'their hair Tyed their Shoes Cleaned, & at all times they appear Dressed in a Decent Manner.'[73]

Many orders mandated hygienic practices in camp. On 15 October 1780, at Morne Fortune, Boycott ordered:

> The Lieut. Colonel finding that the men are So inattentive to orders, & Regardless of their own health, as to make a Common Practice of Easing themselves behind & near the huts, which renders the Camp not only offensive but Unwholesome, Orders, that a doller Reward Shall be given to the man who will Inform the Serjeant Major of any Soldier that Shall in future disobey the order given out Some time ago & repeated that no Soldier shall Ease themselves in any place near the Camp but the Necessary.'[74]

In setting up camp, the preparation of sanitary facilities represented one of the highest priorities, as is reflected in orders such as one given on 1 September 1776: 'Necessary Houses to be immediately made – the Qr. Masters are to be answerable that they are regularly chang'd & cover'd.'[75] Commanding officers also gave orders that were aimed at preserving a supply of good water, as when Loudoun directed, 'no person is to pollute the Stream in the Rear of the Camp, the Women are to Wash and the Horses to be wattered at the Lower part of the Brook.'[76]

Reviewing orders and correspondence, it is apparent that there were health issues that interested some officers more than others. Some worked to limit the spread of venereal disease. Brigadier-General John Forbes was among these, and during the march to Fort Duquesne in 1758 he ordered, 'Any woman suspected to be infected with the Venial Distemper are to be sent to the Hospittal, to be examined & those who are found disordered are either to be kept in the Hospital till Curd or Turnd out of Camp.'[77] More generally, officers sought to curb the consumption of spirits by the troops. Gage himself coordinated such a campaign. But while some officers strove to limit drinking, others were less inclined to confront the problem, even though alcohol abuse was widely seen as a threat to health.[78] The alcohol problem was exacerbated by the practice of troops selling or trading provisions for liquor. Hoping to prevent them from doing so, a number of officers tried to enforce regular messing.[79] Orders might also specify how the mess was to prepare food. Howe addressed this issue and the value of messing in monitoring troops in an order of September 1775:

> [T]he Commanding Officers of Corps will Order the messes of their Regiments to be Visited, to See that the men boil their pots, as many are accused of Selling their provisions. It is recommended by the Hospital, not to Suffer the Pork to be fried, being very Prejudicial to the mens health.[80]

Howe's order reflects the importance of the hospital in fostering campaigns relating to health. By and large, commanding officers heeded the advice of high-ranking hospital personnel, even when they had reservations. In April 1762, Major John Beckwith of the 44th Foot informed Gage that a hospital physician had told him that it was 'absolutely Necessary to have a Regimental Ospital which I was rather against,' but that he had in any case established it.[81]

Those in command not only affected the advice of hospital officers, but also exalted their authority. Most of them had a high opinion of hospital surgeons and physicians. Regimental surgeons and mates, however, they considered quite limited in ability, and they attempted to subordinate them. Howe manifested this bias when he ordered, in September 1775, 'No Amputation or other intricate operation to be undertaken by any of the Surgeons, without Consultation first held with the Surgeons and Physicians of the General Hospital and a proper Number of them to be always present whensoever any Operation is performed.'[82] The prospect of relying entirely on regimental personnel to treat the troops was sufficiently daunting to prompt Gage to challenge and attempt to evade the directive by the War Office in 1764 to reduce the hospital.[83]

The impact of officers on health matters was compromised by the fact that orders were often disregarded, and indeed they were frequently repeated in tandem with the commanding officer's complaint that earlier ones had been ignored. Furthermore, some officers were far less sensitive to medical considerations than were others. Andrew Wilson, a physician and reformer, complained that sick troops were 'obliged to do duty as long as they can stand on their legs.'[84] Officers in command tended to respect the hospital as an institution, but their relationship with its leadership could be frosty. In September 1782, Hugh Alexander Kennedy, physician to the hospital in Canada, pleaded with Sir Guy Carleton, his former commander and newly appointed Commander-in-Chief in North America, to take him with him. 'After four years oppressive servitude' under General Frederick Haldimand, complained Kennedy, he had 'experienced ...every species of asperity and unprovok'd neglect.'[85] The attitude of commanding officers toward regimental medical services was sometimes disdainful. Not only did they tend to compare negatively the abilities of regimental personnel to those of hospital officers, but some believed that soldiers who were being treated in infirmaries were not seriously ill and could be called on for duty if the situation so warranted.[86] The poor relationship that some commanding officers had with particular hospital officers, and their tendency to disparage regimental personnel, may have limited their accessibility to advice. Despite these qualifiers, the preponderance of evidence suggests that as a group those in command cared deeply about health issues, heeded medical counsel, and promoted policies that had a decidedly positive impact on the physical well-being of their men.

Reputation and record

Certainly, one can find manifestations of incompetence among the medical officers. There is the case of John Davis, surgeon to the 100th Foot, a regiment that was recruited in the West Indies and served there throughout its brief existence (1761–3). On the evening of 26 March 1762 Davis attempted to treat a captain who had been stabbed by the major-commandant of the regiment. In testimony at the subsequent court-martial of the major, Davis recalled, 'When the Deponent came, he found [the captain] near his Tent, lying on his back; he ordered him to be brought into his Tent, where he examined his Wounds; he found him speechless, and attempted to bleed him, but he bled a very small quantity and soon expired.'[87] Venesection was indeed a technique commonly used to revive patients who were suddenly rendered speechless, as by apoplexy, but a practitioner was also expected to use discretion in applying it. To bleed a patient who was already suffering from extensive loss of blood, as Davis did, would have been regarded as ill-advised, if not incomprehensible.

When we move beyond such displays of ineptitude, however, what is striking in the evidence is how well, by and large, the medical officers served the army. In judging performance of the medical services, there are three criteria to consider: (1) how effective were the services in preventing disease or reducing its spread?; (2) was disease treated competently in terms of contemporary practice?; (3) did the medical men 'do no harm'?

Regarding the first issue, one might again mention the campaigns to improve sanitation and hygiene. These were overseen by commanding officers, but they were often undertaken at the behest of medical writers or personnel. Moreover, they were only aspects of a broad-based effort to prevent disease. The scope of this effort was far broader than can be covered in a brief essay, but major components may at least be noted.

The value of medicine to the army is nowhere more obvious than in the campaigns against two major diseases: smallpox and scurvy. The use of inoculation to manage smallpox – giving the patient a mild case to avoid the possibility that he would naturally contract a severe one – gained popularity steadily after it was introduced into England around 1720. There was, however, some opposition to the practice for the balance of the century, especially in the lower classes.[88]

There were a number of inoculation campaigns in the army. They were of two types, voluntary and involuntary. As early as December 1756, Loudoun reported to Cumberland that in the wake of a major smallpox epidemic he was 'preparing to *Innoculate* such as have not had it, & are willing to undergo the Opperation.'[89] Responding to an outbreak of smallpox among the troops besieged in Boston in 1775, Howe ordered, first, the preparation of a list of men in garrison who had not had smallpox.[90] Then, on 1 December, he ordered:

> The Smallpox spreading universally about the Town makes it necessary, for
> the safety of the Troops, that such men as are willing and have not had that
> Distemper, should be inoculated immediately.... Inoculated men are to have
> as little intercourse as possible with those men who refuse to be inoculated.[91]

Other commanding officers did not allow a choice. On 24 June 1776, General Guy Carleton, Commander-in-Chief in Canada, ordered that all men under his command who had not had smallpox be inoculated.[92] In 1783 Haldimand confronted an epidemic in Montreal by ordering inoculation of men, women, and children in all regiments serving in Canada.[93] Owing in large part to the inoculation campaigns, the British suffered few outbreaks of smallpox during the War of Independence.

Officers who ordered inoculation did not necessarily do so at the suggestion of medical officers, but often they did. When smallpox struck Crown Point in the early autumn of 1770, the commander of the fort, Captain Gavin Cochrane, first tried to control the outbreak by isolating soldiers who contracted it, but his orders were ignored. He then moved toward inoculation. The new plan he credited largely to James Latham, surgeon of the 8th Foot, who 'communicated his directions to me, which were so consonant to reason & Nature that they removed all my Scruples as to permitting inoculation; and I thought I would be answerable for the consequences to those whom I deprived of the benefit.' Cochrane consequently offered not only soldiers but all residents living near the fort free inoculation, but most civilians held back, 'pretending a Scruple in Religion.'[94]

Although smallpox was a major health threat, it paled in comparison to scurvy, the greatest killer of troops in North America during the French and Indian War. Virtually every winter during the war, the scurvy problem constituted a crisis for the army. In March 1756, Francis Lewis, the commissary at Oswego, wrote to Loudoun, 'our Numbers are greatly diminishing daily by the Scurvy which proves Mortal among the Soldiers, and those now doing Duty are so imatiated, that they look more like Spectres than Men.'[95] While scurvy was most worrisome in wintertime, it could cost the army dearly even during campaign season, particularly in areas where supplies of fresh produce were limited. On 28 September 1759, ten days after the Battle of Quebec, Brigadier-General James Murray ordered returns 'of such men as are so bad of the scurvy as to render them unfit for any duty.'[96] This was only the prelude to medical disaster, though as was typical scurvy struck primarily in late-winter. In March 1760, Lieutenant Malcolm Fraser noted, 'The scurvy... becomes every day more general. In short, I believe there is scarce a man of the Army entirely free from it.'[97] By late-April, the health crisis stood at its most acute. Only 3,341 men were deemed fit, while 2,312 were ill; 682 had died since 18 September, mostly from scurvy.[98]

The winter of 1759/60 saw perhaps the worst outbreak of scurvy ever to hit the British Army. Winter hit early and was exceptionally harsh. By early-January supplies of greens had been exhausted, and virtually every garrison in Canada, the Ohio Valley, and New York was stricken with scurvy. As governor of Montreal, Gage was besieged with reports from outposts in the region.[99] Travel conditions appear to have improved in late-January, for vegetables and vinegar arrived at most of the outposts. Lime juice was also sent.[100] Improvement was prompt and dramatic. By 16 February, Jonathan Rogers, surgeon to the 30th Foot, was reporting to Gage from Ticonderoga:

> The Roots which were sent were no sooner given to the Men, when they began dayly to grow more healthy, The Scurvy which rag'd in a most extraordinary manner amongst them is now disappearing.... I shou'd have lost numbers had not the Vegitables come to our relief.[101]

The shipments of mid-winter brought only temporary improvement, however. Soon Gage was receiving new reports of outbreaks. Gloomiest of all was Captain Lewis Steiner, who commanded at Onondaga:

> The Doctor... reported to me yesterday that there was Scarce one Soldier more of the Command, who had not actually the Scurvy, & who would be in a few Days intirely unfit for any Duty;... When that time comes, which must be Soon, we Shall have no ressource left, than to Shut the Gates, & wait our Doom.[102]

It was only with the coming of spring that the crisis abated. As Captain William Dunbar wrote to Gage on 2 May, from Oneida, 'the men here begin to recover very fast, owing I imagine to the wild greens we pick up.'[103]

While the army suffered heavy mortality from scurvy during the French and Indian War, there were few significant outbreaks during the War of Independence. The worst came in Boston, while the army was penned up in 1775/6. Given the circumstances, the outbreak was almost inevitable, and even in the early autumn Hope was reporting, 'We are now reduced to salt pork and oatmeal...; how long men can subsist on such food without being destroyed by the scurvy, tis easy to conceive.'[104] Scurvy also continued to be a problem on long voyages. In August 1779, a fleet arrived in New York bearing more than 600 sick, many of them scorbutic.[105] And there were a few men hospitalised for the disease each winter.[106] Nevertheless, the contrast from the previous war was dramatic, and it reflected the ability of medical personnel and line officers to co-operate in a concerted campaign against disease.

Fresh greens had long been valued as antiscorbutics, and from the earliest months of the French and Indian War it was common policy to combat scurvy by sending sick troops to New Jersey, where vegetables were plentiful.[107] This was not feasible for troops at outposts in the interior, however, and as the war moved further inland the scurvy threat increased. To combat it, some commanders in frontier areas sought to augment their supply of produce by planting gardens. In February 1756, Colonel James Mercer wrote from Oswego,

> This Garrison begins to be sorely afflicted with an Inveterate and Obstinate Scurvey... and our Surgeons say nothing but Vegetables can avail, I must therefore, beg of You, to send on purpose to the German Flatts, for Cabbage Turnips, & other Seeds, and if they are to be had, some Cabbage Plants, I shall have the Ground ready for them.[108]

The High Command began to coordinate efforts to combat scurvy. Already, by late in the summer of 1758, Major-General James Abercromby, the Commander-in-Chief, noted that scurvy was spreading among the men, and in the anticipation of impending calamity he acted with uncharacteristic vigour, ordering Napier to provide fresh vegetables to the troops in lieu of part of their meat ration.[109] In late-autumn, the Commissary visited various outposts, bringing supplies of onions and other vegetables. Haldimand, at Fort Edward, was told:

> [Y]our Battalion will suffer less from the Scurvy, than any other Regt that has been there is Garrison, as they had had already above 100 Barrells of vegetables, besides [produce] from the Gardens at Fort Edward, & more will be Sent.[110]

Nevertheless, the annual visitations of scurvy continued. In the wake of the devastating outbreak of 1760/1, Gage determined to establish a more reliable supply of greens. In March 1761, he ordered commanders at the various outposts to make plans for vegetable gardens, and he also began to send out seed packets.[111] By mid-April the planting was well under way. Dunbar reported, 'I have already a Garden inclos'd & wait only for the seeds as it is ready prepar'd for Sowing – I had by accident a few with me, which I have sown.'[112] Lieutenant-Colonel John Reed, who had written to Gage that he doubted the land at Fort Edward would be productive, was trying to remedy the situation, by having the troops enclose 'a Spot of ground, for a Cabbage Garden, where formerly was a Pen for Cattle. The Garden on the Island is quite wore out, nor is there any Dung to inrich it with; but by converting it into a Pen for Cattle... it will next year produce any thing.'[113] The next winter saw few outbreaks of scurvy, and Gage's programme was probably a major reason for the contrast. Furthermore, he kept up his initiative, encouraging commanding officers to plant gardens at their outposts. On 24 May 1761, Gladwin reported to him from Fort William Augustus:

> [W]e have been employed in planting pease and Indian corn on Dalyells Island; if the seed answers expectation, it will produce sufficient for the garrison; besides, I flatter myself, I shall be able to raise fifteen or twenty thousand cabbages; I have likewise made a pretty garden on the point of this Island, to raise salad, and cabbage plants.[114]

Besides the planting campaign, the army benefited from the introduction of spruce beer, a potent antiscorbutic that had long been popular in Canada. During the French and Indian War it became standard issue for troops serving in the north. Loudoun established this in a general order of 5 July 1757.[115] Spruce beer rations were not automatic during the war, however. In June 1759, Amherst ordered that the beverage be made available to the regiments and provincial units in northern New York, but one year later the men were ordered to make up their accounts and were informed that no more spruce beer was to be given except for cash.[116] The value of spruce beer again became apparent during the scurvy outbreak that attended the siege of Boston, and in January 1776, Howe ordered the hospital to release the beverage to any soldier with 'the least appearance of a Scorbutic Taint.'[117] George III, in early 1777, allotted a half-gallon of spruce beer as a daily ration for every soldier in North America.[118] It also became a common recourse in combating outbreaks of scurvy. In a letter written in the spring of 1777, Hayes reported that a detachment at Isle aux Noix had recently begun to suffer from scurvy:

> The Regt. was to have been changd but a trial first having been made, of fresh provisions & Spruce Beer, an Excellent antiscorbutic peculiar to this Country; it had it's effects; the Men got Better & therefore remained there.[119]

It is more difficult to speak definitively on the second criterion for judging the record of the medical services: whether, by and large, the medical officers competently applied the best in contemporary therapy. The only book published about service in North America is Thomas Dickson Reide's *View of the Diseases of the Army*, which deals mainly with the author's tour in Canada. Reide's practice was heavily influenced by John Millar, the combative physician whose therapeutics, and especially his condemnation of venesection, placed him far from the mainstream. In any case, Reide's book is only one source, and although there are others – the diaries by Forster and Blagden, occasional correspondence – generalising about therapy on the basis of so little data would be risky. Since more books were published by medical men who had served in the West Indies, a slightly better sense of practice emerges from that theatre. But the question of therapy must also be addressed through inference, and in this respect the key role played by senior hospital officers is of primary importance.

The treatment of troops was to some extent regularised by the predominance of the hospital and particularly of the physicians and surgeons. As has been noted, serious cases of disease and surgical problems that were life threatening were supposed to be treated at the hospital, though in various circumstances – the wake of battle, a major epidemic, remoteness of hospital facilities – such cases were often handled by regimental personnel. Hospital physicians and surgeons also had a supervisory function and the hospital had oversight of all medical officers. The favour of a physician or surgeon could help a young medical officer to advance in the army and perhaps when he returned to the civilian world. There was, for this reason, an inducement for him to conform in terms of practice. If he lost several patients after using unorthodox therapies, his reputation and opportunities for advancement would suffer. The hospital had yet another means of influencing practice. Senior staff was responsible for ordering most of the medicine that was used in the army. Before leaving for America, each regimental surgeon was allotted a medical chest by the Apothecary-General, the drugs and quantities being specified by the War Office. During both the French and Indian War and the War of Independence, regimental surgeons were allowed to replenish their medicines from the hospital. They could also purchase drugs, and some did, but this meant dipping into the medicine money that they received from the regiment. If they merely used the drugs obtained from the hospital, they could pocket the money.[120] This inducement gave the hospital considerable leverage in determining which drugs were used by the regiments, and the extensive orders that are extant suggest that the medicines that it requested from Britain were of a pattern paralleling the reformist and progressive tendencies that marked British pharmaceutical literature, especially from the 1740s.

Finally, did the medical officers do no harm? In particular, in cases where successfully treating disease was beyond the ability of contemporary medicine, did they employ treatments that inflicted unnecessary pain and suffering on the patient and reduced his chances for recovery? Undoubtedly there were some who by their ineptitude or indifference harmed patients. Another problem lay in the tendency of practitioners – in the civilian world as in the military – to experiment on patients who were not responding to standard therapy or who appeared to be dying.

The War Office itself encouraged experimentation, especially as regarded the testing of drugs. In August 1756, Barrington informed Major-General James Ross, who commanded the 38th Foot in Antigua, that a forthcoming shipment of drugs included a gross of James's Fever Powders. Barrington added:

> It is His Majesty's Pleasure that you do order the Surgeon to your Regt. to keep an Exact Account in writing of the Effect Dr James's Powders have on the several Patients to whom he shall Administer any part of those Powders, which Accounts are to be sent to me from Time to Time to be laid before H R Hss the Duke.[121]

Adair regularly requested medical officers to share their discoveries with him. To John Weir, garrison surgeon in Jamaica, he wrote, in December 1786:

> You will please to continue Your Observations on the Effect of Vegetable Acid in dressing the Malignant Sores under Your Care. In general these Cases come to England in a very bad State, & too often require Amputation.[122]

Even Hamilton, who inveighed against the mistreatment of troops by medical men, encouraged experimentation, but he added that 'no trial, dangerous to the patient's life, is ever to be risqued.'[123] It appears that by and large this sense of caution prevailed and that medical officers were no more likely to do harm than were their civilian counterparts. Indeed, army practitioners seem to have been at the forefront of the movement toward moderate therapies that characterised British practice during the latter half of the eighteenth century. Most significantly, there was a dramatic move away from venesection and expulsive drugs among medical officers who practised in the West Indies. Jackson, while himself an advocate of venesection, was left to complain that in the Indies, 'A great majority of British practitioners deprecate the use of the lancet.'[124]

Final reckoning

Significant discrepancies among primary sources, as well as gaps, make it unwise to give precise mortality figures, but it appears that during the French and Indian War, about 4,500 British soldiers died in North America, perhaps 7,000 in the West Indies. In the period 1775–83, with significantly larger forces involved, roughly 10,000 died in North America, another 6,000 in the Indies. During the War of Independence, perhaps 2,000 men died in transit between Britain and New World stations, the voyage to and from the Indies accounting for much of the toll.[125]

Not surprisingly, health issues played a significant role in the military history of the West Indies. The conquest of Havana in 1762 was supposed to be a prelude to a co-ordinated assault on New Orleans by forces coming from the south, commanded by Albemarle, and from the north, under Amherst. The plan, however, had to be aborted when Albemarle informed Amherst that not only could he not provide reinforcements for him, but that owing to his manpower crisis he would have to detain the troops that had been sent from North America to help him take Havana.[126] The Kemble expedition of 1780, initially successful in that the British succeeded in their mission to capture Castle San Juan at the entrance of Lake Nicaragua, was aborted seven months later because illness, mainly yellow fever, had reduced the force by more than three-quarters. In North America, too, disease influenced the course of war, playing a definite role in the defeat of Burgoyne and Cornwallis. During the War of Independence the quality and numbers of British recruits declined steadily, and after 1780 they could not make good their losses.

Like historians since, contemporaries worked on the assumption that the vast majority of soldiers who died in these or any eighteenth-century wars succumbed to disease. Hamilton reported, 'it appears from registers kept of the mortality produced by fevers of various kinds in military life, that eight times more men were lost by these [during the War of Independence], than fell immediately of their wounds, or in battle.'[127] Such observations tend to suggest that medical officers could do little to save the troops. Coupled with figures on sickness and mortality, and with the problems that the death or incapacitation of troops posed in pursuing strategic aims, the evidence may suggest that medical services were seriously flawed.

This evidence is, however, less than it seems. The proportion of deaths from disease represents a case in point. In fact, during the years of heaviest fighting in North America – 1755, 1758–60, 1775–7, 1780–1 – one-third or more of all deaths resulted either from battle or from accidents. It was mainly the epidemics of the West Indies that drove up the ratios of death from disease. More specifically, it was the ravages of yellow fever, the only common and highly mortal disease that medicine was truly incapable of curing or ameliorating.

The ratios of death from disease as opposed to battle-related mortality were quite different for the German allies of the British. According to the best data, 4,626 Hessians died of disease in America in 1776–84, while only 357 were killed.[128] At least in part, this disparity reflects the fact that the Germans were seldom engaged in fighting after 1777, so the preponderant majority of deaths thereafter resulted from disease. Nevertheless, some observers believed that the quality of medical services exposed German soldiers to higher mortality than their British counterparts. Brocklesby asserted, 'The Germans, who speedily recruit their armies, as they happen to moulder away, take very little care of their military hospitals.'[129]

It was not only the British who compared their medical services favourably to those of other armies. James Thacher, the noted American military surgeon and diarist, observed British and German medical men tending to their troops after the capitulation at Saratoga and later reported, 'the English surgeons perform with skill and dexterity, but the Germans, with a few exceptions, do no credit to their profession.'[130] The Americans chose to pattern medical services in the Continental Army on those of the British, and likewise did so as regarded practice and hygiene. Benjamin Rush wrote in 1777, 'I have taken some pains to acquire from a surgeon in General Howe's army a perfect knowledge of the methods of taking care of the sick in the British military hospitals.' Knowing that the quality of British medical services was not solely dependent on medical officers, he noted further, 'I have found, from conversing with the surgeons of the British army as well as from my own observations, that the care of the sick is a matter that engages the attention of even their general officers.'[131] Although Rush and some other prominent Continental medical officers had studied in Britain, the circumstance of war negated any sentimental bias in favour of aping the British. During the War of Independence, Rush himself became something of an Anglophobe. It was simply his sense, and that of his colleagues, that medical services in the British Army represented the best model for the American military to follow.

Works on military medicine had a wide readership and a significant impact on British medicine at large, especially as regarded epidemic disease. The Army tour in the New World, 1755–83, did not produce any work that compared in influence to Pringle's *Diseases of the Army* or several others that grew from the authors' experiences in a European context. Nevertheless, several works relating to army service in the West Indies, especially 1779–83, were influential, most notably John Hunter's *Observations on the Diseases of the Army in Jamaica*.[132] Like Pringle, Hunter came to the military with a significant reputation. Noting the abundance of West Indian plants that might be useful in medicine, John Rollo, a surgeon's mate in the Royal Artillery, commented:

> We look forward with an anxious hope to [Hunter], whose known abilities and industry in this, as well as in every other part of his profession, have fully enabled him to favour the world with satisfactory and important accounts of every medical produce which can possibly be met with in any of the Caribbee Islands.[133]

That individual medical officers earned fine reputations does not of course mean that they represented their colleagues at large. As has been noted, some medical men were incompetent. Many were poorly trained and were too indifferent to take advantage of the opportunities for improvement that army service afforded. But when the record of the medical services is reviewed, when one considers the campaigns to improve hygiene and to combat scurvy and smallpox, even the limited amount of evidence that can be put forward in a brief essay suggests that the services provided a great benefit to the army. If the question were raised, 'Did the medical services materially improve health and reduce mortality?' one might respond emphatically in the affirmative.

Notes

1. New York Public Library, Manuscripts and Archives Division (hereafter, 'NYPL'), 'Papers relevant to Nova Scotia', 20.

2. For further details and references on Adair and his policies, particularly his interest in cost-cutting, see P.E. Kopperman, 'Medical Services in the British Army, 1742–1783', *Journal of the History of Medicine and Allied Sciences*, xxxiv (1979), 449–52. Richard Brocklesby praises Cumberland for having created the hospital board in 1756, but lays the creation of the office of inspector – a negative development, in his opinion – to Barrington:

Oeconomical and Medical Observations, In Two Parts, From the Year 1758 to the Year 1763, inclusive. Tending to The Improvement of Military Hospitals, and to The Cure of Camp Diseases incident to Soldiers (London: T. Becket and P.A. De Hondt, 1764), 30, 33.

3. Local civilian practitioners were sometimes called in to treat military personnel. The Commander-in-Chief often had a personal physician on his staff.

4. Foot regiments who served in America during the French and Indian War had an establishment about one-third larger than during the War of Independence. Some dragoon regiments did include a mate, especially in wartime (e.g., inspection returns for 15th light dns., The National Archives [hereafter NA], War Office [hereafter WO] 27/6; 19th light dns., WO 27/42).

5. Kopperman, *op. cit.* (note 2), 437. By the time of the War of Independence, the position of matron had been largely superseded by that of head nurse; the latter had roughly the same duties, but was paid less and did not rank as an officer.

6. Unless specified otherwise, biographical information noted in this essay is drawn from my data base.

7. Huntington Library, San Marino, California [hereafter HL], Loudoun Papers [hereafter LO] 526.

8. LO 611.

9. LO 2503; the re-issue is in NYPL, 'British Headquarters Papers' (photocopies of originals in the NA), VI, 196, enclosed in Barrington to Gage, 25 September 1775, VI, 195. Another set was sent to Sir Henry Clinton, on 10 November 1775: Clements Library, Ann Arbor, Michigan (hereafter, 'CL'), Clinton Papers, CP 12:6. During the French and Indian War, the instructions were issued to Loudoun, in July 1757, and to Amherst, in December 1758: contemporary marginal notation, WO 26/23/209.

10. Loudoun informed Cumberland of his decision on 25 April: LO 3463B. On 31 December 1756, Dr James Pringle had written to Loudoun to remind him that he had promised himself and the Surgeon-General to appoint Napier as Chief Surgeon: LO 2431.

11. WO 7/96/31; Adair noted that Nooth had referred to the number of mates, apparently with disquiet, in a recent letter.

12. Kopperman, *op. cit.* (note 2), 429, 453.

13. Adair to Matthew Lewis, War Office, 18 December 1779: WO 1/683/335. Other critics of the hospital include: R. Jackson, *An Outline of the History and Cure of Fever, Endemic and Contagious; More Expressly the Contagious Fever of Jails, Ships, and Hospitals; the Concentrated Endemic, vulgarly the Yellow Fever of the West Indies; to Which is Added an Explanation of the Principles of Military Discipline and Economy; with a Scheme of Medical*

Arrangement for Armies (Edinburgh: T. N. Longman, *et al.*, 1798), 393–4; (Sir) J. Pringle, *Observations on the Diseases of the Army, in Camp and Garrison. In Three Parts. With an Appendix, Containing some Papers of Experiments, Read at several Meetings of the Royal Society*, 2nd edn, corr. and enl. (London: A. Millar, *et al.*, 1753), 103–7; Brocklesby, *op. cit.* (note 2), 34–5.

14. WO 4/275/99.
15. On 17 March 1758, Abercromby informed Barrington that he would follow Loudoun's policy of drawing regimental surgeons from hospital mates and also assured him that he would not allow the selling of surgeoncies that had not been bought: WO 1/1/433; cf. Kopperman, *op. cit.* (note 2), 432n21. The War Office had a policy against permitting the sale of hospital surgeoncies: Kopperman, *op. cit.* (note 2), 432.
16. Schools for military surgeons were opened in Hanover (1716), Berlin (1724), Vienna (1781), and Dresden (1784): Erwin H. Ackerknecht and Esther Fischer-Homberger, 'Five made it – One not. The Rise of Medical Craftsmen to Academic Status during the 19th Century', *Clio Medica*, xii (1977), 257. In 1775, five French hospitals were given the task of preparing army and navy medical officers in surgery and anatomy: L.W.B. Brockliss, *French Higher Education in the Seventeenth and Eighteenth Centuries: A Cultural History* (Oxford: Oxford University Press, 1987), 28–9.
17. Some men who entered army service did so after serving apprenticeships with former medical officers; e.g. George Hugonin, who served in a medical capacity (and died) on the Albemarle expedition, had been an apprentice to John Ranby.
18. T. Forster, 'Diary of Thompson Forster: Staff Surgeon to His Majesty's Detached Hospital in North America. October 19th 1775 to October 23rd 1777' (typescript from ms., author's collection), 109, n1.
19. R. Jackson, *A System of Arrangement and Discipline, for the Medical Department of Armies* (London: J. Murray, 1805), 27–33, 76–78; *idem, op. cit.* (note 13), 389–90.
20. J. Bell, *Memorial concerning the Present State of Military and Naval Surgery* (Edinburgh: Longman et al., 1800), especially 6–8.
21. R. Hamilton, *The Duties of a Regimental Surgeon Considered: With Observations on His General Qualifications; And Hints relative to a More Respectable Practice, and Better Regulation of that Department. Wherein are interspersed many Medical Anecdotes, and Subjects discussed, equally interesting to every Practitioner* (London: J. Johnson, *et al.*, 1787), I, viii.
22. *Ibid.*
23. *Memorial , op. cit.* (note 20), 5–6.
24. LO 1152.

25. LO 2669. Oswald asked Loudoun to refer the matter to Huck, with whom McLean had studied.

26. John Macnamara Hayes was appointed physician to the hospital in North America in 1779, although he did not receive his MD (from Rheims) until 1784. His advancement appears to have come through Clinton's favour.

27. F.N.L. Poynter, 'Medical Education in England since 1600', in C.D. O'Malley (ed), *The History of Medical Education* [UCLA Forum of Medical Sciences, 12](Berkeley: University of California Press, 1970), 240. That MDs from more prestigious programs denounced these degrees partly reflected self-interest. Some major medical figures, including Jenner, held degrees from either Aberdeen or St Andrews.

28. W.N.B. Watson, 'Four Monopolies and the Surgeons of London and Edinburgh', *Journal of the History of Medicine*, xxv (1970), 313. In July 1788 Adair informed George Stewart, the Surgeon-General of Ireland, that although he opposed extending the right to examine to Edinburgh he would undertake 'that the respect to be paid to the College of Surgeons in Dublin, & that their Examination shall be admitted here': WO 7/96/226.

29. Barrington gave this choice to John Scott, War Office, 16 March 1756: WO 4/51/276.

30. Beinecke Library (Yale University), New Haven, Blagden Diaries, vol. I.

31. Bell, *op. cit.* (note 20), 18, 20.

32. J. Ring, *Reflections on the Surgeons' Bill: In Answer to Three Pamphlets in Defence of that Bill* (London: Hookham and Carpenter, 1798), 32–8.

33. W.N. Boog Watson, 'Thomas Robertson, Naval Surgeon, 1793–1828,' *Bulletin of the History of Medicine*, xlvi (1972), 134.

34. Royal College of Surgeons, London, ms. 'Examination Book with Index 1745–1800', 278.

35. Wellcome Library, London, ms. RAMC 1037: 'Regimental Practice: Or A Short History of Diseases common to His Majesties own Royale Regiment of Horse Guards when abroad (Commonly called the Blews)'; this quotation is drawn from an unpaginated fragment that accompanies the journal.

36. Letter to Miss Rogers, 30 October 1770: NA 30/39/1.

37. These figures are extracted from the returns in the National Archives of Canada, Fraser Papers, Vol. 35.

38. S. Jackman (ed.), *With Burgoyne from Quebec: An Account of the Battle of Quebec and of the Famous Battle at Saratoga* (Toronto: Macmillan, 1963), 77. Anburey added, however, that Canadians were often consumptive.

39. Except where noted otherwise, data in this essay that is based on returns is extracted from my database.

40. LO 6258.

41. Representation of field officers regarding troops, [Charleston,] 2 December 1757: S.K. Stevens, Donald H. Kent, Autumn L. Leonard (eds), *The Papers*

of Henry Bouquet (Harrisburg: The Pennsylvania Historical and Museum Commission, 1972), I, 248.

42. Bouquet to Col. John Hunter, Charleston, 16 October 1757: *ibid.*, 211.
43. Bouquet to Loudoun, 21 October 1757, Charleston: *ibid.*, 224.
44. Bouquet to Peters, *ibid.*, 226.
45. Lieut. Daniel Doyley to Bouquet, Charleston, 2 December 1757: *ibid.*, 246.
46. Bouquet to Stanwix, Charleston, 21 February 1758: *ibid.*, 309.
47. G. Washington, 'Biographical Memoranda' in J.C. Fitzatrick (ed.), *The Writings of George Washington* (Washington, D.C.: U. S. Government Printing Office, 1931), xxix, 44.
48. 'Journal of Cholmley's Batman,' in C. Hamilton (ed.), *Braddock's Defeat: The Journal of Captain Robert Cholmley's Batman, The Journal of a British Officer* [and] *Halkett's Orderly Book* (Norman: University of Oklahoma Press, 1959), 32.
49. Letter to Charles Mellish, Nottingham University Library, Mellish of Hodsock Mss., 132/111/5.
50. Entry for 18 September, 105–6.
51. Bouquet to Stanwix, Charleston, 23 June 1757: Stevens, *op. cit.* (note 41), I, 121.
52. Letter of 2 May: WO 34/55/139.
53. Manuscript account, composed Havana, 17 August 1762: WO 34/55/181.
54. WO 34/55/193; enclosed in Albemarle to Amherst, 18 August 1762: WO 34/55/185.
55. WO 34/55/235.
56. WO 34/55/228.
57. Brocklesby, *op. cit.* (note 2), 6.
58. *A New and General Biographical Dictionary: Containing an Historical and Critical Account of the Lives and Writings of the Most Eminent Persons of Every Nation; Particularly the British and Irish* (London: T. Osborne, *et al.*, 1767), xii, 378. Some line officers, perhaps most notably John Forbes, were in fact men with medical training.
59. *An Inquiry into the Causes which Produce, and the Means of Preventing Diseases among British Officers, Soldiers, and Others in the West Indies. Containing Observations on the Mode of Action of Spirituous Liquors on the Human Body; On the Use of Malt Liquor, and on Salted Provisions; With Remarks on the most proper Means of preserving them* (London: J. Murray, 1791), 3–4. This author should not be confused with the John Bell who wrote *Memorial concerning the Present State of Military and Naval Surgery*.
60. Order of 29 July 1777: Massachusetts Historical Society, OB, 1st Bn. Marines, Halifax.
61. CO 5/56/98; Amherst to Gage, Crown Point, 2 October 1759.
62. The halting days were 30 June and 5 July; note 'Captain Orme's Journal,'

W. Sargent, *The History of an Expedition against Fort Duquesne in 1755. Under Major-General Edward Braddock* [Pennsylvania Historical Society, *Memoirs*, 5] (Philadelphia, 1855), 345, 350..

63. Gage to Barrington, 11 October 1766; *The Correspondence of General Thomas Gage 1763–1775*, C.E. Carter (ed), (New Haven: Yale University Press, 1931), II, 382.

64. Gage to Barrington, 6 October 1767; *ibid.*, 434.

65. Order dated July 5: CL, OB 2, Boycott.

66. Order dated 15 September: National Army Museum, London, OB, 19th Foot (ms. 6807/160).

67. Order for 27 June 1775: B.F. Stevens (ed.), *General Sir William Howe's Orderly Book, at Charlestown, Boston and Halifax, June 17 1775 to 1776 26 May* (London: B.F. Stevens, 1890), 23.

68. Hope to Sukey Needham; NA 30/39/1/[6].

69. Jackson, *op. cit.* (note 13), 372. While it was common for writers on military medicine to encourage exercise, some, like Pringle and Donald Monro, cautioned against overextending the troops or forcing them to exercise in the heat of the day: Pringle, *op. cit.* (note 13), 92, 116–7; D. Monro, *Observations on the Means of Preserving the Health of Soldiers: And of Conducting Military Hospitals: And on the Diseases incident to Soldiers in the Time of Service, and on the same Diseases as they have appeared in London*, 2nd edn (London: J. Murray and G. Robinson, 1780), I, 74–6.

70. CL, CP 42:1.

71. *Medical Advice, for the Use of the Army and Navy, in the Present American Expedition: Intended for the Perusal of Private Gentlemen as Well as Medical Practitioners* (London: F. Newbery, 1776), 24.

72. See for example, W. Blair, *The Soldier's Friend: or, The Means of Preserving the Health of Military Men* (London: Murray, 1798), 76–83. Writers who were not medical men made the same points; eg. B. Cuthbertson, *A System for the Compleat Interior Management and Oeconomy of a Battalion of Infantry* (Dublin: B. Grierson, 1768), 127–36.

73. Order of 3 January: Scottish Record Office, Rose of Kilravock Muniments (GD 125), Box 34/7.

74. Four days later, he felt compelled to repeat the order: 'Any man that is found Easing himself near the Hutts or tents, Except at the Proper place appointed for that purpose, Shall be Immediately Confined & Severely Punished': CL, OB 2, Boycott.

75. Order of 1 September: HL, HM 617. On 1 July 1757, Loudoun ordered, 'The Necessary Houses Belonging to ye Several Regtts to be Emmediately fill'd Up & New Ones Dug Six feet Deep & about 100 yards in ye Front of ye Respective Encampments. Each Regt Every Evening to cover ye Bootom of them over with Fresh Earth – & New ones to Be Dug Every Wheek & ye

Old ones to Be fill'd Up — The Commanding offr of Each Regt to Be Answerable to ye Genll that this order is Strictly Obayed', in W. Seward Webb (ed.), *General Orders of 1757, Issued by the Earl of Loudoun and Phineas Lyman in the Campaign against the French* (New York: Dodd Mead, 1899), 34.

76. Order of 2 July 1757: LO 3576.

77. Order of 4 October 1758: Library of Congress, George Washington Papers, Forbes OB. Similar efforts are noted in P.E. Kopperman, 'The British High Command and Soldiers' Wives in America, 1755–1783,' *Journal of the Society for Army Historical Research*, lx (1982), 17.

78. Efforts to limit drinking, and the reasons why they were not more intensive and consistent, are discussed in greater detail in P.E. Kopperman, '"The Cheapest Pay": Alcohol Abuse in the Eighteenth-Century British Army', *The Journal of Military History*, 60 (1996), 455–8, 465–8.

79. *Ibid.*, 451, note 20.

80. Order of 20 September: Stevens (ed.), *op. cit.* (note 67), 94.

81. CL, Gage Papers, American Series (hereafter designated 'GP').

82. Order of 1 September: Stevens (ed.), *op. cit.* (note 67), 82–3. Similarly, in November 1779 the secretary at war, acting on Adair's recommendation, subordinated the regimental infirmaries in Jamaica to the hospital physician there: Adair to Sir Charles Jenkinson, Argyll Street, 23 November 1779; [Jenkinson] to General John Dalling, n.d., enclosing 'Instructions for the Conduct of the General Staff serving with the Troops in Jamaica': WO 1/683/317, 319, 323.

83. Kopperman, *op. cit.* (note 2), 448.

84. A. Wilson, *Rational Advice to the Military, When Exposed to the Inclemency of Hot Climates and Seasons* (London, 1780), 5.

85. Shropshire Records and Research Centre, Shrewsbury, Sandford Collection, Kennedy Papers, No. 352.

86. Kopperman, *op. cit.* (note 2), 449.

87. WO 71/48, 187.

88. An extended treatment of this issue would go far beyond the bounds of this paper. One might note, however, the comment by John Heysham, that 'so great is the prejudice against the salutary practice of inoculation amongst the vulgar, that few, very few, can be prevailed upon either by promises, rewards, or entreaties to submit to the operation': *Observations On the Bills of Mortality, In Carlisle, for the Year 1779* (Carlisle: J. Milliken, 1780), 6.

89. Letter of 22 November–26 December 1756: S.M. Pargellis (ed.), *Military Affairs in North America 1748–1765: Selected Documents from the Cumberland Papers in Windsor Castle* (New York and London: D. Appleton-Century Co., 1936), 280.

90. Order of 18 November: *Journals of Lieut.-Col. Stephen Kemble*, New-York

Historical Society, *Collections*, xvi (1883), 255.

91. *Ibid.*, 266.

92. J.M. Hadden, *A Journal Kept in Canada and upon Burgoyne's Campaign in 1776 and 1777, by Lieut. James M. Hadden, Royal Art.; Also Orders Kept by Him and Issued by Sir Guy Carleton, John Burgoyne and Major-General William Phillips, in 1776, 1777, and 1778*, Horatio Rogers (ed.), (Albany: J. Munsell's Sons 1884), 193.

93. T. Dickson Reide, *A View of the Diseases of the Army in Great Britain, America, the West Indies, and on Board of King's Ships and Transports, from the Beginning of the Late War to the Present Time: Together with Monthly and Annual Returns of the Sick, and Some Account of the Method in Which They were Treated in the Twenty-Ninth Regiment, and the Third Battalion of the Sixtieth Regiment* (London: J. Johnson, 1793), 28. Reide later inoculated the entire garrison at Niagara, on the order of Major Archibald Campbell: *ibid.*, 34.

94. 10 February 1771: CL, GP.

95. LO 841.

96. J. Knox, *An Historical Journal of the Campaigns in North America for the Years 1757, 1758, 1759, and 1760*, Arthur G. Doughty (ed), Champlain Society, *Publications*, ix (1915), 158.

97. *Extract from a Manuscript Journal, relating to the Siege of Quebec in 1759, kept by Colonel Malcolm Fraser, then Lieutenant of the 78th (Fraser's Highlanders,) and Serving in that Campaign* (Quebec: Literary and Historical Society of Quebec, 1866), 29.

98. *Ibid.*, 29. Thomas Mante claims that 1,000 died of the scurvy and an additional 2,000 were occasionally hospitalised: *The History of the Late War in North America and the Islands of the West Indies, including the Campaigns of MDCCLXIII and MDCCLXIV against His Majesty's Indian Enemies* (London: W. Strahan and T. Cadell, 1772), 283.

99. Letters illustrating the scurvy outbreak include: Lieutenant-Colonel William Eyre to Gage, 26 January, 1760; Lieutenant-Colonel William Haviland to Gage, Crown Point, 22 January 1760; Colonel John Campbell to Gage, Ticonderoga, 25 January 1760; and Captain Lewis Steiner to Gage, Onondaga Falls, 24 January 1760: all CL, GP.

100. Captain John Foxon to Gage, 1 March 1760; Steiner to Gage, 14 March: both CL, GP.

101. CL, GP.

102. CL, GP.

103. CL, GP. On 15 March, Dunbar had written to Gage that he hoped that the coming availability of wild greens would relieve the problem: CL, GP.

104. Hope to Miss Rogers, 9 October 1775: NA 30/39/1/[7].

105. Hayes to Mellish, 4 September 1779: Mellish of Hodsock Mss, 111/16.

106. Reide, *op. cit.* (note 93), 80.

107. S.M. Pargellis, *Lord Loudoun in North America* (New Haven: Yale University Press, 1933), 328.

108. Mercer wrote to Captain Archibald Williams, but Loudoun received the letter: CO 5/47/334.

109. Abercromby to Napier, 2 September 1758: WO 34/64/67; Napier to Abercromby, 12 September1758: HL, Abercromby Papers, AB 646.

110. Major Alexander Monypenny to Haldimand, 28 January 1759; British Library, Additional Mss 21,661, f. 11. Related letter Robert Leake to Monypenny, 11 December 1758, f. 3.

111. References to his instructions are included in Dunbar to Gage, 15 March 1760: CL, GP; references to seeds also in John Reed to Gage, 1 April 1760: CL, GP.

112. CL, GP.

113. CL, GP. Eyre set off 'a large Piece of Ground for a Garden with Palisades'; letter to Gage of 8 May: CL, GP.

114. CL, GP.

115. LO 3576.

116. *Orderly Book and Journal of Major John Hawks on the Ticonderoga-Crown Point Campaign, Under General Jeffrey Amherst 1759–1760* (New York: The Society of Colonial Wars, 1911), 13, 77.

117. *Journals, op. cit.* (note 90), 282.

118. Order of 2 May 1777: Massachusetts Historical Society, OB, 1st Bn. Marines, Halifax.

119. Letter to Mellish, n.d. (approximate dating inferred from contents), Mellish of Hodsock Mss, 111/3c.

120. Kopperman, *op. cit.* (note 2), 445–6.

121. WO 4/52/162.

122. WO 7/96/193.

123. Hamilton, *op. cit.* (note 21), II, 102.

124. Jackson, *op. cit.* (note 13), 280–1. Likewise, a number of medical officers who served in the West Indies came to argue against the extensive use of purgatives and emetics in treating diseases there, notably yellow fever; note, eg., Thomas Dancer, *A Brief History of the Recent Expedition against Fort San Juan, So far as it Relates to the Diseases of the Troops; together with Some Observations on Climate, Infection and Contagion; and Several of the Endemical Complaints of the West-Indies* (Kingston: D. Douglas & W. Aikman, 1781), 47–8; B. Moseley, *A Treatise on Tropical Diseases; on Military Operations; and on the Climate of the West-Indies*, 2nd ed., enl. (London: T. Cadell, 1789), 429–30, 433–4. I attempted to place such arguments in context in a talk that I delivered at the 37th International Congress on the History of Medicine in September 2000, entitled 'The Drive toward More

Moderate Therapies in British Medicine, 1750–1800'; this paper will be published in the proceedings of the Congress.

125. According to one set of figures, during the years 1775–9, the total number of British soldiers who died in North America, whether of wounds or of illness, totaled 6,046: Sir N. Cantlie, *A History of the Army Medical Department* (London and Edinburgh: Churchill Livingston, 1974), I, 156. Other data conflicts somewhat. The high mortality associated with the Cornwallis expedition boosted the death toll for 1780–81. Of 8,437 men who sailed from Britain to the West Indies between October 1776 and February 1780, 931 (11 per cent) died in passage: P. Mackesy, *The War for America 1775–1783* (Cambridge, MA: Harvard University Press, 1964), 526.

126. Albemarle to Amherst, Havana, 18 August 1762: WO 34/55/185.

127. *Duties, op. cit.* (note 21), (1794 edn), II, 262.

128. E. Kipping (trans. and ed.), *The Hessian View of America 1776–1783*, (Monmouth Beach, New Jersey: Philip Freneau Press, 1971), 39.

129. *Oeconomical, op. cit.* (note 2), 86. Not all British writers deprecated the medical services of foreign armies. Ring wrote, 'It is the height of imposition to pretend, that the great mass of surgeons attending the allied armies on the Continent, were educated in England: nor is it an easy task to convince us, that those German Princes who take so much care to procure good surgeons, wish to destroy their wounded men, in order to avoid the expense of maintaining them': *Reflections on the Surgeons' Bill*, 48.

130. *Military Journal of the American Revolution, from the Commencement to the Disbanding of the American Army: Comprising a Detailed Account of the Principal Events and Battles of the Revolution, With Their Exact Dates, and a Biographical Sketch of the Most Prominent Generals* (Hartford: Hurlbut, Williams & Co., 1862), 112.

131. Letter to Richard Henry Lee, Philadelphia, 14 January 1777: L. H. Butterfield (ed.), *Letters of Benjamin Rush* [American Philosophical Society, *Memoirs*, xxx] (Princeton: Princeton University Press, 1951), I, 129.

132. This author should not be confused with the great anatomist and surgeon of the same name.

133. *Observations on the Diseases which Appeared in the Army on St Lucia, in December, 1778; January, February, March, April, and May, 1779: To Which are Prefixed, Remarks Calculated to Assist in Ascertaining the Causes, and in Explaining the Treatment, of Those Diseases; With an Appendix, Containing a Short Address to Military Gentlemen, on the Means of Preserving Health in the West-Indies*, 2nd edn, rev. (Barbadoes and London: Charles Dilly, 1781), 7.

4

Disease and Medicine
in the Armies of British India, 1750–1830:
The Treatment of Fevers and
the Emergence of Tropical Therapeutics[1]

Mark Harrison

The East India Company's extensive medical establishment was noted for innovation and experimentation, it tested economical mass remedies. The service's control of its patients was significant, prefiguring the birth of the clinical anatomical medicine of Paris of the 1790s. The unique environment created a distinctive medical discipline: the medicine of warm climates. This chapter focuses on fever in particular; attention was focused on malfunction of the liver and the favoured treatment was purgation via mercury. The dominance of this method resulted partly from senior military officers imposing their views on the juniors.

During the eighteenth century, the East India Company became embroiled in a series of conflicts with the French and with Indian polities such as Mysore and the Marathas, who owed their power to the disintegration of the Mughal Empire. The source of these conflicts was two-fold: the Company strove to protect and extend its trading privileges in India while, at the same time, becoming involved in wars of European origin, such as the War of Austrian Succession (1740–8) and the Seven Years War (1756–63). Although the Company received assistance from the Royal Navy and the British Army from the 1740s, it was the Company's three armies based in Madras, Bombay and Bengal that bore the brunt of these campaigns. These were composed of a nucleus of Europeans (Germans, Dutch, Swiss, and even French served alongside the British) and a large number of Indian troops known as 'sepoys'. Although Indian troops predominated, the armies were officered by Europeans.

By the end of the eighteenth century, the Company possessed one of the largest armies in the world. Between 1789 and 1805, the number of men in the Company's armies rose from 115,000 to 155,000; in the Bengal Presidency, which succeeded Madras as the main centre of British power in the second half of the eighteenth century, around forty per cent of the Company's annual income went on military expenditure.[2] The Company was undergoing a rapid transition from a purely commercial organisation to a territorial power; beginning with the *de facto* annexation of Bengal in 1757, it went on to acquire more territory following wars against Mysore and the Marathas. By the turn of century, India under the Company had become, to all intents and purposes, a 'garrison state'.[3]

The Company's transition from a commercial organisation to a military–fiscal state had a considerable impact upon the development of British medicine. Firstly, it dramatically expanded the number of openings for surgeons and, to a lesser extent, physicians, who had trained in Britain, particularly after the formation of medical departments for the three presidency armies in the mid-1760s. By 1785, the peacetime medical establishment of all three medical services was 234 surgeons, and this had risen to 630 by 1824;[4] in addition, there were surgeons in the Company's marine service, although the number employed in the marine establishment has yet to be calculated. The sheer size of the medical establishment in India – both Company and Crown – gave it a certain degree of independence, possibly greater even than that of the West Indies.

Like the medical services of the British Army and the Royal Navy, those of the Company tended to attract young surgeons who had attended Edinburgh University or one of the London anatomy schools. However, a position with the Company was more highly prized, and thus harder to obtain, because it was potentially more remunerative.[5] Although the basic salary of an assistant-surgeon barely covered subsistence, military surgeons could earn extra from the allowances allocated for the purchase of drugs and medical supplies, from trade, speculation and from prize money awarded after military campaigns.[6] Sometimes, this could amount to a considerable sum: Joseph Hume, appointed as an assistant-surgeon in 1799, resigned in 1808 having amassed a fortune of £40,000.[7] There was also the prospect of a lucrative private practice among the Company's civilian employees or of promotion to one of its senior medical posts – the three members of each presidency medical board earned between £1,500 and £2,500 per annum.[8]

The medical institutions attended by those entering the Company's service were among the best in Europe; they also attracted students from poorer or dissenting families who were barred from Oxbridge and the inner circles of medical power in London.[9] It is hardly surprising, then, that the Company's medical services, like those of the Army and Navy, were noted for innovation in theory and practice.[10] The Company's military and naval hospitals in Madras, Bombay, and Calcutta provided an environment in which innovation could flourish. Lacking the humanistic orientation of the metropolitan medical elite, surgeons employed by the Company and the armed forces professed an experimental and empirical approach to medicine. One of the most important advantages enjoyed by Company surgeons, in this regard, was the constant supply of fresh corpses for dissection, which enabled them to ground their clinical practice much more firmly upon post-mortem examinations. In Britain itself, the organ-based pathology of the Paduan anatomist G.B. Morgagni (1682–1771) was not widely known until the end of the eighteenth century. Most civilian practitioners knew little of morbid anatomy until the publication of Mathew Baillie's *Morbid Anatomy of Some of the Most Important Parts of the Human Body* in 1793. But, by this time, morbid anatomy was already a prominent feature of medical practice in British India. In the same year that Baillie's book was published, there appeared *A Paper on the Prevention and Treatment of the Disorders of Seamen and Soldiers in Bengal,* by the Company surgeon John Wade, in which he described a system of therapeutics that had been built explicitly upon morbid anatomy. By 1793, post-mortem examination of those who died in the Company's hospitals was the rule rather than the exception.

The prominence of morbid anatomy was not a uniquely Indian phenomenon and it was evident to some degree in military and naval medicine across Europe and throughout the European colonies.[11] Military and naval surgeons found it far easier to obtain corpses for dissection than their civilian counterparts, and this was especially true of tropical colonies like India or the West Indies where the death rate was many times higher than at home. Thus, developments within the armed forces prefigured those normally associated with the 'birth' of clinico–anatomical medicine at the Paris hospitals in the 1790s;[12] as with the indigent sick of the Paris infirmaries, there were no families to claim the bodies of European soldiers in India and few cared about the fate of what Robert Clive referred to as 'the scum and refuse of England'.[13]

Certain other features of 'hospital medicine' are also evident in the Company's service: systematic bedside observation, the statistical analysis of cases, and the testing of what were presumed to be economical mass remedies. These developments implied, and contributed to, the objectification of diseases and patients.[14] Another thing that Company medicine had in common with hospital medicine in Paris was its iconoclastic empiricism: in Calcutta, as in Paris, Bacon and Locke were the guiding lights. But there were important differences, too. While Parisian medicine was known for its individualistic approach to the treatment of disease, the military structure of the Company's medical establishment produced more conformity in therapeutic practices. The anatomico-pathological medicine of Paris was also rather different from the morbid anatomy of British India in that it came to be based increasingly on the tissue pathology of Xavier Bichat (1771–1802). Pathology in British India remained very much organ-based until the 1830s. Nevertheless, the comparison is instructive because it demonstrates that the military context could provide conditions for innovation in medical theory and practice not unlike those which obtained in Paris after 1789.

Most of the observations made above could apply equally to the armed forces medical services in other colonies, but there were also some aspects of medical practice in the Company that were distinctively 'Indian'. The encounter with India's unique disease environment and, to some extent, with non-European medical traditions fostered a distinctive medical culture.[15] Yet similarities between India and other tropical environments enabled the Company's medical practitioners to contribute to what was rapidly becoming – in the eighteenth century – a distinct branch of medicine: the medicine of 'warm' or 'tropical' climates. This chapter traces the development of this branch of medicine by exploring a hitherto neglected aspect: therapeutics; and in particular, the treatment of fevers. It begins by looking at the incidence of fevers in the Company's armies and then at the theories advanced to explain their seasonal and clinical features. The remainder of the chapter charts the development of a distinctively Indian approach to the treatment of fevers, its spread to other tropical colonies, and its eventual demise.

The incidence and aetiology of fevers

While on active service, Company surgeons were called upon to treat a variety of injuries sustained in battle, ranging from sword thrusts and slashes, through to projectile wounds. However, the vast majority of work, both on active service and in times of peace, concerned the treatment of disease, which was responsible for the vast majority of deaths and admissions to hospital among European troops. It is well known that mortality rates in India and other tropical stations were far higher than among soldiers garrisoned in Britain: a fact easily explained by the prevalence of diseases such as malaria and dysentery. Though lower than the mortality rates of the West Indies and West Africa, those for British troops in India, at the beginning of the nineteenth century, were at least double those in Britain. The data assembled by Philip Curtin show that the likelihood of death in Bengal – regarded as the least healthy province of British India, on account of the prevalence of fevers in the Ganges delta – was six times greater than at home.[16]

Curtin's data, which are taken from regular medical reports, provide a reliable indication of mortality among British troops after 1800, but for the eighteenth century it is impossible to state the incidence of disease with any certainty, since regular records of sickness and mortality were not kept. Apart from the impressions of European soldiers and medical men in India, the only indications of levels of morbidity and mortality are to be found in the few hospital returns that have survived from this period. The only records that exist for Bengal – upon which I shall concentrate in this chapter – are the returns of the military hospital at Fort William in Calcutta;[17] sepoys were not included in these returns, as they were treated in a hospital of their own.[18] Unfortunately, only three admission returns appear to have survived: the records for 1752, 1763, and 1767.[19] In these years there were no major military or naval engagements, and so the casualties admitted were almost exclusively cases of sickness. The data contained in these returns refer mostly to troops from the Fort William garrison, although sailors in the Company's service were also admitted. Some of the latter would have arrived directly from overseas or from Indian ports like Madras. Although the inclusion of men from outside the garrison muddies the waters, we can gain an impression of the chief causes of sickness in Bengal and their seasonal incidence. A brief analysis of hospital admissions for the year 1767 will suffice to give an impression of patterns of sickness among Europeans in Bengal during the eighteenth century.

The most common causes of admission to hospital in 1767 were fevers and fluxes, in that order, and from the evidence available this appears to have been typical of most years in Bengal. In most cases the term flux – sometimes entered as 'bloody flux' – probably referred to dysentery of some sort. The term 'fever' was sometimes entered without further specification and so may have covered an extremely wide range of complaints. But there are often entries for remittent and intermittent fevers or ague, indicating that much of this fever was probably malarial. Although the ancient three-fold division of fever into remittent, intermittent and continual was commonly used in the East Indies, many practitioners simply entered such cases as 'fever' because they believed that each had the same cause and that one could easily mutate into another. Furthermore, within this system of classification, there was considerable room for variation. There were several recognised types of intermittent fever, for example, including tertian fever, which was reckoned to be the most common type of intermittent fever in hot climates. Continual or 'continued' fever was also divided into three classes: inflammatory, nervous, and putrid or 'malignant' fever.[20]

The malarial origin of many of the cases recorded as fever is further suggested by the seasonal incidence of this disease. The year 1767 is typical in that fevers were prevalent in the months during and immediately after the monsoon, when there were plenty of breeding pools for mosquitoes. The admission records of the Fort William hospital are thus in accord with the writings of Europeans stationed in Bengal, who were unanimous in proclaiming the rainy months of August and September to be the most unhealthy time of year, closely followed by the hot season, which lasted from

Table 4.1

Admissions to hospital, European Troops, Fort William, Calcutta, 1767.

Disease	Quartile				Total
	1st	**2nd**	**3rd**	**4th**	
Fevers	11	27	140	105	283
Flux	33	7	60	17	117
Pains	24	21	12	-	57
VD	7	15	5	-	27
Injury	6	7	4	-	17
Gravel	4	2	-	-	6
Sunstroke	-	3	-	-	3
Boils	-	3	-	-	3
Dropsy	1	-	1	-	2
Ulcers	1	-	1	-	2
Lunacy	-	-	2	-	2
Mordechien*	-	-	1	-	1
Obstruction	-	-	1	-	1
Delirium	1	-	-	-	1
Illegible	6	2	2	-	10
Totals	94	87	229	122	532

*Probably either cholera or severe dysentery.
Source: Bengal Army Muster Rolls and Cavalry Returns, L/MIL/10/130/Part IV, Oriental and India Office Collection, British Library.

April to the end of June. The naval surgeon James Lind (1716–94) reckoned Bengal to be the most lethal of all the English factories and identified the months of July to October as the unhealthiest of all, especially for those newly arrived in India.[21] This was confirmed by many subsequent visitors to Bengal, including John Clark, a surgeon on the Indiaman *Talbot*, who worked in the province from 1768 to 1771. Clark observed that putrid remittent fever and dysentery were especially prevalent in the wet season, and were often fatal to newcomers.[22] Indeed, Clark declared that 'During the sickly seasons at Bengal, the uncertainty of life is so great that it frequently happens that one may leave a friend at night in perfect health, who shall not survive the following day.'[23]

While some of the sickness among Crown and Company troops in India was attributed to intemperance, the principal or underlying cause of diseases such as fever and flux was thought to be climate. During the eighteenth century, the military and naval medical services were the vanguard of a neo-Hippocratic medicine – adumbrated by Thomas Sydenham (1624–89) – which emphasised the role of climate and other environmental factors in the production of disease. The British Army physician John Pringle (1707–82) epitomised this trend. While continuing to acknowledge that intemperance, diet, and other individual variables were exciting causes of disease, Pringle paid more attention to what he believed to be the environmental causes of diseases such as dysentery and fever.[24] Most practitioners in the Company's service were favourably disposed to Pringle's theory that atmospheric conditions and 'putrid air' – air corrupted by vapours from rotting matter and the exhalations of the sick – were responsible for many of the diseases commonly met with in the armed forces.[25] Indeed, the supposed putrid tendency of fevers in the East Indies had been remarked upon for many years before the publication of Pringle's *Observations on the Diseases of the Army* (1752), originating in the writings of the Dutch physician Bontius (1592–1631) in the early-seventeenth century.[26]

When medical writers referred to putrid fevers, they were occasionally referring to the putrescence causing the fever – the process of decay that gave rise to miasma – but more usually to the symptoms of the disease itself. As the Company surgeon John Clark explained, the term putrid, when applied to fevers, meant that there were 'symptoms of putrefaction... such as foetid breath, haemorrhage, offensive stools, livid blotches, and great prostration of strength.'[7] Putrescence could be easily discerned by close observation at the bedside but it might also become apparent during post-mortem examinations; such examinations were conducted by Bontius in the early-seventeenth century and were routinely conducted in the Company's hospitals throughout the eighteenth.[28]

Despite increasing criticism of the doctrine of putrefaction by followers of the Edinburgh professor William Cullen,[29] the majority of surgeons working in India continued to uphold it, at least to 1800. But Pringle's medical experience was confined to Europe and practitioners in the tropics attached even greater importance to the role of climate than did Pringle himself. The tropics produced more intense combinations of heat and moisture than other lands, accelerating putrefaction and producing more of the vitiated atmospheres that were thought to cause disease.[30] These climatic extremes were also deemed directly injurious to the 'unseasoned' European constitution. The Company surgeon John Clark expressed a common belief when he wrote that 'A warm climate relaxes the solids, dissolves the blood, and predisposes to putrefaction.'[31] The diseases, too, seemed quite different from those in Europe; even familiar complaints such as dysentery and ague could exhibit different symptoms and have different causes. The surgeon

Charles Curtis was also impressed by the 'illusive and varying forms under which the symptoms of known diseases present themselves in this climate,' and he became convinced that 'European nosology and definitions would, in India, prove but uncertain and fallacious guides.'[32]

One apparently unique feature of fevers in the tropics, in India especially, was that they originated in some malfunction of the liver. The liver was regarded as the organ most adversely affected by exposure to hot climates, and extreme heat was supposed to make it overactive, stimulating a copious secretion of bile. [33] This biliary theory of fevers was quite compatible with the putrid theory, since bile that could not be used up in the normal process of digestion could easily become putrid.[34] From the 1770s, most fevers were attributed to the combined action of bile and putridity but, by the end of the century, increasing emphasis was placed upon hepatic disorders alone.[35]

There are several possible reasons for this. The most obvious is that post-mortem dissections commonly revealed enlargement and discolouration of the liver in those who had died of fevers. Although it was true, as some sceptics were later to claim, that much of this damage could be attributed to the abuse of alcohol, inflammation of the liver is a common symptom of malaria – a disease which probably increased in the late-eighteenth century due to the silting-up of parts of the Ganges delta. This would have stagnated the flow of water, producing conditions suited to the breeding of mosquitoes and hence to the transmission of malaria.[36] The increasing emphasis upon the liver in theories of fever can also be explained by the fact that so many Company employees suffered from impaired digestion, which was generally attributed to some derangement of biliary secretion. Because of the frequency of such complaints, the liver – as the source of bile – became the seat of a general 'tropical' pathology: a chronic condition that was referred to simply as 'the bile'. Although some medical men were wary of attributing too much to biliary disorders, they were generally thought to be the cause of most diseases suffered by Company employees.[37] Certainly, most varieties of fever in India were thus attributed to what Curtis referred to as 'a superabundance and acrimony of bile'.[38] These aetiological shifts, as we shall see, had a significant effect upon therapeutic practices, but though therapeutic fashions changed, the belief that fevers required different forms of treatment than in Britain remained constant.

Tropical therapeutics: the treatment of fevers in British India

There is little doubt that most practitioners in India and other tropical colonies believed that the diseases of these localities were distinctive to some degree, though there is still some disagreement over how far this was so.[39] The history of therapeutics sheds further light on this matter as it is in this branch of medicine that the distinctiveness of tropical practice is most clearly shown. From the middle of the eighteenth century, the Company's surgeons began to reject prevailing views on the treatment of fevers in Britain and to insist that the different varieties of fever found in India required different forms of therapy. The history of therapeutics in British India reveals other aspects of professional identity, too. Most obviously, perhaps, it reveals the empirical ethos of the Company's practitioners, who claimed to base their practice on observation – both at the bedside and post-mortem – rather than on the teachings of respected medical authorities at home. Yet, like many avowed empiricists, their practices sometimes suggested the opposite and even bordered on the dogmatic. Furthermore, the hierarchical structure of the Company's medical services may have compounded any tendency towards uniformity that was based on intellectual conviction.

One distinctive feature of the treatment of fevers in the Company's armies was the growing tendency, during the late-eighteenth century, towards heroic forms of treatment such as violent purging. Such practices were based upon certain assumptions about the nature of fevers in India and may have also reflected the military ethos of the Company's service. Military surgeons considered themselves men of action – tough, practical, and resourceful – and were prepared to take drastic action if this seemed appropriate.[40] The need to preserve manpower, and the rapidity with which fevers claimed their victims, no doubt encouraged such heroic intervention. Also significant is the fact that most of the patients were in no position to object to such treatments. Though not compelled to undergo treatment, most soldiers in the Company's armies had little option but to accept what was on offer or forego professional intervention altogether. Only the most senior officers had the benefit of personal physicians. The existence of such a large population under military discipline enabled the Company's surgeons to conduct mass testing of remedies in a way that was impossible in most civilian contexts.[41] But standardisation was never complete, no matter how desirable it might have been militarily and economically.[42]

From bleeding to bark: therapeutics and the putrid theory of fevers

In the mid-eighteenth century, bleeding was still one of the most popular remedies for fevers such as ague. The therapy was based on Galenic medical theory and was supposed to work by drawing off peccant humours. Although the humoural theory had been partly discredited, many of the practices associated with it – such as purging and bleeding – were rationalised in terms of mechanical and other new conceptions of the body. Thus, blood-letting still had an important place in the therapeutic repertoire of the Leiden professor and iatromechanist Herman Boerhaave (1668–1738), whose students included John Pringle. Like his teacher, Pringle recommended blood-letting as a way of diminishing the violence of remittent and intermittent fevers. Indeed, he believed that bleeding was 'indispensable' and should be carried out before any medicines were administered.[43] Until the 1760s, most British practitioners in India would have agreed with him,[44] as would the Portuguese, who were enthusiastic advocates of blood-letting and even recommended it as a prophylactic. Their enthusiasm stemmed from the belief that the gradual depletion of 'European' blood would 'Indianise' their constitutions thus giving them immunity to the diseases of that country.[45]

By the middle of the eighteenth century, however, some British practitioners began to doubt the wisdom of blood-letting in hot climates. One of the first appears to have been the Calcutta-based surgeon Mr Bogue,[46] who cautioned against bleeding in cases of fever and prescribed, in its stead, a course of emetics followed by purgatives and large doses of Peruvian bark.[47] Much better known, both at the time and subsequently, were the opinions of the naval physician James Lind (1716–94), who believed that blood-letting was both inadequate and dangerous, especially during the most humid months. In his *Essay on Diseases Incidental to Europeans in Hot Climates* (1768), Lind averred that hot climates reduced the body's vitality and that further depletion through bleeding could be fatal, especially in Europeans who had just arrived in hot climates. Instead, he favoured a therapeutic regime that relied heavily on Peruvian bark administered in wine (a stimulant), to the quantity of an ounce and a half every ten to twelve hours. In addition, he used tartar emetic and antimonial medicines to purge the body of putrid substances.[48] The only illness for which Lind was prepared to countenance bleeding was dysentery, and then only with 'extreme caution'.[49] Following Lind, bark became one of the most popular remedies among British practitioners in India for the treatment of intermittent and remittent fevers. It was thought that the substance worked by checking the putrid tendency of fevers, which seemed to be particularly marked in the tropics.[50] However, it was seldom used exclusively and other remedies were employed to counteract the other symptoms of fever. One popular medicine was opium, which not only induced sleep but, expelled noxious substances by inducing perspiration.[51]

The aversion of Company surgeons to blood-letting is demonstrated in one of the most significant British–Indian medical publications of the mid-eighteenth century – John Clark's *Observations on the Diseases in Long Voyages to Hot Climates* (1773). Clark was the surgeon of the *Talbot*, an East-Indiaman, and worked in the Company's hospitals from 1768 to 1771. When he arrived in India, Clark followed Pringle's advice and resorted to copious bleeding in the treatment of remittent fevers, only to find that many of his patients were unable to bear it. His experiences in India therefore convinced him that blood-letting was too usually dangerous to be used in hot climates:

> Encouraged by the familiarity of the Bengal fever to that of the marshes described by Sir John Pringle, without paying regard to the difference of climate, I thought the violence of the fever required at least one blooding.... The consequence was, the first [patient] did not bear evacuation, his pulse flagged, and he was very delerious in the ensuing fit, the remissions were very insensible, and the exacerbations were only to be known by his delerium. The other two were seized very suddenly, and fell down in a delerium; on opening a vein they returned to their senses; but before five or six ounces of blood were taken, they became feint, and the feverish paroxysm ran higher than in those who did not suffer the evacuation. For the future I was determined to be very cautious in blood letting; and, since that period, have laid it aside in every fever in warm climates... unless accompanied by tropical inflammation.[52]

Instead of bleeding, Clark came to favour a variety of other therapies including antimonials, tartar emetic, mercury-based preparations, and bark.[53] In his advocacy of these remedies – especially bark – Clark's recommendations were in keeping with those of Lind; he maintained that 'The bark being antiseptic, cordial, and never suppressing any critical secretion, is well adapted for the cure of fevers in hot climates.'[54] Clark was apparently not alone in holding this opinion, for he declared that:

> Since the days of the judicious Dr Morton,[55] the use of the bark has been greatly limited; but it must give every one a sensible pleasure, that in opposition to every prejudice, the exhibition of this valuable medicine is becoming every day more general. Physicians now prescribe it liberally in every species of remitting and intermitting fever.[56]

The prejudice of which Clark wrote stemmed principally from the fact that bark – which had no purgative or emetic effects – did not conform to Galenic humoural theory.[57] However, several influential figures, including John Pringle, had put forward explanations for its apparent effectiveness in the treatment of intermittent and putrid fevers. In a series of papers read before the Royal Society during 1750–2, Pringle announced the results of experiments that appeared to show that Peruvian bark possessed attributes that counteracted putrefaction;[58] he was followed by several British physicians who compared the efficacy of bark with other remedies in a clinical setting. In addition, Clark was aware of at least two practitioners in India – the Company surgeon James Lind – not the more famous naval surgeon of the same name – and one Dr Broderick, formerly a surgeon of the *Nottingham* East-Indiaman – who had written on the treatment of putrid fevers with bark.[59]

Even though enthusiasm for bark was far from universal, opposition to bleeding united the majority of practitioners in India until the 1820s. Thus Major John Taylor, writing of his visit to India in 1789, warned prospective travellers that bleeding ought never to be resorted to in cases of fever owing to the delicacy of European constitutions in hot climates, and recommended a mixture of bark, antimonials and purgatives instead.[60] The naval surgeon Charles Curtis declared that he saw no reason to bleed, except in cases of acute hepatitis, and boasted that he had never whetted a lancet during thirty years in India.[61] The followers of the Edinburgh practitioner John Brown (1735–88) also shared this aversion to bleeding. Brown, the so-called Scottish Paracelsus, was a student of William Cullen's and, like Cullen, saw the nervous system as the key to understanding disease. But, unlike his teacher, Brown believed that all sickness was caused either by too much nervous excitement (the sthenic condition) or too little (the asthenic). According to the condition, Brown prescribed either sedatives or stimulants. Thus, followers of Brown, such as the Company surgeon Charles Maclean (1788–1824),[62] were implacably opposed to bleeding, denouncing it as 'gross and barbarous'[63] and as 'little better than butchery'.[64] Brown believed that most fevers were the result of diminished excitation and that measures such as venesection would serve only to worsen the disease.[65]

Mercury and the biliary theory of fevers

As mentioned earlier, the putrid theory of fevers was being eclipsed, from the 1780s, by an increasing emphasis on the liver as the origin of nearly all Indian diseases. One consequence of this was that Peruvian bark, which had hitherto been valued for its antiseptic properties, fell into virtual disuse in India, the chief aim of therapy in cases of fever now being to remove the 'superabundant and vitiated bile' that was thought to cause these diseases. Accordingly, purgatives came back into vogue and were used far more extensively than hitherto. The most common of these was mercury, which came virtually to dominate the treatment of fevers in British India from 1790 to 1830. In this respect, again, the therapeutic practices of British India were clearly distinguished from those in Britain itself, where mercury was rarely used in the treatment of fevers. Although some practitioners in Britain came to see mercury as a panacea, its use in medicine was largely confined to the treatment of syphilis and, to a lesser extent, of dysentery.[66]

From around the middle of the eighteenth century, Company surgeons began to administer mercury in the form of calomel pills to patients suffering from inflammatory diseases. In these pills, calomel (mercurous chloride) was often mixed with gum arabic and ipecacuanha – an established medicine for dysentery. These were generally given every three to four hours, until the patient's urine turned pale,[67] or sometimes in sufficient quantities to make the patient salivate. One of the first to advocate mercury in the treatment of Indian diseases was the Company surgeon John Clark, who recommended it in cases of inflamed and obstructed liver:

> In cold climates, the cure, as in all other inflammations, depends on plentiful bleeding, antiphlogistic purges, and the application of a blister to the part affected. But in the East Indies, this method being found unsuccessful, and the disorder in general proving soon fatal, the most experienced practitioners in that part of the world prescribe mercury as a specific. They apply it externally upon the part, and give it internally in such doses as excite a general salivation.[68]

However, Clark remained uncertain about the efficacy of mercurial preparations in cases of fever and he warned that the profuse sweating caused by large doses of mercury could actually prove injurious in the putrid fevers of hot climates.[69]

The earliest British–Indian writer to recommend mercury for the treatment of fevers seems to have been the Calcutta-based physician Dr Francis Balfour.[70] Balfour was one of a number of practitioners in British India who wrote on sol-lunar influences on fever and he attempted to devise a therapeutic regimen in accord with the lunar cycle.[71] He appears to have placed increasing reliance on mercury throughout his career. His first monograph – *Treatise on the Influence of the Moon in Fevers* (1784) – advocated a mixture of treatments, in which mercurial therapies did not figure largely.[72] But mercury was far more in evidence in his later *Treatise on Putrid Intestinal Remitting Fevers* (1790), in which Balfour's favoured method of treatment was to expel putrid matter with a mixture of emetics and purgatives; of the latter, he believed calomel to be especially valuable.[73]

Mercury occupied an even more important place in the pharmacopoeia of the Company surgeon John Wade, who wrote at length on its use in the treatment of fevers in his *Paper on the Prevention and Treatment of the Disorders of Seamen and Soldiers in Bengal* (1793). In common with many other British practitioners in India, he believed that vitiated bile was the cause of intermittent fevers and many other 'tropical conditions'. This seemed to be confirmed by Wade's post-mortem examinations of patients who had died of fever and which usually showed that the liver was more damaged than other organs.[74] Since it was now normal to treat hepatic disorders with mercury preparations – mercury having deobstruent, antibilious, and purgative qualities – it seemed logical to apply these in cases of fevers apparently linked to some derangement of the liver.

99

Wade had been converted to the biliary theory of fever by one Dr Paisly,[75] who worked at the Company's establishment at Madras. Although little is now known about Paisly, who appears to have published nothing during his lifetime, he apparently had a very high reputation and was visited at his place of work – the hospital of Fort St George – by sick Europeans from all over India. Paisly was one of the first to expound the biliary theory of fevers and was an enthusiastic advocate of mercury as a treatment of all disorders stemming from a deranged or obstructed liver. He recommended an initial purge with castor oil, followed by the gradual administration of mercury pills.[76] In a letter to a young surgeon on the Bengal establishment – which was probably Wade – Paisly declared that:

> Mercury, in judicious hands, is a safe and tractable medicine, and it is the only safe and powerful deobstructant in glandular obstructions, it is of consequence the only medicine to be depended upon in those latent defects of the system, which entail diseases or impede recovery; however, it often requires assistance from other medicines, from exercise, from spas, or from medicated aqueous medicines.[77]

Wade was convinced of the efficacy of Paisly's remedies and believed that his knowledge of liver complaints was second to none. The successful treatment of liver disorders, he claimed, 'has long been understood in the honourable company's settlements in the East Indies, and perhaps there only.'[78] Indeed, Wade thought that the use of calomel and other purgatives to treat fevers amounted to a 'therapeutic revolution': an opinion that is borne out by the many eminent British–Indian practitioners who came to advocate its use. Some of these – like the military surgeon George Ballingall – were even stronger advocates of mercury than Wade, ascribing to it almost miraculous powers.[79] Another fan of mercury was the naval surgeon James Johnson (1777–1845), who pronounced strongly in its favour in his widely read book, *The Influence of Tropical Climates*, which was first published in 1813. From then, until the 1830s, scarcely anyone in India doubted the 'absolute necessity of mercurializing every patient affected with fever, dysentery or hepatic affections.'[80]

Mercury was now 'lord paramount' of all the remedies administered in the hospitals of British India, but its use in the treatment of fever had spread beyond India to the West Indies and to practically everywhere where the British Army was stationed. [81] One of its early advocates in the West Indies was Colin Chisholm, author of *An Essay on the Malignant and Pestilential Fever* (1801).[82] This disease, more commonly known as yellow fever, was also thought to be a putrid bilious fever – like many of the fevers in India – even though the symptoms, most notably yellow staining of the skin, marked it out as different to some degree. The black vomit that was characteristic of the later stages of the disease seemed to suggest that the victim's bile had putrefied; hence the apparent suitability of a purgative like mercury. Indeed, all other treatments were subordinated to the removal of the vitiated bile that was supposed to be the hallmark of tropical fevers.

By 1804, the treatment of yellow fever with mercury was already well established among British Army surgeons in the West Indies, according to the French military surgeon J. Mabit.[83] Eight years later, when Robert Jackson took charge of the Medical Department of the British Army in the West Indies, the practice generally adopted in fever was still to 'saturate the system with mercury'.[84] By the 1790s, a number of doctors in Britain itself had also come to recommend purgation with mercury,[85] but the profession in Britain still tended to recommend such remedies as bark and stimulants in cases of fever. One institution in which purgation with mercury made very little headway was in the Royal Navy, with the exception of those naval surgeons who were based for any length of time in India. The Grenada-based military surgeon, Colin Chisholm, declared that there was a 'powerful prejudice' against the practice in the medical department of the Navy.[86] One reason for this may have been that Cullenian ideas had been popularised in the Navy by such influential naval practitioners as Thomas Trotter (1760–1832).[87] Furthermore, the treatment of fevers with mercury appears to have been a purely British pre-occupation. While some foreigners who had visited India – such as the French naturalist Pierre Sonnerat – subscribed to the biliary theory of fevers, and probably to mercurial treatment,[88] French practice in the West Indies appears to have tended more towards blood-letting, although by no means exclusively so.[89]

The sovereignty of mercury in British India clearly owed much to widely held assumptions about the climate and its effects on the human body, but its dominance was also due to the robust way in which its advocates dealt with contrary viewpoints. Although most advocates of mercury were wary of excessive salivation, and seldom relied on mercury alone, they took pains to denounce rival systems of treatment. Wade argued that hitherto common therapies, such as treatment with Peruvian bark, were of little use in India. He could accept that bark was 'a medicine occasionally applicable to the various modifications of fever... as they occur in Europe' but maintained that such occasions were 'very infrequent in warm climates', even in the case of intermittent fevers which were generally thought to respond well to this treatment.[90] Stimulants such as wine were also of little use in the tropics, he claimed, and in some cases they had been positively detrimental because they had been given in enormous quantities. Those who advocated such practices, he argued, had usually little experience of fevers in India.[91]

Indeed, Wade insisted that surgeons arriving in India dispense with any 'prejudices acquired at the university or at the shop',[92] and warned that 'the diseases of warmer latitudes differ very materially from such as afflict the inhabitants of cold climates, and the methods of treating them should consequently vary.'[93] His cautionary remarks applied not only to the teachings of university professors, but to the methods espoused by John Brown, which were then being popularised in Calcutta. Several endorsements of Brown's system of healing – and of the efficacy of regulating the body with liberal doses of stimulants or sedatives – had appeared in Calcutta newspapers during 1788 and 1789, and were attributed to surgeons in the employ of the Company.[94] The extent to which Brunonianism gained support in India has yet to be determined, but it did make some distinguished converts, including the Company surgeon and author of several influential tracts on plague, fevers, and quarantine, Charles Maclean. Maclean, who arrived in Bengal in 1792, was not an uncritical admirer of Brown but he held him in very high esteem, referring to him as the 'Hippocrates of the Eighteenth Century'.[95] Maclean had been exposed to Brown's teaching in Edinburgh but claimed not to have become a convinced Brunonian until discovering, in the East Indies, that treatment based on Brunonian principles worked far better than the usual regime of purging and evacuation in cases of fever. He, and his colleague at the Calcutta General Hospital, William Yates, came to believe that *all* diseases were diseases of deficient excitement and that they should be treated by stimulants. The stimulants used most often by Maclean and Yates were mercury and opium, although they used mercury in smaller quantities than those – like Wade – who employed it as a purgative.[96]

Though it relied heavily on mercury, few of Maclean's colleagues approved of the therapeutic regime at the Calcutta General Hospital: it was the system rather than the therapy, which offended the sensibilities of medical practitioners in British India. Maclean wrote of the widespread 'prejudice' that existed against Brunonian ideas in India during the 1790s and his publications were intended largely to dispel this. Certainly, some Company surgeons – such as John Wade – publicly denounced Brunonian ideas:

> Doctor Brown's practice may possibly apply to some circumstances of low fever in Europe, but the occurrence of such fevers will be found very rare in the meridian of Bengal, particularly in the upper provinces, where most acute disorders have, what would be deemed in Europe, and according to Doctor Moseley in the West Indies, an inflammatory aspect, and are also characterised by larger secretions of bile.[97]

Antipathy to Brunonian ideas was also evident in later British–Indian writings, such as Johnson's *Influence of Tropical Climates*.[98] Johnson's high reputation in India and Britain, and his powerful connections,[99] ensured that Brunonian practitioners were marginalised during the 1810s and 1820s, despite the fact that some surgeons would have been taught by Maclean in England, after he found employment in 1809, as the Company's lecturer in the diseases of hot climates.

The career of Brunonianism in the tropics is a subject that deserves a separate article and it is not possible to reflect at greater length upon it here, except to suggest reasons why some Company surgeons may have denounced Brunonian ideas. Company surgeons were not unusually sensitive to accusations of quackery and empiricism and, indeed, prided themselves on the latter, often espousing theories unfashionable in Britain, such as the sol-lunar theory of fevers. They were therefore unlikely to have been afraid of being branded 'mere empirics' by the physician elite in Britain. More plausible reasons for the prejudice encountered by Maclean are that Brunonianism negated the importance of morbid anatomy, which had come to play such an important part in British–Indian medical practice, and that the Brunonian system was regarded as too speculative and reductive, despite its pretensions to empiricism.[100] Yet, this very reduction may also have appealed to some tropical practitioners. As Maclean pointed out:

> In climates and countries where the transition from health to disease, and from disease to death, is often alarmingly rapid, and health always precarious, the knowledge of a doctrine, which reduces the practice of medicine to a degree of certainty hitherto unknown, cannot but be attended with great and evident advantages.[101]

But any popularity which Brunonianism might have enjoyed in the 1790s, may have been offset by its associations with political radicalism. Although the French were no longer a direct threat in India during the 1790s, the beginning of the Revolutionary War opened up the possibility of an alliance between revolutionary France and warlike Indian polities such as Mysore. Maclean, himself a Radical, was expelled from India in 1798 by the incoming Governor-General, R.C. Wellesley (the brother of the future Duke of Wellington) for his intemperate criticism of one of the Company's magistrates.[102]

The denunciation of rival systems of medicine, such as that of Brown, shows that a new orthodoxy had emerged in British–Indian medical practice – grounded in the biliary theory of fevers, and manifest in the over-riding emphasis on mercury as a therapy. Although the military context provided many of the conditions necessary for innovation in medical practice, and though military surgeons prided themselves on their empiricism, it also enabled senior medical officers to impose their views upon juniors. This could be done to some extent through the exercise of patronage, without which the aspiring surgeon had no chance of appointment to the Company or the armed forces medical services, or of advancement through the ranks. Once in the service, surgeons and physicians in charge of hospitals were in complete control of the purchase of medicines and were in a position to regulate their use. Above these surgeons came the Inspectors and deputy Inspectors-General of Hospitals and the Medical Boards – in India there was one for each presidency – that had the power to enforce certain practices on pain of disciplinary action. Some medical officers viewed the powers wielded by these individuals as tyrannical. In a tract of 1810, in which he criticised the Army Medical Department, Charles Maclean, who had been employed in both the Army and Company medical services, declared that 'The Inspectors and Deputy Inspectors of Hospitals seem invariably to consider themselves as entitled to interfere in the practices of all inferior Officers.'[103]

There is at least one well-documented case of a medical officer falling foul of the Indian medical authorities for pursuing practices at variance with the official line: that of the British Army surgeon Thomas Clark. Clark's *Observations on the Nature and Cure of Fevers, and of the Diseases of the West and East Indies* (1801) is unusual in that it was written not so much to communicate new ideas, as to vindicate its author, who had recently been accused of malpractice in the military hospital at Colombo. Clark joined the Army as an assistant surgeon at the end of 1790 and was sent immediately to Canada. In August 1793, he was dispatched to Barbados and served there, and on several islands in the West Indies, before purchasing a surgeoncy with the 113th Regiment in Ireland. In October of that year, the Regiment embarked for India and Clark arrived in Madras in November 1796. Shortly afterwards, he was ordered to Ceylon to take charge of the military hospital at Colombo. When Clark arrived in the East Indies, he was a very experienced surgeon and had learnt much about the diseases of warm climates; his approach was flexible and empirical, in the best tradition of British military medicine. While at Colombo, however, he fell foul of the Medical Board in Madras and, in particular, of Dr Ewart, the Inspector-General of Hospitals. Ewart – a British Army physician – appears to have had authority over both Crown and Company hospitals, and issued orders that applied to both.[104]

One such order was that all surgeons working in hospitals had to fill in casebooks describing the patient's symptoms and the treatment given; a rule that was generally flouted owing to competing claims on surgeons' time. Clark was one of the few who carried out these orders and, though ill himself, ordered his assistants to complete the forms. They did this for one month and, towards the end of 1798, Clark dispatched the form to the Inspector-General as requested.[105] Shortly afterwards, Ewart replied to Clark enclosing 'a long and elaborate dissertation upon his Case-Books, in which he was pleased totally to reprobate the Medical Practice Reported in them.'[106] Ewart even went so far as to accuse Clark of killing one of his patients by using inappropriate treatments. Unfortunately, Clark did not specify which treatments Ewart complained of in his letter, and the latter's 'dissertation' was lost by Clark when returning from India. However it is clear from Clark's writings, and the subsequent actions of Ewart, that they disagreed fundamentally about the causation of diseases like fever and dysentery and about their treatment.

Whereas Ewart subscribed to the conventional British–Indian view that fevers and dysentery originated in disorders of the liver, and were most effectively treated with mercury, Clark believed that both fevers and dysentery – while often connected with liver disorders – could develop independently. Clark further believed that the primary cause of all these diseases was the 'sedative' action of tropical climates, which checked perspiration, causing the body to overheat and the heart and arteries to become over-excited. Heat also led, he believed, to a marked 'determination' of the blood from the skin towards the thoracic and abdominal organs, causing them to become distended and inflamed; this – rather than superabundant bile – was the cause of fevers, dysentery and hepatic disorders. In Clark's opinion, all these complaints could be treated effectively by bleeding, as it reduced the quantity of blood and diminished inflammation.[107] Clark's advocacy of blood-letting in these diseases was clearly at odds with British–Indian practice, which was to prescribe mercury. As he later pointed out, Ewart was of the opinion that 'fever, and likewise dysentery, were almost always occasioned by the state of the liver',[108] thus their respective approaches to the treatment of these diseases necessarily differed.

However, Clark did not advocate bleeding to the exclusion of all other treatments. In cases of fever, bleeding was followed by the administration of large doses of calomel, or Dr James' or antimonial powder.[109] The latter would have been acceptable to Ewart and the Medical Board, but Clark's primary course of bleeding was not; nor was his insistence on ipecacuanha – rather than mercury – as the chief remedy for dysentery. When Ewart visited Colombo in November 1798, shortly after having sent his comments to Clark, he took over the running of the hospital and immediately abolished the use of ipecacuanha.[110] Shortly after this, Clark was arrested and threatened with a court-martial for disobeying orders, on the grounds that his assistants were no longer keeping a log of treatments. However, given that most surgeons regarded this as an 'intolerable piece of drudgery'[111] and refused to comply with Ewart's orders, it seems likely that the charge was merely a pretext to exclude Clark from practice. Ultimately, Clark did not face trial but was kept under arrest for around three months, during which his health deteriorated further. After his release, in 1799, he was forced to leave Ceylon and to return to Britain, where he wrote his extraordinary vindication.

Although mercury therapy never became totally dominant in British India, the treatment of fevers came to display a certain amount of rigidity and uniformity. Any tendency to conformity arising from convictions about the uniqueness of the Indian disease environment was compounded by the hierarchical organisation of the military medical services and the boards that regulated military and naval hospitals. Heroic treatments such as purgation with mercury also befitted a military service and suggested a worldly, no-nonsense approach to those who had fallen sick. To many in the Army and Navy, sickness seemed rather ignoble and was closely associated with poor discipline; indeed, many illnesses were ascribed, in part, to disorder or intemperance. Back in the seventeenth century, Bontius had written of the need to 'restrain the fury of rioting morbific matter' in cases of bowel disease,[112] and analogies between putrefaction and social decay abound in the literature on Indian fevers in the eighteenth century.[113] In fact putridity and biliousness became metaphors for Indian society: the subcontinent's great heat, according to the physician William Falconer, had caused its people to secrete an excess of bile and it was this that accounted for their 'aversion to motion' and 'indolence of disposition'.[114] What would happen to Europeans – particularly those of lax moral fibre – if they remained in India's enervating heat? By the end of the eighteenth century, the Company's historian Robert Orme, among others, feared that the British might go the way of previous conquerors, and become 'Indianised' to such a degree that they would become indistinguishable from the peoples over whom they ruled.[115] Given such anxieties, and the low esteem in which British soldiers were held, it may well have been that vigorous purging had a disciplinary element: a subconscious desire to purge Europeans of any harmful alien elements.

All these factors may help to explain the prevalence of mercury therapy for fevers in late-eighteenth and early-nineteenth century India, but it is likely that the resort to large quantities of mercury was indicative of desperation as much as anything. In one of his first letters home, the Company surgeon Francis Maxwell told his father – who seems to have possessed some knowledge of medicine – that:

> You would be surprised, and, I'll venture to say, so would every Medical man in Glasgow, at the quantity of Mercury we give in Feveres [*sic*], Fluxes, etc., for diseases here are such that if we do not stop them soon by vigorous

remedies, they will save us trouble by killing the patients. As you are a bit of a doctor, you may form some idea of your practice when I inform you I frequently give a man 70 or 80 grains of Calomel in 24 hours, and perhaps continue the same for some days.[116]

However, patients often took some convincing that mercury therapy was in their best interests, as George Cormack, a cornet in the Bengal Army, recalled when recovering from an attack of bilious fever:

The fatigue I underwent brought on a Bilious Fever and this is the first letter I have written since my recovery. The Fever did not annoy me above five days, but the Doctor, a cabbage headed West Country Medicine Pounder, crammed me with such a quantity of Calomel as salivated me completely for 25 days. I had no use of either gums or teeth.[117]

The demise of mercury and the return to blood-letting

The unpleasant side-effects of mercury and its failure, in many instances, to arrest the progress of disease, induced many practitioners in India to turn against it. By the 1830s, indiscriminate and excessive mercurialisation was denounced by two of the most influential figures in British–Indian medicine: William Twining,[118] an eminent practitioner at the Calcutta General Hospital, and H.H. Goodeve,[119] the Professor of Medicine at the newly established Calcutta Medical College. They challenged the biliary theory of fever on the basis of new findings in pathology and pointed to the efficacy of new drugs, such as quinine, in the treatment of intermittent fevers.[120] But the most significant turning point was the return to blood-letting, which had previously been rejected by the majority of practitioners in British India.

The return to blood-letting that occurred in India during the 1830s amounted to a second revolution in British–Indian therapeutics; indeed, the treatment of fevers had turned full circle and returned to the position which obtained prior to 1750. One of the strongest new advocates of bleeding was Twining, who based his treatment of fevers upon post-mortem examinations of soldiers and civilians who had died in the Company's hospitals. These showed that one of the characteristic features of fever was engorgement of the viscera with blood, while previous findings, which appeared to show a preponderance of liver disease, were explained away as the consequence of intemperance in food and alcohol.[121] Twining followed the French pathological anatomists in identifying, not simply the organs affected by particular diseases, but specific tissues, such as the 'cellular structure' lining the duodenum.[122] His findings seemed to agree with observations made of fevers in other tropical countries, including the notorious yellow fever of the West Indies. Twining declared that:

> The recent practice of bleeding in Intermittents... not only accords with the acknowledged pathology of that class of Fevers; but seems to bring our system of therapeutics... within the limits of those established principles adapted to the treatment of other fevers [eg. yellow fever].[123]

Twining followed the Jamaica-based military physician Robert Jackson in recommending bleeding in the early stages of fever. Jackson had begun to advocate the treatment three decades before, despite the fact that the majority of the profession was then opposed to bleeding.[124] This was still the case in 1812, when he took charge of the Medical Department of the British Army in the West Indies, but once in that position he was able to influence many military surgeons to abandon mercury in favour of the lancet. Jackson and his followers in the West Indies made much of the fact that their treatment was in accord with the latest findings in pathology; investigations which they themselves had conducted.[125] They were unanimous in condemning old ideas of putrefaction as a vestige of humoural pathology; they attributed fevers and dysentery, not to the obstruction or corruption of bodily fluids, but to diminished vitality of the nervous system. It was this diminished vitality – in the form of a weakened pulse – that seemed to explain the congestion of blood in the organs of patients who had died from fever.

The emphasis upon the nervous system in the writings of Twining and Jackson owed much to the theory of fever developed by Cullen in the late-eighteenth century, and possibly something to the theories of Brown and Erasmus Darwin. But they differed from Cullen in their enthusiasm for blood letting. Cullen generally recommended restorative treatment for fevers, and blood-letting only to relieve a spasm. Certainly, most of Cullen's disciples believed that blood-letting could lead to debility or death, especially in hot climates.[126] Thus, this new fashion in tropical therapeutics was again quite distinct from common practice in Britain, although, by the 1820s, Jackson had apparently convinced many in Britain itself that bleeding could be useful in the treatment of fever.[127]

Conclusion

The treatment of fevers with mercury, and opposition to blood-letting, were among the most distinctive characteristics of medical practice in British India from around 1750 to 1830. Both were predicated on the assumption that India was a very different disease environment from Britain and other temperate countries: Indian fevers were widely regarded as more likely to be putrid or bilious in nature, and therefore to require treatments that checked these tendencies. The Indian environment posed a challenge in another sense, too. The suffocating humidity of the hot and rainy seasons seemed to enfeeble the European constitution and it was widely believed that it could not bear further depletion through bleeding. This led the Company's surgeons and physicians to abandon bleeding – which was still recommended by many European authorities in the treatment of certain forms of fever – and to develop treatments which seemed to be in conformity with diseases as they appeared in the tropics. The most distinctive of these was the treatment of fevers with large doses of mercury: a practice that was rare in Britain itself. This was predicated on the assumption that Indian fevers – like other tropical fevers – were diseases of abundant or vitiated bile: the liver being the organ least able to withstand the tropical heat.

The biliary theory of fevers and their treatment with mercury were peculiarly Indian innovations, originating among surgeons and physicians in the employ of the East India Company. However, they later spread throughout the British Army – though apparently not the Royal Navy – to other tropical colonies, such as the West Indies, where they came for a time to dominate medical practice. This demonstrates that the Company's medical services played an important part in the development of what was increasingly recognised as a distinct branch of medicine: the medicine of 'warm' or 'tropical' climates, even though the biliary theory and mercury therapy were subsequently challenged. As Charles Maclean observed, the sheer scale of the medical establishment in British India encouraged it to develop independently of medical opinion in Britain:

> The great independence of mind, which prevails among the faculty in the East and West Indies, but more especially in the former, from the superior organisation of the East India Company's extensive medical establishments... not only admit[s] of, but even enjoin[s], an increased freedom of investigation; of which a more efficacious, as well as a more discriminating practice are the inevitable result.[128]

The medical services of the Company thus emerge, along with those of the Army and Navy, as important sites of innovation in eighteenth- and early-nineteenth-century medicine. Military service brought medical practitioners into contact with new disease environments, and their experiences led them to abandon or to adapt much of what they had learned in Britain. The readiness with which military surgeons abandoned 'prejudices acquired at the university, or in the shop', as the surgeon John Wade put it,[129] can also be attributed to the mentality of those who joined the services. The Company's medical services, like those of the Army and Navy, attracted a disproportionate number of young men who had been trained at Edinburgh and London surgical establishments: men who were often from dissenting backgrounds and barred from entry into the medical elite. Furthermore, military and naval practitioners had certain practical advantages over their civilian colleagues. Military hospitals provided a steady supply of fresh corpses for dissection – especially in tropical stations – and this allowed surgeons to base their practices to an unusual extent on morbid anatomy. The military environment also enabled the Company's surgeons to experiment with new remedies to a degree that would have been impossible in most civilian contexts.

It would, however, be a mistake to exaggerate the licence enjoyed by the Company's medical practitioners. Although many forms of medical practice were tolerated, therapeutic practices began to harden into a new orthodoxy. Those, like Charles Maclean and Thomas Clark, who doubted the wisdom of the prevailing system of medicine, and who advocated remedies – or systems – of their own, were denounced and even reprimanded. The establishment of regulatory boards, the power wielded within hospitals by senior surgeons, and competition for lucrative civil appointments, all served as further incentives to toe the line. Yet British–Indian medical practice did not become so ossified that it was incapable of change: therapeutic fashions, including that of mercury, came and went, and medical practice was influenced both by developments in Europe and in the other tropical colonies. But the medical officers of the Company, and later those of the Crown, remained adamant that climate was the most important factor in the causation of disease and that Indian diseases required different forms of treatment than those in Europe.[130]

Notes

1. I am grateful to Bill Bynum for information on eighteenth-century theories of fevers, and to Michael Worboys for his helpful comments and criticisms on an earlier draft of this paper. I also wish to thank those who commented on an earlier version of this paper, read at the Wellcome Symposium on British Military Medicine before 1800.
2. C.A. Bayly, *Indian Society and the Making of the British Empire* (Cambridge: Cambridge University Press, 1988), 85.
3. See D.M. Peers, *Between Mars and Mammon: Colonial Armies and the Garrison State in Early Nineteenth-Century British India* (London & New York: I.B. Tauris, 1995).
4. D. Arnold, *Science, Technology and Medicine in Colonial India* (Cambridge: Cambridge University Press, 2000), 58.
5. L. Rosner, *Medical Education in the Age of Improvement: Edinburgh Students*

and Apprentices 1760–1826 (Edinburgh: Edinburgh University Press, 1991), 20–1.

6. Francis Maxwell to his father, 19 January 1801, Letters from Dr Francis Maxwell, Bengal Medical Establishment, 1798–1805, Mss. Eur. C.101, Oriental and India Office Collections [hereafter OIOC].

7. D.G. Crawford, *A History of the Indian Medical Service, 1600–1913,* Vol. 2, (London: Thacker & Co., 1914), 78.

8. Crawford, *ibid.,* Vol. 1, 365.

9. W.F. Bynum, 'Cullen and the Study of Fevers in Britain, 1760–1820', in W.F. Bynum and V. Nutton (eds), *Theories of Fever from Antiquity to the Enlightenment, Medical History Supplement No.1* (London: Wellcome Institute for the History of Medicine, 1981), 135–48; D. Harley, 'Honour and Property: The Structure of Professional Disputes in Eighteenth-Century English Medicine', in A. Cunningham and R. French (eds), *The Medical Enlightenment of the Eighteenth Century* (Cambridge: Cambridge University Press, 1990), 138–64.

10. P. Mathias, 'Swords and Ploughshares: The Armed Forces, Medicine and Public Health in the Late Eighteenth Century', in J.M. Winter (ed.), *War and Economic Development* (Cambridge: Cambridge University Press, 1975), 91–102; U. Tröhler, 'Quantification in British Medicine and Surgery, 1750–1830, with Special Reference to its Introduction into Therapeutics' (PhD thesis, University of London, 1978); Bynum, 'Cullen and the Study of Fevers,' *op. cit.* (note 9); N.A.M. Rodger, 'Medicine and Science in the British Navy of the Eighteenth Century', in C. Buchet (ed.), *L'Homme, La Santé et la Mer* (Paris: Champion, 1997), 333–44.

11. See for example, L. Brockliss and C. Jones, *The Medical World of Early Modern France* (Oxford: Clarendon Press, 1997), 689–700; O. Keel, 'The politics of Health and the Institutionalisation of Clinical Practices in Europe in the Second Half of the Eighteenth Century', in W.F. Bynum and R. Porter (eds), *William Hunter and the Eighteenth-Century Medical World* (Cambridge: Cambridge University Press, 1985), 207–58.

12. On pathology and Paris medicine see: E.H. Ackerknecht, *Medicine at the Paris Hospital, 1794–1848* (Baltimore: Johns Hopkins Press, 1967); D. Vess, *Medical Revolution in France, 1789–1796* (Gainesville: University Presses of Florida, 1975); R.C. Maulitz, *Morbid Appearances: The Anatomy of Pathology in the Early Nineteenth Century* (Cambridge: Cambridge University Press, 1987); R.C. Maulitz, 'The Pathological Tradition', in W.F. Bynum and R. Porter (eds), *Companion Encyclopedia of the History of Medicine* (London: Routledge, 1993), 169–91.

13. Quoted in R. Harvey, *Clive: The Life and Death of an Emperor* (London: Hodder & Stoughton, 1998), 66.

14. This was one of the characteristic features of military medicine as it developed during the eighteenth century. See M. Harrison, 'Medicine and the Management of Modern Warfare', *History of Science*, 26 (1996), 379–410; C. Lawrence, 'Disciplining Disease: Scurvy, the Navy and Imperial Expansion', in D. Miller and P. Reill (eds), *Visions of Empire* (Cambridge: Cambridge University Press, 1994), 80–106.

15. In this chapter I will not have the opportunity to examine this dimension of medical practice in British India, but the dialogue between European and Indian practitioners is discussed in M.N. Pearson, 'The Thin End of the Wedge: Medical Relativities as a Paradigm of Early Modern Indian–European Relations', *Modern Asian Studies*, 29 (1995), 141–70; R. Grove, 'Indigenous Knowledge and the Significance of South-West India for Portuguese and Dutch Constructions of Tropical Nature', *Modern Asian Studies*, 30 (1996), 121–44; P. Boomgaard, 'Dutch Medicine in Asia, 1600–1900', in D. Arnold (ed.), *Warm Climates and Western Medicine* (Amsterdam: Rodopi Press, 1996), 42–64; M. Harrison, 'From Medical Astrology to Medical Astronomy: Sol-Lunar and Planetary Theories of Disease in British Medicine, c.1700–1850', *British Journal for the History of Science*, 33 (2000), 25–48; M. Harrison, 'Medicine and Orientalism: Perspectives on Europe's Encounter with Indian Medical Systems' in M. Harrison and B. Pati (eds), *Health, Medicine and Empire: Perspectives on Colonial India* (New Delhi: Orient Longman, 2001).

16. P.D. Curtin, *Death by Migration: Europe's Encounter with the Tropical World in the Nineteenth Century* (Cambridge: Cambridge University Press, 1989), 24.

17. During this period there were two hospitals at Fort William. The first was established in 1707/8 but was destroyed after the sack of Calcutta by the Nawab of Bengal in 1756. From 1757 to 1769, the hospital was re-established in a fairly dilapidated building within the bounds of the old fort. It moved to new and improved premises in the suburbs in 1769. Crawford, *op. cit.* (note 7), Vol. 2, 422–3.

18. *Ibid.*, 422.

19. For 1752 and 1763 see: 'Account of the Military sent to the Hospital, July–December, 1752', Bengal Army Muster Rolls and Cavalry Returns, L/MIL/10/130/Part II, OIOC; Bengal Army Muster Rolls and Cavalry Returns, L/MIL/10/130/Part III, OIOC.

20. J. Clark, *Observations on the Diseases in Long Voyages to Hot Climates, and Particularly on Those which Prevail in the East Indies* (London: D. Wilson & G. Nicol, 1773), 118–120.

21. J. Lind, *An Essay on Diseases incidental to Europeans in Hot Climates with the Method of Preventing their Fatal Consequences*, 6th edn (London: J. & J. Richardson, 1808; first published 1768), 91.

22. Clark, *op. cit.* (note 20), 51–2.

23. *Ibid.*, 53.

24. Sir J. Pringle, *Observations on the Diseases of the Army* (London: A. Miller *et al*, 1768, 6th edn.; first published in 1752), 79–98, 184–5.

25. See for example: J. Lind, *Treatise on the Putrid and Remitting Marsh Fever, which raged at Bengal in the Year 1762* (Edinburgh: C. Elliot, 1776); F. Balfour, *A Treatise on Putrid Intestinal Remitting Fevers* (Edinburgh: W. Smellie, 1790). The James Lind mentioned above is not the famous Royal Navy surgeon but a Company surgeon attached to the Drake Indiaman.

26. J. Bontius, *An Account of the Diseases, Natural History, and Medicines of the East Indies*, trans. anon (London: T. Noteman, 1769; first published in 1645); H.H. Goodeve, 'A Sketch on the Progress of European Medicine in the East', *Quarterly Journal of the Calcutta Medical and Physical Society*, 2 (1837), 126; M. Harrison, *Climates and Constitutions: Health, Race, Environment and British Imperialism in India 1600–1850* (New Delhi: Oxford University Press, 1999), 37–8.

27. Clark, *op. cit* (note 20), 122.

28. See Bontius, *op. cit.* (note 26), 85–100; Clark, *op. cit.* (note 20), 134–5; C. Curtis, *An Account of the Diseases in India, As they Appeared in the English Fleet, and in the Naval Hospital of Madras, in 1782 and 1783, with Observations on Ulcers and the Hospital Sores of that Country* (Edinburgh: W. Laing, 1807), 148–9.

29. William Cullen (1710–90), Professor of the Institutes of Medicine at Edinburgh University from 1773 to 1790, rejected the hydrodynamic system of the Leiden professor Hermann Boerhaave (1668–1738) and stressed the primary role of the nervous system in the production of disease. In so doing, he abandoned the old humoral pathology, holding that all diseases could be attributed to disorder of the nervous system. See Bynum, 'Cullen and the Study of Fevers in Britain', *op. cit.* (note 9); L.G. Wilson, 'Fevers', in W.F. Bynum and R. Porter (eds), *Companion Encyclopedia of the History of Medicine* (London: Routledge, 1993), 282–411. One of Cullen's main champions within the armed forces was the naval physician Thomas Trotter (1760–1832), who criticised putrefaction as the 'last remnant of Humoral Pathology' and welcomed Cullen's 'more rational and refined investigation of a vital principal'. See T. Trotter, *Observations on the Scurvy, with a Review of the Opinions lately advanced on that Disease, and a new Theory Defended, on the Approved Method of Cure, and the Induction of Pneumatic Chemistry* (London: T. Longman, 1792; first published 1785), 1.

30. For a fuller discussion of the 'diseases of warm climates', see the essays in Arnold, *op. cit.* (note 15), Harrison, *op. cit.* (note 26).

31. Clark, *op. cit.* (note 20), 269.

32. Curtis, *op. cit.* (note 28), xvi, xix.

33. J.P. Wade, *A Paper on the Prevention and Treatment of the Disorders of Seamen and Soldiers in Bengal* (London: John Murray, 1793), 47; Clark, *op. cit.* (note 20), 267.

34. See W. Falconer, *Remarks on the Influence of Climate, Population, Situation, Nature of Food, and Nature of Country, Way of Life, on the Disposition and Temper, Manners and Behaviour, Intellects, Laws and Customs, Forms of Government, and Religion, of Mankind* (London: C. Dilly, 1781), 13.

35. Goodeve, *op. cit.* (note 26), 133, 142.

36. P.J. Marshall, *Bengal: The British Bridgehead. Eastern India 1740–1828* (Cambridge: Cambridge University Press, 1987), 4–5, 20; Harrison, *op. cit.* (note 26), 155–7.

37. A. Burt, *A Tract on the Biliary Complaints of Europeans in Hot Climates; Founded on Observations in Bengal and Consequently Designed to be Particularly useful to those in that Country* (Calcutta: John Hay, 1785), 15–18.

38. Curtis, *op. cit.* (note 28), 120.

39. Michael Worboys argues that differences between tropical and non-tropical diseases were seen as differences of degree rather than of kind ['Tropical Diseases', in W.F. Bynum and R. Porter (eds), *Companion Encyclopedia of the History of Medicine* (London: Routledge, 1994), 512–36] whereas the present author has argued that these differences were seen as so marked that they required radically different forms of practice, Harrison, *op. cit.* (note 26); M. Harrison, '"The Tender Frame of Man": Disease, Climate, and Racial Difference in India and the West Indies, 1760–1860', *Bulletin of the History of Medicine*, 70 (1996), 68–93.]

40. There are marked similarities in this respect between military surgeons and the medical practitioners of ante-bellum America. See J. H. Warner, *The Therapeutic Perspective: Medical Practice, Knowledge and Identity in America, 1820–1885* (Princeton: Princeton University Press, 1997), 11–36.

41. See also Brockliss and Jones, *op. cit.* (note 11).

42. The physicians-general of the British Army had a long history of resisting demands for complete standardisation of treatment. H.J. Cook, 'Practical Medicine and the British Armed Forces after the "Glorious Revolution"', *Medical History*, 34 (1990), 1–26. Although treatments did become more standardised in the course of the eighteenth century, they never became universal.

43. J. Pringle, *Observations on the Diseases of the Army*, 6th edn (London: T. Cadell, D. Wilson, T. Durham & T. Payne, 1768; first published 1752), 241–44.

44. Goodeve, *op. cit.* (note 26), 126.

45. Harrison, *op. cit.* (note 26), 47.

46. There is no trace of Bogue in Crawford's *Roll of the Indian Medical Service.*

He was probably employed by the Company as a ship's surgeon.

47. Editorial, *India Journal of Medical Science*, n.s., 2 (1837), 305.
48. Lind, *op. cit.* (note 21), 78–9.
49. *Ibid.*, 267.
50. Goodeve, *op. cit.* (note 26), 129.
51. *Ibid.*, 130.
52. Clark, *op. cit.* (note 20), 136–7.
53. *Ibid.*, 137, 145.
54. *Ibid.*, 145–6.
55. Clark is probably referring to Richard Morton (1637–98), author of the widely read treatise on physic, *Opera Medica* (1697), which went through several editions until its last publication in 1737. This, and Morton's other works, discuss inflammatory fevers and their treatment.
56. Clark, *op. cit.* (note 20), ix.
57. A.-H. Maehle, *Drugs on Trial: Experimental Pharmacology and Therapeutic Innovation in the Eighteenth Century* (Amsterdam: Rodopi, 1999), 284.
58. *Ibid.*, 260–2.
59. Clark, *op. cit.* (note 20), viii–ix. I have been unable to trace the Dr Broderick referred to by Clark.
60. J. Taylor, *Travels from England to India, in the Year 1789* (London: S. Low, 1799), Vol. 2, 80.
61. Curtis, *op. cit.* (note 28), 132.
62. Maclean was a student at Edinburgh during the mid-1780s, when Brown's influence was at its height. He began his medical career as a surgeon on an East-Indiaman but in 1792 settled in Bengal, where he took charge of the European general hospital in Calcutta. He was expelled from India by the Governor-General R.C. Wellesley after criticising a magistrate in a local newspaper. He afterwards returned to Britain where he made a name as a critic of quarantine and an opponent of smallpox vaccination. In 1809/10, he found a position as the East India Company's lecturer on the 'diseases of hot climates', which is surprising in view of the fact that Maclean's views were somewhat at odds with those of the medical profession in India; M. Harrison 'Charles Maclean (*fl.*1788–1824)', *Oxford Dictionary of National Biography* (Oxford: Oxford University Press, 2004), found on the web at: http://www.oxforddnb.com/view/article/17649.
63. C. Maclean, *Results of an Investigation Respecting Epidemic and Pestilential Diseases* (London: Thomas & George Underwood, 1817), Vol.1, 52.
64. Maclean, *op. cit.* (note 63), Vol. 2, 413.
65. *Ibid.*, 394, 467, 467.
66. See Maehle, *op. cit.* (note 57), 15–17; W.F. Bynum, 'Treating the Wages of Sin: Venereal Disease and Specialism in Eighteenth–Century Britain', in W.F. Bynum and R. Porter (eds), *Medical Fringe and Medical Orthodoxy*

1750–1850 (London: Croom Helm, 1987), 5–28; L.J. Goldwater, *Mercury: A History of Quicksilver* (Baltimore: York Press, 1972), 239–48.

67. Goodeve, *op. cit.* (note 26), 145.

68. Clark, *op. cit.* (note 20), 269.

69. *Ibid.*, 139.

70. Francis Balfour (d.1767) obtained an MD at Edinburgh University in 1767 and joined the Company's Bengal service as an assistant-surgeon in 1769; he resigned his combat commission on promotion to surgeon in 1777 and he became head surgeon in 1786. In 1788 Balfour gained a prestigious post as a member of the medical board, on which he sat until 1796; he was re-appointed to the board in 1800 and remained a member until he retired in 1807. In addition to the works cited in this article he was the author of *Dissertatio de Gonorrhea virulenta* (1767), *The Forms of Herkern* (1781) and a lost translation of the *Seir-I-Mutakherin*. D.G. Crawford, *Roll of the Indian Medical Service 1615–1930* (London: Thacker & Co., 1930), 15.

71. See Harrison, 'From Medical Astrology', *op. cit.* (note 15).

72. Francis Balfour believed that the s- called 'Pucca Fever' of Bengal could not be cured with anything but bark, which checked the process of putrefaction; see his *Treatise on the Influence of the Moon in Fevers* (Calcutta: C. Elliot, 1784), 17–20. Balfour was in correspondence with Pringle and was aware of the latter's experiments which appeared to show that bark had an antiseptic quality. However, Balfour allowed that purely bilious fevers could be cured simply through evacuation, 21.

73. Editorial, *India Journal of Medical Science*, n.s., 2 (1837), 306; Balfour, *op. cit.* (note 25), 111–12, 129–30.

74. Wade, *op. cit.* (note 33), 116–117, 129.

75. There is no record of a Dr Paisly or any practitioner of similar name in Crawford's *Roll of the Indian Medical Service*. He was most likely a surgeon in the Company's marine service.

76. Wade, *op. cit.* (note 33), 155. Wade spells his mentor's surname without an 'e' but elsewhere it is sometimes written as 'Paisley' or 'Pasly'.

77. Paisly quoted *ibid.*, 162.

78. *Ibid.*, 112.

79. Ballingall served in India for seven years as assistant-surgeon to the 2nd Battalion of Royal Scots and was a great advocate of mercury in cases of dysentery. See G. Ballingall, *Practical Observations on Fever, Dysentery, and Liver Complaints, as they occur amongst the European Troops in India* (Edinburgh: David Brown & A. Constable & Co., 1818), 81.

80. Goodeve, *op. cit.* (note 26), 147.

81. *Ibid.*, 145.

82. C. Chisholm, *An Essay on the Malignant Pestilential Fever Introduced into the West Indian Islands from Boullam, on the Coast of Guinea, as it Appeared in*

1793 and 1794 (London: C. Dilly, 1795), 163.

83. J. Mabit, *Essai sur les Maladies de l'Armée de St.-Domingue en l'an XI, et principalement sur la Fièvre jaune* (Paris: École de Médicine, 1804), 17.

84. J. M'Cabe, *Military Medical Reports; Containing Pathological and Practical Observations illustrating the Diseases of Warm Climates* (Cheltenham: G.A. Williams, 1825), 13.

85. Wade mentions a number of practitioners including one Dr Lyssons of Bath and the London practitioner Sir William Fordice, *op. cit.* (note 33), 52–3.

86. Chisholm, *op. cit.* (note 82), 163.

87. For Trotter's views on yellow fever see his *Medicina Nautica: An Essay on the Diseases of Seamen: Comprehending the History of Health in His Majestey's Fleet, under the Command of Richard Earl Howe* (London: T. Cadell & W. Davies, 1797), 334–6.

88. P. Sonnerat, *Voyage aux Indes Orientales et à la Chine, fait par Ordre du Roi, depuis 1774 jusqu'en 1781* (Paris: Privilege of the King, 1782), Vol. 2, 75.

89. Mabit, *op. cit.* (note 83), 17–18.

90. Wade, *op. cit.* (note 33), 59.

91. *Ibid.*, 62–3.

92. *Ibid.*, 48.

93. *Ibid.*, 50.

94. *Ibid.*, 68. The armed forces medical services were probably one of the main conduits for the dissemination of Brunonian ideas. See M. Barfoot, 'Brunonianism under the Bed: An Alternative to University Medicine in Edinburgh in the 1780s', in W.F. Bynum and R. Porter (eds), *Brunonianism in Britain and Europe, Medical History Supplement No. 8* (London: Wellcome Institute for the History of Medicine, 1988), 23.

95. Maclean, *op. cit.* (note 63), 54.

96. C. Maclean and W. Yates, *A View of the Science of Life; Or, the Principles established in the Elements of Medicine, of the Late Celebrates John Brown, M.D., with an Attempt to Correct some Important Errors of that Work; and Cases in Illustration, Chiefly Selected from the Records of their Practice at the General Hospital, at Calcutta* (Philadelphia: William Young, 1797); C. Maclean, *A Treatise on the Action of Mercury, upon Living Bodies and its Application for the Cure of Diseases of Indirect Debility* (Philadelphia: William Young, 1797); C. Maclean, *Practical Illustrations of the Progress of Medical Improvement, for the last Thirty Years: Or, Histories of Cases of Acute Diseases, as Fevers, Dysentery, Hepatitis and Plague, treated according to the Principles of the Doctrine of Excitation, by Himself and other Practitioners, chiefly in the East and West Indies, in the Levant, and at Sea* (London: for the author, 1818).

97. Wade, *op. cit.* (note 33), 67.

98. J. Johnson, *The Influence of Tropical Climates, more especially of the Climate of India, on European Constitutions* (London: J.J. Stockdale, 1813), ix, 27, 94.

117

99. Johnson spent only three years in India (1803–6) but in that short time he gained a reputation as an expert on the diseases of warm climates. On returning to Britain in 1814, after naval service in other parts of the world, he established a private practice in London and became a royal physician. See M. Harrison, 'Tropical Medicine in Nineteenth-Century India', *British Journal for the History of Science*, 25 (1992), 299–318.

100. Brunonianism was opposed for these reasons in Britain, too. See C. Lawrence, 'Cullen, Brown and the Poverty of Essentialism', in Bynum and Porter, *op. cit.* (note 94), 1–22.

101. Maclean and Yates, *op. cit.* (note 96), 27.

102. Harrison, *op. cit.* (note 62). From 1793 to 1815, the Calcutta government became increasingly secretive and concerned with political agitation, keeping radicals and potential traitors under close surveillance. There were fears of a world-wide republican conspiracy. See C.A. Bayly, *Empire and Information: Intelligence Gathering and Social Communication in India, 1780–1870* (Cambridge: Cambridge University Press, 1996), 146.

103. C. Maclean, *An Analytical View of the Medical Department of the British Army* (London: J. Stockdale, 1810), 90.

104. T. Clark, *Observations on the Nature and Cure of Fevers, and of Diseases of the West and East Indies, and of America: With an Account of Dissections performed in these Climates and General Remarks on Diseases of the Army* (Edinburgh: Bell & Bradfute, 1801), vi.

105. *Ibid.*, vi–vi.

106. *Ibid.*, vii.

107. *Ibid.*, 18–19, 30–34, 39.

108. *Ibid.*, 234.

109. *Ibid.*, 19.

110. *Ibid.*, 234.

111. *Ibid.*, vii.

112. Bontius, *op. cit.* (note 26), 27–8.

113. Harrison, *op. cit.* (note 26), ch. 2.

114. Falconer, *op. cit.* (note 34), 13.

115. Harrison, *op. cit.* (note 26), 102.

116. Maxwell to his father, undated c. August 1798, Letters from Dr Francis Maxwell, Mss. Eur. C.101, OIOC.

117. Letter from George Cormack, 17 November 1804, in Alexander Allam Cormack (ed.), The Mahratta Wars 1792–1805: Letters from the Front by Three Brothers – Nicholas, George and Thomas Carnegie of Charleton, Montrose, RAMC 715/6, Contemporary Medical Archives Collection, Wellcome Library.

118. William Twining (1790–1835) was born in Nova Scotia and died in Calcutta. He gained the MRCS in 1806 before spending two years as a

hospital mate in the Royal Navy. He joined the Army Medical Department in 1812 and in 1814 became an assistant-surgeon. In 1821 he was sent to Ceylon to serve the Governor, Gen. Sir Edward Paget, and accompanied him to India, in 1824, when he was appointed Commander-in-Chief. After arriving in India, Twining joined the Company's Bengal service and eventually took charge of the Calcutta General Hospital. He played a prominent part in the Calcutta Medical and Physical Society. In addition to the work cited below, Twining was author of *Diseases of the Spleen* (1826) and *Epidemic Cholera* (1833). Crawford, *op. cit.* (note 70), 86.

119. H.H. Goodeve (1807–84) became an MRCS in 1828, and took an MD at Edinburgh the following year. He became an assistant surgeon in the Company's Bengal service in 1831 and a surgeon in 1848; he retired in 1853. After retirement, Goodeve went on to become an FRCS in 1844, MRCP (Lond.) and FRCP (Lond.), both in 1860. He was best known as Professor of Medicine at the new Calcutta Medical College (founded 1835) and as author of *Hints on Children in India* (1844). Crawford, *op. cit.* (note 70), 103.

120. Goodeve, *op. cit.* (note 26), 152–4; W. Twining, *Clinical Illustrations of the more important Diseases of Bengal with the Result of an Inquiry into their Pathology and Treatment* (Calcutta: Baptist Mission Press, 1835).

121. *Ibid.*, 570.

122. *Ibid.*, 672.

123. Twining, *op. cit.* (note 120), xvii–xix.

124. R. Jackson, *An Outline of the History and Cure of Fevers, Endemic and Contagious* (Edinburgh: Mundell & Sons, 1798), 271–3.

125. R. Jackson, *A Sketch of the History and Cure of Febrile Diseases; More Particularly as they Appear in the West Indies among the Soldiers of the British Army* (Stockton: T. & H. Eeles, 1817), ch. 7; M'Cabe, *op. cit.* (note 84).

126. M'Cabe, *op. cit.* (note 84), 12.

127. *Ibid.*, 13.

128. Maclean, *op. cit.* (note 63), xiii.

129. Wade, *op. cit.* (note 33), 59.

130. See I. Klein, 'Cholera Theory and Treatment in Nineteenth-Century India', *Journal of Indian History*, 58 (1980), 35–51.

5

Who Cared?
Military Nursing during the English Civil Wars and Interregnum, 1642–60

Eric Gruber von Arni

Very little work has been done on nursing prior to the nineteenth century; this chapter offers an examination of the profession in the mid-seventeenth century. Commonwealth Exchequer papers from the Long Parliament's Committee for Sick and Wounded Soldiers are used. The numbers treated, the nature of contemporary military treatment by surgeons and physicians, and the extant evidence for medical and nursing practice at these hospitals are detailed, and it is suggested that the quality was far superior to that assumed by many historians.

Background

Military nursing is now recognised as a distinct speciality within the wider body of the profession, with its own unique fund of knowledge and experience. Although this reality has been generally accepted for many years, the concept has only recently been given sound academic support with the establishment of a service-based Masters degree programme for serving military nursing personnel of the British Army, Royal Navy and Royal Air Force. A similar format has also been adopted by the Republic of South Africa's Defence Forces. Such developments provide a stark contrast with former times when this branch of the profession was, sadly, neglected, frequently undervalued, and ignored by historians and nurses alike.

A common misconception holds that the period between the sixteenth-century closure of monastic establishments and the mid-nineteenth-century arrival of Florence Nightingale formed a black void in which nursing existed only in parody.[1] Indeed, Granshaw claims that the nursing reformers of the second half of the nineteenth century went out of their way to vehemently stress the darker side of earlier nursing in order to emphasise the need for reform. Real or imaginary cases of drunkenness, dishonesty, immorality, corruption, and laziness among nurses were rolled out, tarring all with the same brush.[2] As a direct result, widespread ignorance of earlier practices has prevailed for much of the twentieth century. The work of military nurses of earlier times has been inexorably excluded from the literature of warfare.[3] A search for appropriate imagery among contemporary literature and drama offers little guidance, albeit this comment is equally valid when applied to the study of sick-nursing in general. In 1907, Nutting and Dock placed seventeenth-century nursing firmly in the 'dark ages' while in 1919, Alice Clark commented that seventeenth-century sick-nurses were recruited from the lowest classes of women who only undertook the work as a means of earning their food.[4] Even Dr Margaret Pelling, writing in 1998, has remarked that 'on the present basis, it is quite difficult to decide whether the early modern sick-nurse existed in England at all before the late-seventeenth century.'[5] Is this true?

This chapter examines the nursing care provided during the English Civil Wars and Interregnum, 1642–60, as a test case. Remarkably, in the preface to his *magnum opus, The London Dispensatory,* written in 1649, Thomas Culpeper, the renowned seventeenth-century apothecary and herbalist provides a contrasting picture when he dedicates his work as follows:

> Not the least of all my respects kind Gentlewomen to you who freely bestow
> your pains, brains and cost, to your poor wounded and diseased neighbours.
> [You] must not be forgotten. I humbly salute you with many thanks and
> present these, the beginnings of my labours at your feet.[6]

This was a glowing tribute in an age when the College of Physicians and the Company of Barber–Surgeons were heavily committed to increasing their influence on health care and suppressing the traditional role of carers and healers. In lauding the work of nurses, Culpeper was acknowledging the reality that nurses had provided the primary source of hands-on health care in most rural and poor communities for many hundreds of years and continued to do so.

Unfortunately, Henry VIII's Dissolution of the Monasteries had destroyed the medieval facilities that had provided hospital-based health care to all-comers. Subsequent changes in the concept of hospitality and the public provision of charity were associated with a concomitant degrading of the status of nursing. Whereas many nursing nuns had formerly been recruited from the rich, noble and merchant classes, by the mid-sixteenth century when the major poor hospitals were re-established, considerations of cost and supply became paramount.

By the eve of the Civil Wars, most nurses working in the London poor hospitals probably shared the same deprived background as that of their patients. However, the widespread nature of the fighting brought people of all classes into contact with the sick and wounded. Fortunately, large numbers of citizens came to regard the task of caring for the needy as a patriotic duty. Examination of the surviving evidence appears to indicate that those men and women who struggled to provide care and comfort to the victims of the fighting adopted a manner no less genuine than their equivalent representatives today. Carlton has compared the overall casualty figures for war-attributed deaths during the Civil Wars with those of the two World Wars of the twentieth century. Expressed as percentages of the total population, 11.5 per cent compared with 3.04 per cent and 0.64 per cent respectively, statistically the impact of the Civil Wars on the general population would appear to have been, potentially, greater than any other conflict in British history, including the two World Wars.[7] Given these figures, the non-recognition of the achievements of those who cared for military casualties during those unsettled times is surprising to say the least. In truth, the Civil Wars elicited a dramatic improvement in facilities afforded to the sick and wounded and stand as a major milestone in the history of military nursing.

Compared with Parliamentary sources, documentary evidence for the provision of nursing care to Royalist forces is relatively scarce. Throughout the Wars the King's attitude towards his army's casualties was ambivalent at best. Lackadaisical administrative paperwork was followed by wholesale destruction of documents following the surrender of Oxford. Even contemporary Royalist sources conceded that their enemy's medical services were far superior to their own.[8] Their enemies adopted a much more positive approach towards its sick and wounded, and therefore, this work will concentrate on the facilities afforded Parliamentary troops.

Parliament's military hospitals

On the field of battle, casualty care starts at the point of injury. Contemporary armies were accompanied by soldiers' wives and camp followers who, it is frequently assumed, provided what little on-the-spot succour was available to their injured menfolk. However, then as now, a nursing presence on the battlefield during active combat was of limited value. It was important to remove casualties to a secure and stable environment as soon as possible in order to provide definitive nursing care.[9] Although both sides were constantly stretched to find sufficient funds with which to provide adequate care, Parliament's control of London, with its wealthy and influential City merchants, facilitated the use of various fund-raising schemes to advantage. In October 1642, the wounded from Edgehill who had returned to London with the Earl of Essex, together with those from the skirmish at Brentford, lay scattered all over the western suburbs of London and throughout the City. A Committee for Sick and Maimed

Soldiers was established and, on 13 November, Parliament identified the Savoy Hospital as the central treatment facility for military casualties. Here, each morning between eight and nine o'clock, a physician and surgeon were present at a daily 'sick-parade' for the dressing of wounds and other treatments.[10] The Savoy, a medieval establishment founded by Henry VII, had survived the Dissolution albeit in a parlous financial state. The first and most significant of the various hospitals dedicated to the care of Parliament's military casualties, it filled rapidly and many of the wounded continued to be lodged in other buildings in and around the city. Four 'nursing sisters' remained from the original civilian staff and were instructed to care for the soldiers admitted to the hospital under the orders of a newly appointed overseer. Their identity is unconfirmed but financial accounts compiled in 1649 mention the continuing presence of Sister Collyns, Sister Ann, Sister Bird and Sister Maud whereas all other nurses are given the title 'nurse'.[11] At least twelve nurses were eventually employed to staff the four main wards sited in the 'dorter', (or dormitory), a large, cruciform building over two hundred feet long and thirty feet wide. Long Ward was sited in the nave, Chapel Ward in the chancel, and Newbury Ward and Reading Ward were arranged in the two transepts, the latter two names being wartime innovations to commemorate Parliamentary victories.[12]

Throughout the war London's civilian hospitals also received a steady flow of wounded soldiers. However, significant as their contribution was, these hospitals handled only a small proportion of military casualties. With their continuing responsibilities towards the capital's population, and with most of their funds committed by statute to specific charities, they could not be relied upon to provide all the hospital requirements of the army. By March 1645, a second military hospital had opened in the western suburbs of the city and functioned effectively for eighteen months.[13] Frustratingly, apart from identification as 'the hospital at Parson's Green', this hospital's exact location is not identified in contemporary documents, but the premises must have been reasonably substantial as over seventy patients were admitted at one time. There were only three buildings in the Parson's Green and Fulham area large enough during the 1640s: Fulham Palace, the seat of the Bishop of London; Parson's Green House, owned by the family of the Earl of Peterborough; and thirdly, the house of Sir Nicholas Crispe in Fulham.

The last named property, leased from the Bishop of London and ideally situated alongside the Thames between Fulham and Hammersmith, exceeded eighty-six acres in extent and lay approximately one mile from Parson's Green village. The grounds extended from Bridge Road, Hammersmith in the north to the orchard known as Crabtree in the south. Crispe was a wealthy Royalist merchant who fled London in January 1643 when it became known that he had been secretly sending money to Royalist funds in Oxford. On 24 September the following year the Commons issued orders for Crispe's town house at Lime Street in the City to be sold to raise money for the care of Essex's defeated army that had recently returned from the disastrous Cornish campaign.[14] It is not unreasonable to assume that as part of Crispe's estate had already been sold and the profits used for the benefit of Parliamentarian wounded, his remaining property in Parson's Green was also put to similar use. Additional weight is given to this premise by the local parish accounts of St. Paul's, Hammersmith which contain several entries relating to disbursements for maimed soldiers as well as a payment of 2s 4d to the sexton for seven graves for soldiers that had died in Crispe's house.[15] It has also been reported that human bones, described as the remains of Parliamentary soldiers, were discovered in the Crabtree area of Crispe's former estate during Victorian times and therefore, in the absence of adequate primary source confirmation, the weight of secondary evidence points unwaveringly towards Crispe's house as the most likely site for the military hospital.[16]

The Overseer's account book for Parson's Green hospital, which provides almost the sole surviving documentation relating to the work of this facility, shows that the number of nurses employed varied according to the workload. For the majority of the time the staff consisted of four ladies with an occasional reduction to three as the workload varied and an increase to five when admissions peaked in November and December 1645 after the storming of Basing House. The hospital closed in September 1646 when its remaining in-patients were transferred to the Savoy.

Ely House, a former palace for the Bishops of Ely, off High Holborn, had lain unused for many years but, since 1643, had been rented for service as a prison for Royalist prisoners of war.[17] On 14 April 1648, following the sale of Bishops' lands, these buildings were transferred to the Commissioners for Sick and Maimed Soldiers for conversion into a military hospital. From then until shortly after the Restoration, Ely House remained the centre of military hospital administration and welfare provision.[18] Fortunately, patient bed occupancy figures for the two main military hospitals are available for October 1648 and these are shown in Table 5.1, overleaf.

The newly opened Ely House became effective towards the end of September and filled rapidly over a period of two to three weeks. By comparing these figures with those recorded by the Treasurers for Sick and Wounded Soldiers at St Bartholomew's and St Thomas's during the same period we can see that the two service hospitals undertook by far the greater proportion of military casualty work.[19]

Table 5.1

Patients in hospital, October 1648.

Week	Savoy	Ely House	St Bart's	St Thomas's
1	N/A	48	N/A	22
2	200	71	57	N/A
3	213	127	63	23
4	202	119	61	27
5	205	112	45	28

N/A = Figure not available

Source: The National Archive [hereafter NA], SP28/141B, *Accounts of the Treasurers for Sick and Maimed Soldiers*, fo. 4.

The nurses

On 15 November 1644, the Committee for Sick and Maimed Soldiers issued their 'General Rules and Regulations for the Governance of Patients and Nurses'.[20] This important document, a highly significant artefact in the history of British military nursing, is probably the earliest surviving set of British military hospital rules. The contents were designed to provide a disciplinary framework which delineated the pattern of patients' lives, the environment within which care would be conducted, and established guiding principles for nurse selection, terms of employment, conduct and practice. Although austere and prescriptive, these rules represented a first step on the ladder of progress towards today's recognition of the unique role and function of the military nurse whilst, coincidentally, recognising their position as falling within the military organisation.

Candidates for appointment to nursing vacancies in military hospitals were chosen primarily from soldiers' widows experienced in the ways of the army, and therefore, resilient characters used to living within a disciplined environment yet capable of using their own initiative when required.[21] Such women would have been reliable when carrying out instructions and unlikely to leave an environment that offered security and familiar surroundings. Like their civilian counterparts, military nurses were expected to conform to a code of conduct that imposed both restrictions and responsibilities upon them.

The regulations clearly imply that the perceived duty of a nurse was to care for and succour the patients in her charge and that the care given was to be kindly, free from coercion and bullying, and in the patients' best interest. Nurses who were found to be negligent in their duties, failed to give adequate attention to their patients, were bad tempered or indulged in brawling or other disturbances would, for the first offence be fined 2s, for the second lose a week's pay, and for a third be expelled from the hospital. Contemporary attitudes to religion ensured that the personal behaviour of both nurses and patients was also addressed and the regulations imposed strict religious tenets and moral standards. Nurses were accommodated separately from their area of responsibility and segregated as far as possible from all but professional contact with men. Ward doors were locked at eight o'clock each evening and re-opened at seven o'clock next morning during the winter months. These times were adjusted to 9pm and 6am in the summer. Although these regulations may appear harsh, military nurses were well-provided-for in comparison with contemporary standards elsewhere.

Nurses in the military hospitals were paid 5s weekly but forfeited their 4s widow's pension so Parliament obtained their labour for a mere 1s extra to its existing commitment. Their pay was, however, enhanced by the permanent nature of their employment and, as with their civilian counterparts, boosted with the addition of free food and accommodation and ready access to expert medical care. This level of remuneration compared very favourably with that of nurses in civilian employment at St Bartholomew's where the top weekly rate of 3s 6d included a special payment of 6d for additional work involved in caring for military patients. Even nurse selection differed from civilian practice. Unlike St. Bartholomew's and St Thomas's hospitals, where the matrons were responsible for selecting newly appointed nursing staff, military nurses were selected by a minimum of two Committee treasurers who had to signify concurrence and approval before an appointment or dismissal was confirmed. Equally, there is no clear evidence that the supervisory and regulatory role of the Matron at St. Bartholomew's and St. Thomas's hospitals was replicated at the Savoy and Ely House where the main wards were sub-divided into smaller areas, each in the charge of a head nurse, assisted by additional nursing staff in varying numbers.[22] In October 1648, shortly after the opening of Ely House, the nursing staff for the two London military hospitals was as shown in Table 5.2, overleaf.

During busy times, sickness, or staff shortages, temporary assistants known as help-nurses were employed to maintain adequate staff levels. In addition, the Treasurers occasionally employed and paid for similar temporary personnel to work in St Bartholomew's and St Thomas's Hospitals caring specifically for military patients. Their knowledge or experience was not defined, nor was their background and yet, as their weekly pay varied from 2s 6d to 5s, this must have reflected their varied abilities to some degree. Payments made by the hospital Overseer during the ten days from

Table 5.2

Nursing staff employed at the Savoy and Ely House, October 1648.

Week	Savoy		Ely House	
	Nurses	Help Nurses	Nurses	Help Nurses
1	8	0	N/A	N/A
2	7	0	13	4
3	8	0	13	4
4	8	0	14	3
5	7	1	13	3

N/A = Figures not available.
Source: NA, SP28/141B, *Accounts of the Treasurers for Sick and Maimed Soldiers*, fo. 4.

25 April to 4 May 1658 show that during this short period staff sickness and pressure of work resulted in the employment of 'help-nurses' on eight different wards for the equivalent of eleven working days, while seven wards contained patients who required nightly observation.

The normal expenses of a hospital ward at this period were many and varied. Candles cost 6s a dozen and were usually bought in quantities of twenty or thirty dozen at a time. Coal was bought at £1 14s a chaldron or 5s 4d for individual sacks. Clothing was provided for the in-patients at the state's expense and the purchase of a total of two hundred and eighty shirts and thirty-five shrouds during the period December 1653 to March 1654 reflects a significant patient turnover at that time.[23] The hospital nursing staff were equally fortunate in their access to the provision of a wide range of necessary items. In January 1654 a hospital labourer, 'Old Dundee', was provided with a pair of spectacles, a surgeon provided Nurse Horne with two stockings on 12 April, two weeks later Nurse Wild was granted 2s 6d to buy shoes, probably for medical reasons as another account entry recorded that a patient received shoes made to the doctor's own design.[24] With regard to another important aspect of patient care, the laundering of clothes and bedding, whereas these articles were washed by ward sisters in civilian hospitals, this does not appear to have been the case in military hospitals where the nurses seem to have been accorded a higher social status, and washerwomen were specifically employed.

It is also evident that military nurses were afforded some individual responsibilities involving expense, planning, and representing the needs of their patients.[25] A degree of authority was granted them to make general

Table 5.3

Nurse Bedwyn's bill for expenses, 28 April 1654.

Item	Cost
One kettle	8s.
One small kettle	3s.
One plain skillet	3s.
One small skillet	2s.
One small iron pot	2s.
Two washing tubs	3s.
Two iron candlesticks	8d.
For mending kettles	1s 2d.
Exchanging kettles and skillets	8s.
Total	£1 10s 10d.

Source: NA, SP24. n.f.

incidental purchases for the better running of their wards, especially for the repair or renewal of cooking equipment. The items purchased by Nurse Bedwyn on 28 April 1654 is typical of one nurse's routine expenses, shown in Table 5.3.

The total amount reimbursed to the nurses of Ely House for incidental expenses during 1654 amounted to £24 2s 2d, with the monthly payment varying between £2 10s and £3 10s. Table 5.4, overleaf, provides a list of typical payments made to nurses at the Savoy in a typical week, that of 16–23 June 1654.[26]

Treatments

Quackery and charlatanism were prevalent in contemporary health care provision and it was extremely difficult for the layperson to distinguish good from bad advice. Many publications that purported to offer advice and recipes for self-administered cures commonly included 'cures' that appear extremely unpleasant, even loathsome, to modern readers. Such odious products continued to feature in popular lay medical books until the late-eighteenth century, despite the fraud involved in many of the examples. This was probably due to their ability to shock or titillate rather than any inherent efficacy they might offer and the practice of exploiting the gullible public continued even into the twentieth century when country fairs frequently brought the travelling quack selling noxious patent 'miracle cures'. Unfortunately, the tendency of some writers to concentrate on the more

Table 5.4

Payments to the nurses of the Savoy Hospital in reimbursement of expenses,
23 June 1654.

Nurse	Payment
Nurse Blessingham	11d.
Nurse Cole	1s 3d.
Nurse Cooke	10d.
Nurse Davis	1s 4d.
Nurse Gibbs	1s 6d.
Nurse Godolphin	1s.
Nurse Hastings	1s 4d.
Nurse Jackson	1s 3d.
Nurse Palmer	10d.
Nurse Tims	9d.
Nurse Titmus	1s 2d.
Total	12s 2d.

Source: NA, SP Dom 18, ff. 104a and 104b.

lurid side of seventeenth-century medical products has frequently obscured the considerable amount of efficacious advice and treatments recommended by more reliable texts.

Seventeenth-century military surgeons were greatly influenced by the work of the Frenchman Ambroise Paré (1510–90), who had revolutionised the treatment of battle casualties during the wars of religion in the previous century. In place of the drastic cauterisation formerly advocated, Paré's teachings substituted the application of egg-yolk, oil of roses, and turpentine to gun-powder burns with the precise application of ligatures to arrest haemorrhage. He had also developed several innovative surgical instruments and prosthetic limbs. It is distinctly probable that Thomas Trapham, senior surgeon at the Savoy, followed Paré's teachings and methods, but sadly, there is no surviving record of his operating methods. Fortunately, Richard Wiseman, a Royalist surgeon with wide personal experience of treating combat injuries in England, the West Indies, and the European theatres of war, published several notes and books intended to provide comprehensive advice to fellow surgeons.[27] From basic definitions of wounds, through signs, symptoms, and prognoses, he described every stage of treatment with particular remarks added to cover specific problems and, in the main, Wiseman followed Paré's teaching closely. Trapham was a contemporary of Wiseman and, like him, had also worked with Molins and Hollyer, two of the most eminent London surgeons of the day. It is not, therefore, unrealistic to assume that Trapham used similar operative techniques to Wiseman.

Recommended suturing techniques were straightforward whilst particular attention was paid to methods of wound dressing: the nature, type, material, and style most suitable to each case for wound closure. Bandages were made from good, strong, evenly woven white cloth, that was clean and soft without hems, seams or loose threads in widths of six inches for shoulders, five inches for thighs, four inches for lower legs, three inches for arms, and one inch for toes and fingers. Red flannel is known to have been used for bandages at the Savoy and Ely House. Very large quantities of soft tow were used with up to 3 lb being used for each surgical procedure and post-operative dressing.

Normal or light diets were prescribed to post-operative patients according to the individual's situation and requirements. Light diets were indicated for patients whose wounds were inflamed or who were weakened by blood loss. For these patients Wiseman recommended broths and jellies, but was also quick to point out that consideration should also be given to the patient's normal life-style and diet.[28] During his military service he had developed a deep understanding of his soldier and sailor patients and, despite his own life-long abstention from alcohol, his experiences had taught him to be realistic. He commented that he had often seen seamen, who drank extraordinarily and were full of drink during sea battles, who could 'scarcely be treated without an allowance of wine' and recommended that it was better to allow such men the hair of the dog rather than entirely deprive them of drink, as their chances of survival would be enhanced thereby.[29] He did, however, add what he termed 'vulnerary' drinks to their fluid intake as an aid to wound healing.[30] These included decoctions of comfrey, ladies mantle, wild tansy, vervaine, valerian and red roses, mostly made by boiling in white wine and honey.

Gunshot wounds were particularly difficult to treat as the indiscriminate path of the missile caused widespread tissue damage, and the extraneous material, such as clothing, carried into the wound by the missile resulted in multiple complications.[31] The timing of surgery after war injuries was, and remains, critical. As with late-twentieth-century practice it was deemed essential that extraction of bullets and extraneous material, followed by wound toilet, cleansing and dressing, with excision of dead tissue or amputation where necessary, should be undertaken as quickly as possible after injury, delay resulting in excessive pain for the patient thus making bullet extraction and wound surgery more difficult for the surgeon.

At variance with modern practice, after the wound had been dressed the patient was given a 'clyster' [or enema] using for preference extracts of mallow, violets, linseed oil or bay and juniper berries. If these were not available, then a readily available alternative could be made from meat broth, camomile, sugar, egg yolk, a little salt, butter or oil. In an age before the availability of intravenous infusion the treatment was potentially beneficial as the patient could thereby absorb nourishment and gain fluid replacement. Unfortunately, despite Harvey's recent description of the circulation of the blood, the recommended post-operative care also included bleeding the patient, despite their existing blood loss. According to Galen's teachings, this was believed to offer some benefit if conducted on the same side as the injury. Others advocated the use of the opposite side.[32]

During the first post-operative day the patient was kept warm, offered drinks, cordials 'to refresh the spirits', and a light diet such as barley gruel, a thin broth or a poached egg. The cordials recommended included distilled essence of lemon syrup, cinnamon, gillyflowers, roses, borage, crocus root and the herb ox-tongue or 'bugloss'. For the common soldier, a drachm of 'London treacle' or mithridate dissolved in wine was said to be an adequate prophylactic against infection, as were other tonics chosen from a comprehensive list of recommended recipes contained in Culpeper's *Physical Directory*.[33]

On the second day after operation, the patient was purged using a mixture that included cassia bark, tamarind, rhubarb and rose water taken in whey or a 'ptisan'.[34] The wound was usually inspected daily, with suitable poultices applied dependant on the appearance of the wound and the amount of pain experienced, until the seventh or ninth day after surgery. Successful progress was judged by the satisfactory separation of a wound slough and the presence of 'laudable pus', an almost universal sequel to surgery prior to the development of modern antibiotics.

Whilst the surgeons held sway at the Savoy, the physicians were pre-eminent at Ely House where they treated a wide variety of conditions including infective, systemic, and psychiatric disorders.[35] The opening of a ward known as the hot-house was a novel experience for the soldier–patients and was probably inspired by the work of Peter Chamberlen, a physician of some influence who, in 30 September 1648, was granted sole right:

> [T]o make artificial baths and bath stoves with their appurtenances of cisterns, waterworks, engines, hammock beds, hammock sleds, hammock chairs, hammock couches (for the safe and easy sitting, lying or conveying of weak and sickly persons)...[36]

He could then install them in public baths within any city and town of England or Wales, for a period of fourteen years. The 'sweating treatment' was used particularly for those suffering from venereal infections and there appears to have been a refreshingly non-judgmental approach to the needs of these patients.[37] Similar facilities existed in St Thomas's Hospital where two wards, then known as the 'Sweating Wards' were established, one for male patients and the other for females, for the treatment of syphilis.[38] These wards were kept so busy that, on 8 February 1647, the sisters in charge were instructed to notify the hospital officers of the number of available beds prior to the Monday morning admission session.[39] At Ely House, two male nurses supervised the soldiers who sat or reclined in cubicles whilst smoking from issued clay pipes, and wearing special caps and heavy baize coats in the atmosphere of a Turkish bath created by a copper bath stove from which heat was channelled to each cubicle. No expense was spared in running this facility – in one week alone one hundred and ten sheets and many towels were sent for laundering – and, on Sunday 26 June 1654, a dozen linen drawers were purchased at a cost of £1 16s together with three long coats at £1 12s for use in this department. Other regular provisions for the hot-house included the liberal supply of claret wine and sugar.

The drugs and medicaments used on the wards were dispensed for both military hospitals from a central pharmacy at Ely House where the patients of physician, Dr Barksdale, were located and where the apothecaries, Mr Leadbetter and, latterly, Mr William Day, conducted their business. At the Savoy, where the patients were mostly surgical cases, Mr Kirk Bond was employed to dispense drugs previously made up by the apothecaries at Ely House. Unfortunately the specific ingredients used by Leadbetter, Day and their colleagues have been deliberately obscured as a protective measure against revealing their 'mysteries'.[40] In their bills, items were listed under basic generic terms, such as 'a cordial' or 'a purging potion', just as, until recently, modern pharmacists labelled pill boxes and bottles as 'the tablets' or 'the tonic' rather than specify the product's correct pharmaceutical name. A typical apothecary's bill for items supplied for the use of patients in the Savoy Hospital, such as that for the month of October 1644, included various medicines in the form of pills, cordials and juleps, diet drinks, purging potions, pectoral syrups, liquorice juice, powders, sweating potions, emetics, ointments, gargles, and for the surgeons, cataplasms, fomentations, styptics and precipitators.

The most expensive single item recorded in the hospital accounts was the provision of spa water treatment. Mineral water had been noted and held in high regard for its curative properties since Roman times, especially from the source and hot springs at Bath in Somerset. As early as August 1645 the treasurers paid £4 5s for soldiers to travel to Bath for treatment and significant groups of sick soldiers also visited the city at public expense during 1647 and 1648. However, after Dr John French became the senior physician at Ely House in 1649, his enthusiasm for using mineral waters in the treatment of a wide variety of conditions led to the organised visits to

Table 5.5

Annual payments for soldiers to go to Bath for treatment.

Year	Amount
1647	£103 13s.
1648	£44
1649	£452 2s.
1650	£430 10s.
1651	£517
Total	£1,547 5s.

Source: NA, SP 28/141A, ff. 2 and 5 after 410 and SP 28/141B, pt 3.

Bath by patients from the Savoy and Ely House becoming an annual event.[41] Between 1647 and 1651 the treasurers spent over £1,500 in providing spa treatment to soldier patients.[42] The annual costs of these visits are tabulated in Table 5.5.

Despite increasing financial stringency these annual spa trips continued and even increased following a re-organisation of the military hospital administration in 1653. In 27 May 1653 – only one week after announcing the establishment of a committee to investigate and audit the affairs of the Committee for Sick and Maimed Soldiers – the Council of State approved an allocation from the excise to enable two hundred and twenty soldiers, accompanied by a surgeon, a physician, and an apothecary of Ely House, to travel to Bath to assist their recovery and effect their cure. A bill for £400 was drawn by the Overseer of the Savoy, Richard Malbon, who travelled in charge of the party.[43] The costs involved in the undertaking were to rise dramatically above the figure originally intended and appear quite exceptional. Approximately £1,600 was made available for the venture, an extraordinary sum even though part was arranged as letters of credit.[44] Why was Parliament prepared to commit such a huge sum of money to such an undertaking? Any response to this question can only be speculative. Altruism and the desire to provide the most up-to-date treatment available are considerations but, in terms of hard cash, a reduction in overall expenditure would, inevitably, have resulted from a rapid cure in Bath compared with expensive on-going in-patient care at the Savoy or Ely House.[45]

Whatever the motivation behind such expeditions, the soldier patients appear to have been remarkably well-behaved and appreciative of the care they received. In 1650, when the city was visited by six wagon-loads of sick and wounded soldiers seeking treatment, a Member of Parliament who lived nearby wrote to Richard Malbon, the Savoy Overseer in charge of the party, to compliment the visitors on their behaviour and enclosed £20 for the soldiers' use. In glowing terms he also expressed approval of Parliament's concern for the soldiers' well-being in arranging their journey and accommodation:

> It has been a fault condemned in many states and persons, for casting off their faithful servants without reward or regard, when those servants have been dis-enabled to do them any more service, but it is not so with you, or the persons under your charge, who have cause to bless God, and thank those that have taken more care of them. I had this day intelligence from some that came to my house from the City of Bath, that there came last week to that City, four wagons loaded with sick and maimed soldiers, where they were to abide one month in expectation of some comfort and relief by those waters, (which I pray God send them), that the men were frugal and careful in their expenses, civil and pious in their deportment, and that they had good allowance from the Parliament to maintain them whilst they made use of the Bath.... I have sent them by my servant a token of my love, the sum of twenty pounds, which I pray you to distribute equally amongst them, for though I am informed their allowance is very good which the Parliament have appointed and provided for them, yet I know well that sickness and lameness cannot be attended and accommodated with an ordinary expense, and if, before they go off, you shall inform me that either some or all of them shall need a further assistance, I shall most readily supply them with the like sum.[46]

This extraordinary unsolicited letter encapsulates the hopes, aspirations, concepts, and inherent belief in fellow man that the Commonwealth aspired to. It cannot be bettered as evidence of the desire to care for those wounded in the state's service.

Quality of care

We may now pose the question 'Is it possible to assess the quality, availability and effectiveness of the nursing care provided in these establishments in the light of surviving evidence?' On the one hand, it may seem presumptuous to attempt to define acceptable standards for mid-seventeenth-century nursing practice and make comparisons with those of the late-twentieth century, and yet many aspects of nursing practice have remained constant over the centuries.

Contemporary nursing inherited certain attitudes, traditions and regulations from earlier, medieval practice, notably Christ's 'Parable of the

Talents' which formed the basis of the six Christian prerequisites for salvation, also known as the six 'Comfortable or Corporal Works of Mercy'.[47]

> For I was an hungred, and ye gave me meat:
> I was thirsty, and ye gave me drink:
> I was a stranger, and ye took me in:
> Naked, and ye clothed me:
> I was sick, and ye visited me:
> I was in prison and ye came unto me.
>   Matthew 25:35–6.

Post-Dissolution Protestants could inherit and accept these principles without difficulty and later added a seventh requirement, that of giving Christian burial to the dead.[48] These tenets were clearly listed in the original 1515 statutes for the Savoy Hospital and it would not be unreasonable to suggest that the same standards were inherited by the nursing sisters who remained in the hospital in 1642.[49] Equally, there was a continuing adherence to the fundamental principles underlying the six 'non-naturals' incorporated in the *Regime Sanitatis* which emphasised the need to control patients' environment, rest and exercise, evacuation and repletion, diet, sleep, and state of mind.

During recent years, a variety of authors have devised a selection of 'models of nursing' that offer guidelines for determining appropriate nursing practice. In searching for a suitable model that could be adapted to provide a crude, yet valid, assessment of the quality and quantity of nursing care in mid-seventeenth-century military hospitals, I settled upon the Roper, Tierney and Logan model. This tool, which assesses patients' ability to cope with twelve everyday functions known collectively as 'The Activities of Daily Living',[50] seemed the most appropriate, and is summarised in Table 5.6. The model bears obvious close comparison with both the *Comfortable Works* and the *Regime Sanitatis*:

The 'Activities of Daily Living' may also be used to determine the amount of nursing intervention required to assist a patient to fulfil each of these twelve functions. If the nursing skills and facilities provided in the mid seventeenth-century military hospitals are assessed regarding their ability to encompass these functions, it may be possible to arrive at an overall judgement regarding the quality of care provided.

As regards the first of our activities, 'maintenance of a safe environment', attention was certainly paid to the security of the building with the doors being locked at night and a gate guard on duty during the day. On entering either the Savoy or Ely House, the new patient would have found himself comfortably housed in clean surroundings albeit aware of the all-pervading

Table 5.6

'The Activities of Daily Living.'

| Maintenance of a safe environment |
| Mobilisation |
| Communication |
| Breathing |
| Eating and drinking |
| Elimination |
| Personal cleaning and dressing |
| Controlling body temperature |
| Working and playing |
| Expressing sexuality |
| Sleeping |
| Dying |

Source: N. Roper, W.W. Tierney, A.J. Logan, *The Elements of Nursing* (2nd edition, Edinburgh: Churchill Livingstone, 1985), *passim.*

aroma from the burning pitch used to fumigate the wards. He would have been allocated one of the heavy wooden beds that were set around the walls of the wards, each one sprung with cord lacing stretched across the frame and provided with a flock mattress, feather bolsters and pillows, blankets and sheets. Curtains were fitted to the beds, the ward windows were curtained, and screens were available for privacy. Rugs were laid on the floor, mobile patients had chairs and settles to sit on, and benches were set around the dining tables.[51] Hospital appointments and surroundings received regular maintenance and account entries indicate that cleanliness was regarded as a highly important factor in hospital routine. Bed frames were regularly painted with lime-based whitewash, which has mild disinfectant properties, but, when a ward was to be thoroughly cleaned, all the beds and fittings were removed to another area and replaced afterwards. On 26 June 1654, workmen were paid 4s 6d for moving beds from one ward to another and incidental charges, varying from 1s to 2s, were levied for the first cleaning of new areas when additional beds were brought into use. On 29 May, at significant cost, fifty-eight beds were moved out of the Savoy's Long Ward, twenty from Reading Ward and twenty-four from Chapel Ward for airing and re-cording prior to being returned. As the bedsteads were large wooden four-poster structures with curtains and valances that were removed for cleaning, this was a considerable undertaking and attracted significant costs. The safety of individual patients endangered by virtue of their illness, such as epileptic and 'disturbed' patients who required extra attention, was

Table 5.7

William Bradley's carpentry bill, 21 June 1654.

Item	Cost
A pin and straps for William Jones	**1s 6d.**
A pin for Anthony Bacon and another with an iron swivel	2s 1d.
A wooden leg and materials for Thomas Harrison	10s.
A wooden leg and materials for Joe Wilson	10s.
Two pins for Sergeant Courts	1s.
Two pins with six straps for Henry Williams	2s 6d.
Total	£1 7s 1d.

Source: NA, SP/29/104A, n.f.

supervised by 'watchers' hired for the purpose who could summon medical or nursing assistance if required during the dark hours.

In fulfilling the requirements of our second standard, assisting 'mobilisation', requisite treatments, both medical and surgical, were provided, wounds were appropriately dressed, and during a patient's recovery mobilisation was assisted in a variety of ways, including the provision of a rope hoists to assist patients re-positioning themselves in bed.[52] Many of the patients were confined to bed for prolonged periods and for them the essential nursing task of preventing the occurrence of 'bed sores' was well appreciated. In the words of Brugis, written in 1651, it was essential to enable the patient to 'air his back and hips lest they excoriate with too much lying'.[53] Assistance with mobilisation was particularly relevant for those who had lost limbs, for whom prosthetic appliances were supplied and fitted. Ely House became a centre for the supply of these items to both in-patients and out-pensioners, including maintenance and after-care services.

The high incidence of amputations carried out in the surgical treatment of battle casualties was reflected in both the resources and relatively sophisticated equipment provided for the comfort and care of patients who had suffered the loss of limbs.[54] Such cases were nursed under bed cradles supplied by the hospital carpenter whilst their wounds were dressed with red dyed cotton and linen bandages which were frequently washed and re-used. Crutches were supplied in various lengths. For example, in January 1653, an order was placed for 144 crutches, 72 long and 72 short, at a total cost of £5 2s. Wooden splints provided support for fractures whilst hernia cases were fitted with straw-filled trusses. On 20 March 1653, John Fife, a patient on Nurse Godolphin's ward, received a truss valued at 3s. The work of

William Bradley, the hospital carpenter, who was frequently required to provide wooden legs and the associated attachments for them, is illustrated in the bills that he submitted for his work. On 15 May 1654, he charged £2 9s for supplying a pair of legs with straps and buckles for Thomas Swaine, adjusting the wooden legs of seven residents and for supplying two pins for a wooden leg.[55] His bill of 21 June 1654 is summarised in Table 5.7.

This service continued after the patients were discharged from hospital and the resources of the hospital carpenter remained available to those outpatients who required continuing assistance with their prosthetic appliances such as spare parts for their false legs and arms. However, although surgeons and physicians could recommend and prescribe treatments, patients were unlikely to receive their care in a manner conducive to the improvement of their health and wellbeing without the conscientious support and intervention of a dedicated nursing staff.

The third element, 'communication', was clearly facilitated, especially the voicing of patients' grievances. On admission to hospital, soldiers remained subject to military discipline but retained the right to their weekly pension allowance of up to 4s, from which they were able to supplement their diet and purchase additional comforts such as tobacco and extra beer. Unfortunately, in the later years of the Protectorate, pension payments became infrequent and there were several instances of patients petitioning senior officers, such as Sir Thomas Fairfax, who in an age of micro-management, went directly to Parliament for action. As a result, many of these petitions met with recorded and effective response.

As regards the next activity, 'breathing', the frequent fumigation of wards with burning pitch would, almost certainly, have resulted in a thick, heavily laden atmosphere exacerbated by tobacco smoke and the odour of infected wounds, compounded at night by closed windows and the common contemporary belief that the miasmas that accompanied nocturnal air were unhealthy. It is most unlikely that ventilation was adequate, and although expectorants and bronchial medications, including inhalations, were frequently prescribed, the assistance offered to those with respiratory problems cannot be assessed on the surviving evidence.

'Eating and drinking', our next topic, is somewhat complex. The head nurse of each ward was responsible for food preparation for the patients in her charge but little evidence remains of the diet provided for patients in London's military hospitals. However, appropriate source material does survive in papers relating to Heriot's Hospital, Edinburgh, dating from the period of its use as a military hospital under Monck's administration, 1653 to 1659. There, each patient was provided with a pint of gruel or milk for breakfast, and on four days each week, a pint of beer, five ounces of butter, five ounces of cheese, and two pounds of bread. On the other three days the

Table 5.8

Food and calorific values in the Heriot's Hospital diet.

Element	Heriot diet	Recommended daily intake*	Surplus/ deficiency
Calcium	1217.6 mg	700.0 mg	517.6 mg +
Vitamin C	3.7 mg	40.0 mg	36.3 mg -
Iron	27.0 mg	8.7 mg	18.3 mg +
Protein	152.1 mg	55.5 mg	96.6 mg +
Kcal	4189.4 kcal	2250.0 kcal	1839.4 kcal +

*Males 19–50 years: 1990.
Source: Dietary calculations kindly provided by Mrs F. Bowen, Senior Dietician, Frimley Park Hospital.

food remained the same except that one and a quarter pounds of meat were substituted for the cheese.[56] Appropriate quantities of liquid refreshments were available, albeit in the form of ale or other alcoholic beverages which formed the normal contemporary drink in the absence of a potable water supply. Table 5.8 shows a comparison of relative food values between the Heriot's Hospital diet and modern daily recommendations.

This diet compared favourably with normal military rations. Using the garrison accounts of Great Chalfield, Wiltshire and those of Waller's army during 1643, Stuart Peachey has examined the content of average military ration issues, both in a garrison situation or on the march.[57] If Peachey's figures are tabulated alongside those of the Heriot's Hospital regime, as in Table 5.9, we can see that the soldiers' potential for recovery was disadvantaged even before their moment of injury due to their pre-existing lack of essential vitamins, particularly Vitamin C, as well as essential minerals and other dietary elements.

The hospitals' diet may have also gained hidden extras from another source. At their foundation, the grounds of both the Savoy and Ely House had contained large, well-stocked gardens for the supply of both food and medicinal herbs. These gardens were protected and maintained throughout the Civil Wars and Interregnum and there is no reason to suggest that they did not continue to provide a valuable source of fresh produce.[58] Unfortunately, food could occasionally be witheld as a punishment as George Hillyard, a soldier patient in St Thomas's Hospital, found to his cost on 30 January 1645, when, in addition to being threatened with expulsion

Table 5.9

Comparative daily values of hospital, garrison and marching solders' diets.

Item	Heriot's Hospital		Chalfield Garrison	Marching
Bread and biscuit	**2lb.**		**8 ozs.**	**10¹/₂ ozs.**
Peas and beans	**Unrecorded**		**4 ozs dried or**	**3 ozs. dried**
			pint fresh	**or 6 ozs. cooked**
Meat and dairy	**1¹/₂ lb.**		**1 lb.**	**5 ozs.**
produce	**(3 days weekly)**			
Salt	**Unrecorded**		**Unrestricted**	**1 oz.**
Beer	**1 pint**		**2¹/₂ pints**	**¹/₂ pint**
Oatmeal				
(Gruel ± milk)	**1 pint**		**¹/₂ lb.**	**Nil**
Cheese	**5 ozs.**		**2 ozs.**	**Nil**
	(4 days weekly)			
Butter	**5 ozs.**		**Unrecorded**	**Nil**
Fish	**Unrecorded**		**Unrecorded**	**Nil**

Source: NA, SP 28/128, pt. 28, fo. 26; S. Peachey, *Civil War and Salt Fish*, (Leigh on Sea: Partizan, 1988), 7; J.H.P. Pafford, *Accounts of the Parliamentary Garrison of Great Chalfield and Malmesbury, 1645–6* (Devizes: Wilts. Archaeological Society, 1966).

from the hospital for bad behaviour, he was also deprived of his rations for a day on account of his 'surliness'.[59]

'Elimination of bodily waste' was assisted by various laxatives and diuretics prescribed when deemed necessary and a variety of contemporary medical texts show that the importance of maintaining normal bodily functions during periods of bed-rest was well appreciated. The bed-ridden were provided with pewter chamber pots stored in bedside 'close stools' [commodes] and supplied with tow for hygiene purposes. At the Savoy, Goody Swayne was paid 2s weekly to empty the close stools every morning and evening and, presumably, similar offices would have been performed at Ely House. As regards 'personal cleaning and dressing', it was part of each nurses' specific responsibility to ensure that their patients were kept 'clean and sweet smelling'. Weekly laundry lists were compiled by the head nurse of each ward sub-division in both the Savoy Hospital and Ely House and documents covering the year September 1653 to September 1654 clearly demonstrate that in both military hospitals the patients' sheets were laundered weekly along with at least two changes of underwear per week. A summaries of laundry costs is given in Table 5.10, overleaf.

Table 5.10

Summary of Savoy Hospital and Ely House laundry bills,
September 1653 to September 1654.

Item	Savoy		Ely House	
	Total	Weekly average	Total	Weekly average
Sheets	3,864 pairs	92 pairs	3,937 pairs	94 pairs
Underware and Towels				
	9,899 pairs	236 pairs	9,578 pairs	228 pairs
Bedding	328	8	604	14
Cost	£105	£2 7s.	£98	£2 3s. 8d.

Source: NA, SP 28/140A, n.f.

The 'maintenance of ambient and body temperature' was a prominent feature in most treatment regimes. Warming pans heated the patients' beds in winter; coal fires routinely heated the open wards, fed by a man employed specifically to bring coals from the cellar to the wards. When assessing the inclusion of temperature control and its role in the treatment of disease, the use of heat treatment, as previously mentioned, should also be considered.

'Facilitating work and play' is a difficult area to assess. Mobile patients were given general maintenance tasks during the day and some were paid to watch over other patients at night. They could also relax in the spacious, fragrant gardens available in the grounds of both hospitals. As an amusing aside, a pet fox was officially maintained at Ely House for some eighteen months, fed by payments out of hospital funds, possibly as a form of pleasurable relaxation for the patients.

It is an even more complex task to assess the support for enabling patients to express their sexuality. As this function includes the provision of help in shaving and personal grooming it is possible to confirm a positive approach to the task. However, the wider aspects of sexuality were actively repressed throughout contemporary society. In both military and civilian hospitals, marriage between patients and nurses was expressly forbidden because it was regarded as likely evidence of over-familiarity between the sexes and a threat to both discipline and public morality. Such marriages were penalised by immediate expulsion of both parties.[60] The army was at the forefront of a drive to reform social practices that offended puritan morés such as stage plays, morris dancing, cock fighting, bear baiting and all forms of lewdness.[61] The perception of an omnipresent, chastising God led to specific legislation to suppress overt sexuality, especially in public institutions.

Religious observance was mandatory and worship figured largely in the patients' daily lives. In common with earlier medieval practice, patients and staff were expected to attend church and Bible reading on a regular basis. More specifically, the first two paragraphs of the hospital rules stipulated that every soldier who was able was to attend church twice every Sunday and a bible reading twice a day. Failure to attend church at least once on Sunday, without good reason, resulted in the loss of the following week's 4s pension and, for each unauthorised absence from the daily bible readings, a 2s forfeit was imposed. Two ministers, Mr Jessey and Mr Barker, were attached to the hospitals to provide spiritual support, each drawing annual salaries of £20. Religious books were liberally distributed throughout the wards with each patient being supplied with a Bible and spiritual texts. In one purchase, on 23 March 1654, fourteen copies each of the Bible, Apocrypha and John Arnold's book of sermons were purchased at a cost of £4 4s.[62]

If we now progress to examine the next characteristic, 'sleeping', we can assume that this was assisted by the comfortable beds with which the patients were provided. When necessary, sleeping draughts were prescribed and, if undue noise was produced during the hours of darkness, offenders were liable to punishment.

As the great majority of contemporary deaths took place at home, death and dying were familiar concepts, viewed as natural and expected events.[63] Despite the Protestant repudiation of the concept of purgatory, ample evidence survives to demonstrate that, except in the aftermath of battle, soldiers expected and normally received a formal religious burial.[64] Ministers provided spiritual support for the dying, the dead were treated with reverence and respect and legislation was introduced which required the presence of representatives from dead soldiers' regiments at military funerals. The usual practice was to bury the dead in shrouds, and whilst coffins were provided for cadavers dissected post-mortem, the more usual absence of coffins for soldiers' burials was unremarkable as these were deemed an expensive luxury.[65] On a lighter note, it was routine in the military hospitals to invariably provide alcoholic drinks for the deceased's fellow patients after the funeral.[66]

So, although an accurate overall 'quality assessment' as required in a modern hospital cannot be compiled from the limited extant evidence, it is possible to draw significant conclusions from this comparative exercise. Sufficient material evidence remains to suggest that the nursing staff of the Savoy and Ely House military hospitals provided a significantly greater contribution to the work of caring for their soldier–patients than has previously been credited to them. After the Restoration, at a stroke, the care and welfare innovations and improvements introduced during the Wars and Interregnum were swept away. Subsequently, despite the foundation of Royal Hospitals at Kilmainham and Chelsea roughly twenty years later, the perceived status of the nurse in society fell to a very low level. Did two hundred years pass before these workers regained the status and standards of care comparable to those provided in the Parliamentary military hospitals? When writing about the eighteenth-century British Army, Kopperman commented that:

> [Q]uality nurses were probably the exception but those women who served as nurses for extended periods achieved a level of competence that won them the respect of medical men... the patients who were treated by them were lucky indeed, for through knowledge of their duty and conscientious devotion to it these women helped to save many a life.[67]

To paraphrase Rawcliffe, 'although they rarely obtained much in the way of recognition at the time, matrons, sisters, housekeepers and maids have been woefully neglected by historians ever since'.[68] The misconception that nursing Civil War casualties was restricted to the haphazard efforts of camp followers and members of the lowest levels of society ignores a significant body of responsible women and men committed to comforting and caring for their fellows in a manner no less dedicated than that of their modern professional counterparts.

Notes

1. L.R. Seymer, *A General History of Nursing* (London: Faber and Faber, 1954), *passim.*
2. L. Granshaw, 'The Rise of the Modern Hospital in Britain', in A. Wear (ed.), *Medicine in Society* (Cambridge: Cambridge University Press 1992), 209–10.
3. B.C. Hacker, 'Women and Military Institutions in Early Modern Europe: A Reconnaissance', *Signs: Journal of Women in Culture and Society*, vi (1981), 643–71.
4. M.A. Nutting and L.L. Dock, *History of Nursing*, 4 vols, (New York: Putnam's, 1907–12) Vol. 1, *passim*; A. Clark, *Working Life of Women in the Seventeenth-Century* (1919, reprinted London: Routledge and Kegan Paul, 1982), 243–4.
5. M. Pelling, 'Nurses and Nursekeepers: Problems of Identification in the Early Modern Period', in *The Common Lot* (London: Longman, 1998), 179–202.
6. N. Culpeper, *A Physical Directory* (London, 1649) iv–v.
7. Professor C. Carlton has attempted to calculate overall casualty figures for

the opposing armies in England during the years 1642–51. His calculations arrived at the figures of 33,445 Parliamentarians and 41,536 Royalists. The statements made here are based on Carlton's estimates, nevertheless it should be remarked that he qualified them as 'underestimates' and 'inspired guesses': C. Carlton, *Going to the Wars* (London: Routledge, 1992), 203–199; P.J. Haythornthwaite, *The World War I Source Book* (London: Arms and Armour, 1992), 54; J. Ellis, *The World War II Databook* (London: Aurum, 1993), 253.

8. G. Bernard (ed.), 'Life of Sir John Digby' in *Camden Miscellany*, xviii (London: Royal Historical Society, 1910), 67–119; C. Hill and E. Del, *The Good Old Cause* (London: Cass, 1969), 243.

9. F. Nightingale, *Notes on Nursing* [1859] (reprinted, Edinburgh: Churchill Livingstone, 1980), 1–2.

10. *Journal of the House of Commons*, (1643–60) [hereafter *JHC*] ii, 874.

11. Although the title 'Sister' was universal within the civilian hospitals, this is the only known instance of its use in connection with the military hospitals. The term was probably only employed here because it was the one by which the nurses were known prior to the hospital's conversion to a military facility: The National Archives [hereafter NA] SP28/141A, pt. 5, ff. 2, 24, 130, 134 and 401.

12. NA, S.P. Dom 28, Piece 104A.

13. *JHC*, iii, 691.

14. *Ibid.*, 638.

15. Archive & Local History Centre, Hammersmith, Ref. PAF/1/22 St Paul's, *Hammersmith Parish Register*, 41v.

16. The author is grateful to Ms A. Wheeldon, Archivist, Hammersmith & Fulham Local History Centre for drawing his attention to this material: A. Sproule, *Lost Houses of Britain* (Newton Abbot: David & Charles, 1982) 63; L. Hasker, *The Place Which Is Called Fulanham* (London: Fulham & Hammersmith Historical Society, 1981) 32. Unfortunately, both Sproule and Hasker fail to quote their sources.

17. *JHC*, ii , 912.

18. *Ibid.*, v, 30.

19. F.G. Parsons, *The History of St. Thomas's Hospital* , 2 vols, (London: Methuen and Co. Ltd., 1934), Vol. 2, 81–2.

20. NA, Exchequer Papers, S.P. Dom 16/89, pt 2, fo. 199.

21. In 1637, Monro recorded an appropriate comment on the character of soldiers' wives when he claimed that 'no women are more faithful, more charitable, more loving, more obedient or more devout than soldiers' wives as daily experiences doth witness': R. Monro, *Monro – His Expedition with the Worthy Scots Regiment (called MacKeyes Regiment) Levied in August 1626* (London, 1637) pt ii, 27.

22. This arrangement poses remarkable similarities to the modern 'named nurse' concept as defined in the 1991 'Patient's Charter'; Department of Health, Publication Ref, F82/005 1687IP 3.25m, *The Patients' Charter*, 2nd Edition (January 1995).

23. The purchase of these items was probably related to the large numbers of casualties landed along the east coast after the battle of the Texel fought 31 July 1653, some of whom were later transferred to London.

24. NA, SP 28/104, pt i. n.f.

25. In one instance a sister of the Savoy Hospital was instrumental in securing certain payments due to the hospital porter, Goodman Thompson and his wife, and in another, a man named Mr Dorne was released from prison due after similar intervention by a nurse: NA, SP28/141A, fo. 35.

26. NA, SP 18, ff. 104a and 104b.

27. Following the Restoration, Wiseman was appointed Serjeant-Surgeon to Charles II.

28. R. Wiseman, *Of Wounds, Of Gun-Shot Wounds, Of Fractures and Luxations* [1676], J. Kirkup (ed.), (Bath: Kingsmead, 1977) 346.

29. Wiseman, *ibid.*, 346.

30. '*Vulnerary* – An Agent Used to Promote Wound Healing', in *ibid.*, xli; *Dr Samuel Johnson's Dictionary of the English Language* [1834], A. Chalmers (ed.), (London: Studio Editions, 1994), 809.

31. *Ibid,* 409.

32. Wiseman, *op. cit.* (note 28), 414.

33. '*Mithridate* – a mixture of many "simples" or extracts in honey, regarded as a universal antidote against poisons and infectious diseases': Wiseman, *ibid.*, xxxvii; *Dr Samuel Johnson's Dictionary, op. cit.* (note 30), 471; Culpeper, *op. cit.* (note 6).

34 '*Ptisan* – a nourishing medical drink made of barley decocted with raisins and liquorice': *Dr Samuel Johnson's Dictionary, ibid.*, 578.

35. The Order Books of Generals Lilburne and Monck, successively Commanders-in-Chief in Scotland, provide a source of identification for the various ailments suffered by patients admitted to Ely House: Monck's Order Book, Worcester College Library, Oxford, Clarke Mss. fo. 46; NA, SP 28/140A, pt ii, ff. 148 and 171–5.

36. *Historic Manuscript Commission* [hereafter *HMC*] pt. 1, sec i, 230a.

37. This enlightened attitude differs dramatically from that adopted in contemporary France where the nursing communities at the Hotels Dieu, run by the Daughters of Charity, a nursing order of nuns founded in 1633 by Vincent de Paul, barred the admission of syphilitics and patients suffering from other infectious diseases: R. Porter, *The Greatest Benefit to Mankind* (London: HarperCollins, 1997), 240.

38. London Metropolitan Archives [hereafter LMA] Ref H1/ST/A1-5, St

Thomas's Hospital General Court of Governors Minute Book (5 vols) 159.

39. LMA, Ref. H1/ST/A6/1-2, St Thomas's Hospital, *Grand Committee Minute Book* (2 vols), Vol. 1, 63.

40. Fortunately an inventory, compiled in 1657 for the purchase of the stock and equipment for Ely House from Mrs Mary Bateman, the widow of a recently deceased apothecary, survives to illustrate the nature of their department: NA, SP28/140A, n.f.

41. French's influential book which described the beneficial qualities of the natural springs at Knaresborough gave widespread publicity to his water treatment theories: J. French, *The Yorkshire Spaw* (London, 1652).

42. NA, SP 28/141B, pt 3.

43. *Cal. S.P. Dom.1652–3,* 320, 341 and 355; British Library [hereafter BL], Thomason Tracts, E. 605 (1); T. Venner, *The Baths of Bathe* (1650) 1; P. Holland, *Camden's Britannia* (London, 1637) 236 quoted in J. Wroughton, *A Community at War: The Civil War in Bath and North Somerset 1642–1650* (Bath: Lansdown Press, 1992), 36.

44. *Cal. S.P. Dom 1652–3,* 320,332,341 and 355.

45. Bath Record Office, *The Survey of Bath* (Bath, 1641); Wroughton, *op. cit.* (note 43), 36.

46. BL, E.534, *A Perfect Diurnal, 20–27 May 1650,* 5.

47. I am grateful to Dr Carole Rawcliffe of the University of East Anglia for her illuminating work on medieval nursing practices and for directing my attention to this source: C. Rawcliffe, *Medicine and Society in Later Medieval England* (Stroud: Alan Sutton, 1995) 194–215; *idem,* 'Hospital Nurses and their Work' in R. Britnell (ed.) *Daily Life in the Late Middle Ages* (Stroud: Sutton, 1998), 43–64.

48. Rawcliffe, 'Hospital Nurses and their Work', *ibid.,* 44–5.

49. BL Cottonian MS Cleopatra CV, *Statutes of the Savoy Hospital,* 1524, ff. 30–4.

50. N. Roper, W.W. Tierney, A.J. Logan, *The Elements of Nursing,* 2nd edn (Edinburgh: Churchill Livingstone, 1985), 5 *et. seq;* M. Walsh, *Models in Clinical Nursing* (London: Bailliere Tindall, 1991), 53–89.

51. NA, SP 28/140A , n.f., and 140B, ff. 1–5; S.P.28/141A, n.f.; J.J. Keevil, *Medicine and the Navy, 1200–1900, Volume 2* (London: E. & S. Livingstone, 1958), 24–5.

52. T. Brugis, *Vade Mecum, or a Companion for a Chyrurgion* (London, 1651) 176.

53. *Ibid,* 176.

54. NA, SP 28/140A, pt 1, f. 184 and pt 4, fo. 103.

55. *Ibid.*

56. At Heriot's Hospital, where two fires were allowed for cooking – one for roasting and another for boiling, the nurses were not responsible for

preparing the patients' food. Instead, a staff cook and an assistant cook were
employed: J. Thurloe, *Collection of State Papers,* 7 vols (London, 1742) Vol.
6, 525.

57. S. Peachey, *Civil War and Salt Fish* (Leigh-on-Sea: Partizan, 1988), 7; J.H.P.
Pafford, *Accounts of the Parliamentary Garrison of Great Chalfield and
Malmesbury, 1645–6* (Devizes: Wiltshire Archaeological Society, 1966); NA,
SP28/128, pt 28, fo. 26.

58. The state of maintenance of the Savoy's gardens is not known but at Ely
House Parliament had issued specific instructions for the gardens to be
protected and maintained: *JHC,* ii, 912.

59. LMA, Ref. H1/ST/A6/1, *op. cit* (note 39), i., ff. 36.

60. *Ibid.,* i, ff. 44–98.

61. I. Gentles, *The New Model Army in England, Ireland and Scotland,
1645–1653* (Oxford: Blackwell, 1992), 110–1.

62. NA, SP 24, n.f; SP 28/141B ff. 1–5.

63. C. Gittings, *Death, Burial and the Individual in Early Modern England*
(London: Croom Helm, 1984), 8–9.

64. L. Stone, *The Family, Sex and Marriage in England, 1500–1800* (London:
Weidenfeld and Nicolson, 1977, reprinted 1990), 55–65.

65. NA, SP 28/141A, pt 2, fo. 22.

66. NA, SP 28/141A, pt 2, ff. 49 and 229.

67. P.E. Kopperman, 'Medical Services in the British Army, 1742–1783', *Journal
of the History of Medicine and Allied Sciences,* 34 (1979), 428–55.

68. C. Rawcliffe, *Medicine and Society in Later Medieval England* (Stroud: Alan
Sutton, 1995), 212.

6

Privates on Parade:
Soldiers, Medicine and the Treatment
of Inguinal Hernias in Georgian England

Philip R. Mills

Hernias were prevalent among servicemen, typically recruited from amongst the malnourished. Civilian medical practice deemed the rupture incurable, taking a palliative approach. For the military this was unacceptable: wastage rates due to ruptures were high, servicemen were valuable commodities. Examples here are used to illustrate that experimentation was a contentious activity, reliant on the whims of patronage and war-time budgets. Although military hospitals provided a good venue to engage in experimentation it was contested.

Introduction

In May 1766, 'an account of an uncommon large hernia' was published in the *Royal Society of London Philosophical Transactions*.[1] Dr George Carlisle reported brief biographical and autopsy details of ex-serviceman, John Hollowday, who had died in Carlisle of natural causes, aged approximately eighty. Hollowday joined the army as a young man and underwent 'several hardships in the Flanders campaigns under the Duke of Marlborough' during the War of Spanish Succession (1701–13). On returning to England in 1713, he noticed 'a small tumour' in the right side of his groin. Finding this of little inconvenience, Hollowday carefully concealed the hernia 'to avoid the scoffs of his companions'. The hernia increased in size, until adjudged 'unfit to serve', he was admitted as an out-pensioner of the Royal Hospital, Chelsea in 1725, whilst still in his mid-thirties.

Carlisle deemed this hernia remarkable in a number of ways - not least for its size. When Hollowday lay on the mortuary slab the hernia measured fifteen inches from top to bottom, seventeen-and-a-half inches at its widest point and thirty-four inches in circumference, see Figure 6.1 overleaf. Over a fifty-five year period, a large portion of intestines had gradually slipped through the inguinal ring on the right side of his lower abdomen, followed the path of the spermatic cord to form a mammoth scrotal hernia that buried

Figure 6.1

An uncommonly large hernia, by George Carlisle (1766).
© *The Royal Society.*

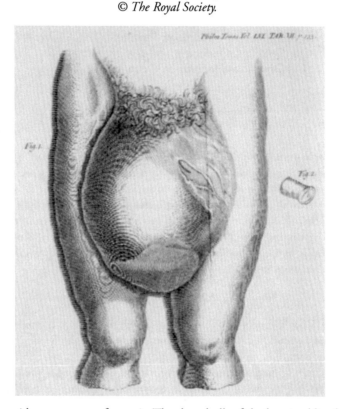

any outside appearance of a penis. The sheer bulk of the hernia obliged the pensioner to have a specially constructed bag attached to the front of his trousers, over which he always wore a leather apron to conceal the deformity. On opening the cadaver, Carlisle discovered that the liver, stomach and pancreas had enlarged and migrated to fill the area vacated by the intestines. Remarkably, apart from the occasional chafing of thigh and scrotum, the hernia caused no discomfort. Both bowel and bladder apparently functioned normally. Even in his dotage, Hollowday was described by his doctor as a stout, strong, 'well-made man', 'not subject to any other complaints than are common at his age'.

Hollowday's case was far from unique. Indeed, its very ordinariness makes it an exemplary illustration of the four major characteristics of eighteenth-century hernia treatment in Britain. First, predominately a male disorder, ruptures were seen as an unmanly ailment that questioned the virility and general health of the afflicted. No glory or cultural kudos, such as that associated in some social circles with gout,[2] could be attributed to hernia. Rather hernia was an embarrassing condition that was, as Hollowday demonstrated, preferably kept secret. Second, hernia was a disability that could be managed by the prevailing palliative procedures but not cured, and was therefore a chronic disorder. Third, Hollowday suffered from an inguinal hernia. This category formed approximately eighty-five per cent of all hernias and over ninety per cent of all male hernias and would have been familiar to the majority of medical practitioners.[3] Fourth, and perhaps most illustrative of contemporary perceptions of the distribution of hernia, Hollowday was male, poor, and a one-time soldier. Alongside labourers, medical practitioners believed that servicemen suffered the largest numbers of hernias. Although sailors were believed to be particularly vulnerable, this paper focuses on the historically neglected health and welfare of soldiers.

A comprehensive examination of British military medical provision in the eighteenth century remains to be written.[4] This is perhaps surprising, since recent historiographical developments have indicated that historians need to pay greater attention to the martial dimensions of Britain's emergence as a 'fiscal–military' state. For Linda Colley and John Brewer, forging a nation and global economic empire by force of arms was the single most significant feature of this period.[5] Both military and medical historians have recognised the importance of medicine to the conduct of warfare.[6] Michel Foucault, for example, suggested that medicine and military activity were closely related. He recognised that the military, along with the medical profession, were among the first managers of 'collective space'.[7] It is also clear from Christopher Lawrence's excellent study of hygiene in the Royal Navy that the naval context was of great significance in the development of medicine's disciplinary role.[8] Likewise, according to pioneering articles by Harold Cook and Peter Mathias, military doctors sought mass 'simple cures' and the implementation of prophylactic measures rather than the individual therapeutics favoured in private practice.[9] Thus, a thorough investigation into army medical provision would provide a useful contribution to our current historical understanding of British military structure.[10] Moreover, as Roger Cooter has submitted, historians of medicine have seldom attempted to understand military medicine in its broader social, economic and political settings, or even in its full medical contexts of the 'long eighteenth century'.[11]

This short article does not attempt to fill this void, but it is hoped that a detailed exploration of this hitherto little-studied disorder, will provide a valuable glimpse into the relationship between medicine and the British Army. Concentrating on mid-century events that culminated in the provision and maintenance of a hospital for ruptured soldiers from 1758 to

1770, I examine the role of experimentation and innovation in the treatment of hernia. The states of peace and war are also important to this story since I argue that they exacerbated the evident tension between military imperatives and medical efficacy.

Soldiers and hernia

General medical publications defined hernia as any unnatural protrusion from the lower abdomen, or, in the words of one early-eighteenth-century medical dictionary, 'a lump on the groin'.[12] The terms 'hernia' and 'rupture' were interchangeable and referred to the swelling rather than the opening through which the protrusion occurred. As a consequence, hernia types were simply distinguished by the 'Name of the Part affected'.[13] Thus, *hernia scrotalis*, for example, derived its name from the swollen scrotum associated with the disorder. The most common ruptures treated by eighteenth-century practitioners were inguinal hernias. They affected both sexes and all ages, although practitioners agreed that inguinal hernia appeared most frequently in men between the ages of twenty and forty. The reasons for this age and gender bias caused a great deal of speculation and argument amongst contemporary medical practitioners. This, in turn, created and sustained inconsistencies in medical theories and practice involving the treatment of hernia throughout the early-Georgian period.

Inguinal hernias attributed to acquired defects alone account for only a small percentage of all ruptures.[14] Straining to urinate or defecate, coughing, and heavy lifting were implicated as causative factors that led to trauma and weakening of the inguinal floor. By the mid-century, surgeon and truss-maker, Thomas Brand could state, without risk of contradiction, that actions as innocuous as: 'a sudden sneeze, a violent fit of coughing, excessive laughter, passion, loud speaking, an epileptic fit, wrestling, jumping, a severe emetic or accidental vomiting, constipation, with the difficulty of expelling indurated faeces, a blow on the part; slipping off the footpath in walking, and by so trifling an exertion as drawing the cork from a bottle [could produce hernia in men].'[15] Recent clinical research has indicated that some hernias, previously only associated with old age, could equally affect the chronically ill, smokers, and malnourished *of all ages*.[16] An association between tobacco smoking and direct inguinal hernia, in particular, has gained scientific credibility. Inhaled tobacco smoke can interfere with the formation of 'connective tissues', reducing collagen elasticity and thus reduce its resistance to rupture.[17] Although this concept was unknown to eighteenth-century practitioners, the causal effects of smoking are relevant in assessing the occurrence of hernias in soldiers, especially since it is readily accepted that Georgian troops consumed large quantities of tobacco.[18] Indeed, regimental surgeon and later founding member of the Royal

Medical Society of Edinburgh, George Cleghorn observed in the 1740s that soldiers were 'so much addicted to the use of Tobacco, as never to be without a Pipe, either in their months or in their Pockets'.[19] Thus, soldiers may well have suffered from some of the degenerative conditions associated with tobacco smoking – including hernia.

Other acquired defects included violent blows or wounding to the abdomen. Soldiers 'shot through the Belly', or kicked by horses sometimes developed hernia through a punctured abdominal wall.[20] Such acquired defects were not exclusive to the armed forces, or even to men. The origin of the 'large umbilical rupture' of Ann Edwards, for example, was attributed to domestic violence. Her husband 'gave her a kick on the belly; and from that she complained of pain, and a Swelling about the Navel, which in time increased to the size of a man's head.'[21] Within days the rupture mortified and the patient died. Besides wounds and injuries, the 'extraordinary exertion' experienced in difficult labour occasionally caused hernia. Although arduous births caused 'happily few'[22] hernias in women, manual workers, on the other hand, were not so fortunate in their labours.[23] It is important to remember, however, that the actions of extreme physical effort alone contributed to only a minute proportion of the total number of male hernias.

The vast majority of inguinal hernias are 'indirect', with congenital origins.[24] Indirect inguinal hernias have their origins in an embryonic phenomenon. The passage of spermatic vessels in men, and *ligamenta uteri* in women, during foetal development, creates the inguinal rings in the lower wings of the abdominal muscles through which, in certain circumstances, viscera can rupture. But this is only possible if any part of the *processus vaginalis* becomes trapped in the rings – a congenital abnormality that has been associated with low birth rate, malnourishment in early childhood, and pelvic deformities common amongst the eighteenth-century poor.[25] Both sexes might have these congenital weaknesses, but the 'rings' are usually much larger in men and are therefore more likely to rupture than those of women.[26]

If congenital weakness allowed indirect inguinal hernias, it was a combination of health and physical action that made them occur. Describing himself as an independent manufacturer of 'mechanical applications', with a lifetime knowledge and experience of hernias and hernia treatment, Timothy Sheldrake proposed that 'relaxed and debilitated' muscles were as much responsible for hernia as any congenital imperfection.[27] Similarly, the renowned surgeon Percivall Pott insisted that in the case of inguinal ruptures, '*the less the natural strength of the subject, the more likely will this be to happen.*'[28] Thus, groin hernias in the eighteenth century were largely viewed as a male disorder that affected specific men – the sickly, malnourished, but physically active.

Little research has been dedicated to the physical condition of service or servicemen in the eighteenth century.[29] This is due to the predominant traditional concerns of military historians with tactics, strategy and leadership rather than with the day-to-day activities of soldiering.[30] Thankfully, some historians have begun to redirect historical investigation in favour of the lower ranks.[31] In particular, investigation of recruitment has elicited some useful information about the individuals who joined the Army.[32] Disclosing ages, heights, and personnel details, recruitment records have added some welcome flesh to the otherwise intellectual dry bones of drum and trumpet history.

The underlying motive for enlistment was material. Barring few exceptions,[33] prospective soldiers were recruited from the migrant unemployed, unemployable, criminal, and vagrant sections of society.[34] As a result the armed forces were the occupation of last resort, employing the undernourished, underdeveloped, and generally unhealthy poor. Aware of this situation, successive governments attempted to counter such shortcomings with legislation. After the Impress Act of 1745, all recruits were screened prior to enlistment.[35] To aid this process, each regiment was issued with sets of recruiting instructions intended to standardise the soldier's size and physique and eliminate the sick, the deformed, and the ruptured. Article three of the recruiting instructions read:

> All Recruits are to be able Bodied, Sound in their Limbs, free from Ruptures, Scald heads, Ulcerous Sores or any Remarkable deformity, None to be Inlisted who cannot wear his hair, who is in knee'd, Splay footed, or Subject to fits.[36]

Unfortunately, despite governmental guidelines, the available recruits did not always match the desired physical requisites. On receiving a draft of new recruits in New York, 1758, General Jeffery Amherst, reported to the Secretary-at-War that he had returned twenty two men, 'on a certificate from the surgeons of the hospital' because:

> No man with a rupture can serve here, for whenever they march, or we are employed in carrying of wood, or making entrenchments in the Summer, it increases it immediately to such a degree, as to make them entirely unserviceable ever after.[37]

In the absence of any organised recruiting service or central depot system, successful enrolment depended on regimental recruitment parties. When competition for recruits was intense, especially in times of war when large numbers of men were sought over short periods of time, physical and moral standards flexed to meet the particular needs of individual regiments. In the midst of an intensive Seven Years War recruitment drive, Lieutenant-Colonel Edward Windus informed his commanding officer:

> We have many [recruits] rather too young and weak at present, but I dont think we have 20 too Old... several who were neither too Old, or too Young, were not thought fit, on Account of being Pox'd, & others having sore Legs, which are often hidden disorders for they don't Acquaint the Surgeon with these things.[38]

In wartime then, quantity took precedence over quality, and, at various times and in certain circumstances, sick, disabled, and ruptured poor entered the Army. Out of twenty-seven soldiers recorded as ruptured by one surgeon in the mid-eighteenth century, five entered the army with hernia, eighteen cases happened on active service, whilst four occurred during post-service old age.[39] But why did over two-thirds of these soldiers become ruptured in service? Could it be that these hernias were undisclosed to the authorities when recruited? Or were they openly accepted into the ranks during a manpower shortage, only to be rejected when they were no longer required? Both these suggestions are highly plausible explanations for some but not all of these hernias. Obviously, something about military service and eighteenth-century warfare contributed to this disorder.

As noted above, obesity could cause hernia, and soldiers, as some contemporaries noted with considerable derision, were all too often overweight. General Henry Hawley, for instance, reflected during a sustained period of inactivity:

> If the peace continues very long, I may see the foot of England carried in waggons from quarter to quarter, for what with their vast size and the idleness they live in, I'm sure they can't march... Take the case of a peasant. He is strong and vigorous when he leaves his village, and his arms are muscular and inured to toil. Soon he is incapable of wielding anything more than his musket. His hands become as delicate as those of a young girl, and are no longer equal to gripping a spade or a pick.[40]

Thus, due to the sporadic nature of eighteenth-century warfare – prolonged periods of peace, long winter billeting, and static garrison duties – it would appear that some soldiers became the living embodiment of an engorged Hogarthian caricature. If commentators like Hawley were to be believed, soldiers were equally susceptible to hernia with the unaccustomed strenuous exertions of a new spring campaign, as they were expected to burst their stretched waistbands with the slightest movement.

155

Poor food and chronic alcoholism further exacerbated this general infirmity.[41] The military 'seven rations' – seven pounds of bread or flour, seven pounds of beef or four of pork, six ounces of butter, three pints of peas, and a half-pound of rice or oatmeal – lacked many essential nutritional elements for a balanced diet. These basic supplies were intended to be subsidised by private purchase and locally-grown products.[42] But this was not always possible. Hostile environments and warfare often precluded these activities. Primitive storage meant that fresh food was condemned as unfit to eat long before it reached the colonies.[43] This had significant repercussions for forces serving outside Europe that were almost totally reliant upon salted and dried imports for sustenance.[44] Even forces stationed in long-established regions of the British Empire regularly faced rationing and food depravation that resulted in, amongst other things, scurvy.[45] The occurrence of scurvy had little relevance to the causes of hernia for contemporary practitioners, but recent clinical research indicates that collagen deficiency, caused by repeated bouts of scurvy, can contribute to a rare form of congenital direct inguinal hernia.[46]

As well as overfed and under-exercised, or malnourished and vitamin-deficient, soldiers were often constipated. Physician-General John Pringle noted that troops disembarking transport ships were sometimes constipated, because of 'the want of exercise on board and the diet, which consisted chiefly in cheese and sea biscuits'.[47] Regimental surgeon John Buchanan, serving with the Royal Blues during the Flanders campaigns of the 1740s, noted that 'costiveness is common amongst us, often proceeding from a natural dry habit of body; living much on salt or smoked meats, drinking too freely Spirituous Liquors.'[48] Analysing the diet of soldiers serving in Minorca, Gleghorn noted that although the soldiers had 'three or four plentiful Meals a Day, they are generally costive; and many in perfect Health, have no Occasion to ease themselves oftener than twice a Week.'[49] For Cleghorn, the proliferation of constipation on the island explained:

> [W]hy Ruptures are so common in this place; for the other Bowels being swelled beyond their natural Size, the Intestines are too much confined; and from the Nature of the [ailment], being frequently distended with Wind, it is not to be wondered at, that they often push through the Rings of the Abdominal Muscles.[50]

Coughing was another well-known cause of hernia, and soldiers were seldom free from coughs. Consumption and bronchial ailments, due to overcrowded living conditions, were virtually endemic in the camps and garrisons of the British Army.[51] It would not have been unusual to find whole regiments coughing and wheezing their way through the winter months.[52]

For experienced army physician Richard Brocklesby, the cough was the first of all soldier's ailments – common throughout the year.[53]

The combination of the day-to-day activities of campaigning[54] - marching, building roads, digging ditches, and repairing fortifications – dietary wants and disease went some way to answering the oft-heard cry: 'Why are our Armies drained, and Hospitals crowded with Soldiers deemed unserviceable by this Distemper?'.[55]

This rather dramatic lamentation has prompted at least one military historian and biographer to speculate that hernia caused 'by far the greatest wastage in the army'.[56] Since the ubiquitous fever contributed to eight out of every nine hospitalised cases, this assessment seems dubious, although it is evident that ruptures were a significant cause of manpower wastage. At least sixteen per cent of Chelsea pensioners between 1715 and 1746 were admitted with hernias.[57] The total percentage of soldiers afflicted with the disorder may have been higher. It would seem that soldiers with hernia could serve in reduced capacity. Even those soldiers who were pensioned could be call upon to serve in an emergency. In an official despatch, as Surgeon-General, John Hunter requested Regimental Surgeon Spencer Pembrook, to examine:

> Out Pensioners [of Chelsea Hospital] who have reducible Ruptures, which in your Judgement, may not incapacitate them from being useful in a Garrison, where there is neither much Marching, nor Exercise, and where proper Attention to such slight Cases can be paid, must be marked down as such.[58]

Indeed, one way or another, many soldiers continued to serve, untreated and unknown to regimental officers and surgeons, preferring, as Hollowday did, to keep the disease secret, 'least it might be the occasion of his discharge, which he dreaded and wanted to avoid'.[59]

'The most insidious disorder'

In its mildest form, a hernia restricted physical activity. Mundane everyday movements, such as sitting, standing, and walking were uncomfortable and tiring. More demanding exertions, such as running, digging, carrying, and lifting, caused excruciating pain, could enlarge the hernia, and increase the risk of strangulation and an agonising death. In all cases, hernia prevented labourers from working and incapacitated soldiers to such an extent that if discovered it could lead to dismissal. In response, orthodox practitioners managed hernias with temporary reparative treatments and the prophylactic application of a truss, rather than attempting to cure the disorder. This approach was a source of much contention. Not only was this practice unsatisfactory for patients wanting to remain employed and employers reluctant to lose experienced workers, it also attracted censure from within medicine. Exploiting both the inherent shortcomings of a practice that admitted its own limitations and the hopes of those affected, medical entrepreneurs and rupture specialists promised much more attractive 'radical cures'. They proved extremely popular, as Pott warned in his preface to his seminal *Treatise on Ruptures*:

> No disease has furnished and supported a more constant succession of pretenders than hernias.... The generality of mankind look upon a rupture as a kind of imperfection in their form, and as a disease which impairs their strength and abilities; and the more modest and bashful are fearful of leaving their disorder known from the mere situation of it... will be glad to be rid of it at almost any expense or trouble: hence the ignorant and credulous are subjected to tedious confinements, painful applications, and hazardous operations, while the timorous and bashful are cheated out of large sums of money for imaginary diseases or pretended cures.[60]

Radical intervention was intended to produce a permanent 'absolute' or 'perfect' cure. There were a number of radical cures in existence in the eighteenth century. None of them achieved universal approval and all were expensive, painful, and potentially fatal.[61] Amongst the more widely-used radical cures were those using escharotics, such as caustics or cautery, and intended to prevent hernia by sealing the inguinal rings with scar tissue. This technique caused excruciating pain, unsightly scars, and occasionally, accidental sterilisation. Even some prominent surgeons, such as Alexander Monro (Primus), advocated the liberal application of 'corrosive agents' in the course of hernia treatment.[62] As the century advanced, however, most medical practitioners viewed such treatments as crude tools of the uneducated empiric that, according to John Hunter, hardly ever succeeded.[63]

Perhaps the most extreme radical cure for hernia was castration.[64] In this procedure, the testicles were removed and the obsolete scrotal skin was used to close the openings through which hernia could enter the scrotum. The humanitarian and therapeutic value of herniary castration had been contentious for centuries.[65] In the late-sixteenth century, for example, learned surgeon, Peter Lowe, considered the castration cure to be 'a heinous sin'.[66] By the eighteenth century, castration was virtually unknown in Britain and outlawed in France.[67] Those who read Pott's 1754 treatise – and many did – were in no doubt that all herniotomies were unnecessary in most, and extremely risky in all, cases. For Pott, escharotics and incisional procedures: 'proved mischievous and inefficacious; the majority of those who have submitted to them, have remained uncured of their rupture; many have been mutilated, and some absolutely destroyed.'[68]

The only herniotomies encouraged were those reserved for emergencies. Strangulated hernias occurred when a restricted blood supply caused inflammation and mortification of the trapped contents of the hernial sac. This was a death sentence, from which the only possible reprieve was surgery. For operations on strangulated scrotal hernias the patients were first purged, bled to induce faintness, and placed 'horizontally on a table with a pillow under the shoulders and the thighs raised by assistants to slacken the parts'.[69] The surgeon placed himself between the patient's knees. Cutting the skin only, the incision ran from an inch above the abdominal ring to the bottom of the hernia. The sac was then opened in order to examine the bowels for damage and mortification. Any obstructing tendons were cut, after which the viscera could be pushed back through the enlarged opening with the finger-tips. If the patient survived the shock of surgery, he seldom recovered from the septicemia that followed. Expensive, specialised, time-intensive, and all-too-often deadly, the operation remained the treatment of last resort.[70]

The preferred everyday treatment of hernias was palliative rather than radical. Rest and diet were central tenets of any palliative programme. Patients were advised to abstain from strenuous activity and avoid 'all flatulent meats' and 'unctious [*sic*] things... such as butter and oyl'.[71] Once the patient had been stabilised by diet and relaxation, the hernia was then reduced. The protruded contents often reduced naturally when the patient lay down. When 'natural reduction' failed, patients were purged and bled as in the pre-operative routine described above. After the body became limp from loss of blood, the hernia was returned to the abdominal cavity by digital manipulation. In cases of stubborn reduction, the distinguished surgeon and then physician, William Hunter, suggested that 'making the Patient stand on his head and throw his legs over the shoulders of a strong man who may give him a shake or two sometimes answers the [problem]'.[72]

After reduction, trusses were applied in order to prevent relapse. Trusses were distinguished between the 'Elastic and Non-elastic, or trusses with or without springs'.[73] The choice of manufacturer and model was as varied as the large numbers of truss-makers in practice. At the turn of the century, patients could choose between a belt truss, 'the old serpent truss', a common truss, 'Egg's Patent truss', 'Patent Self-resisting and Adjusting German Truss, without straps', 'Cole's Trusses', 'Adam's graduated pressure truss', 'Salmon's patent self-adjusting opposite-sided truss', a pipe truss, 'Bellow's Truss', and the 'rack truss' to name but a few, see Figures 6.2 and 6.3 overleaf. Large, long-established, painless hernias that could not be reduced were supported in a 'bag truss', similar to that used by Hollowday.

Figure 6.2

*A front and back view of Salmon's double Truss and applied
for oblique inguinal hernia, by G.S. Acret, see note 73.
Courtesy: Wellcome Library, London.*

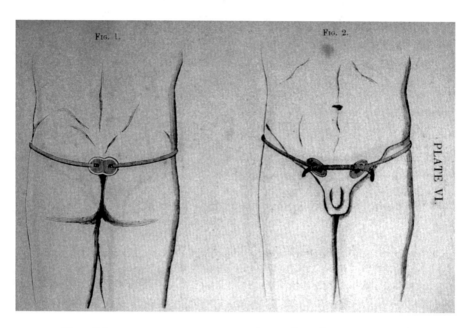

Top-of-the-range trusses were expensive and made-to-measure. They consisted of calfskin and cork cushions, held in place with supple leather straps and strengthened by a metal spring. Few labourers could afford such craftsmanship. Instead, the ruptured poor turned to a thriving second-hand market, or settled for the relatively cheap trusses made from wood, cotton and linen. The lowly and poorly paid servicemen, on the other hand, had even less choice. Trapped in the confines of the military establishment, ruptured soldiers were issued with state-supplied trusses. This was out of a sense of duty rather than charity, and always under the watchful eye of economic restraint. Varying from institution to institution and subject to contractor, military trusses were usually mass-produced fit-all ligatures. Transferring his attention to London, the famous French surgeon, George Arnaud, for instance, promised to relieve hernia sufferers with the same 'universal application' that had left the Military Hospitals of Paris with 'a store-house... filled with trusses which it was impossible to use, because they were only of three different sizes, and only contrived for one kind of

Figure 6.3

*Two figures shewing the application of the Common Truss in direct inguinal
and oblique inguinal herniae, by G.S. Acret, see note 73.
Courtesy: Wellcome Library, London.*

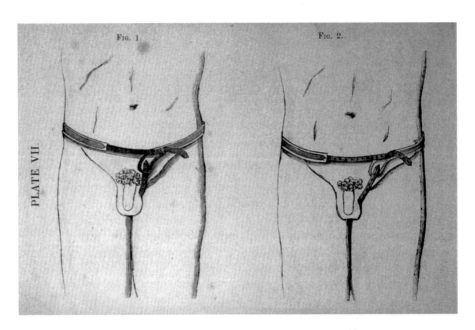

rupture'.[74] Similarly, Robert Brand supplied a 'patent universal truss' – fitting
all ages, sizes and hernias – to the Royal Hospital, Greenwich.[75] Whether
'universal' or not, there can be little doubt that military and naval trusses
were of dubious quality. Especially, when it is considered that 1366 trusses
noted by the Naval Sick and Hurt Board cost only £303 8s in 1748.[76] This
works out at 4s 5d per item, compared with 20s that some truss-makers
charged for their product.[77]

'Fit-all' trusses were far from the ideal. When Alexander Reid asserted
that patients wearing a well-fitting truss were 'enabled to do almost every
office in life equally well with a person who was never afflicted with this
disease,'[78] he was referring to the individually crafted variety seldom, if ever,
available to the poor. In contrast, and with first hand knowledge of the
practical therapeutic power of trusses supplied to the armed forces,
regimental surgeon, Robert Hamilton, assessed ruptures as:

[A] disease which will not admit of those afflicted with it to be continued in the army, as the constant exercise their duty calls on them to perform, must inevitably obviate their cure, and render them always liable to insurmountable difficulties.[79]

Showing a similar absence of faith in trusses, the Naval Sick and Hurt Board[80] was careful to note that ruptured sailors: 'shouldn't be obliged to hand or reef because the pressure they must meet with in that service would be very apt to force the intestines into the scrotum notwithstanding the Trusses'.[81] Finding trusses uncomfortable, embarrassing, and wholly inefficacious, many people opted for discrete and practical alternative solutions. Soldiers, for example, concealed ruptures behind strips of bark, or under a 'pad' of material held in place by means of tight fitting clothing, and continued service undetected.[82] The truss was therefore equally dissatisfactory to both commanding officers and soldiers alike.

Manpower and medical efficacy

There is little doubt that servicemen afforded surgeons a superb opportunity for 'experimental practice'.[83] The medical management of military personnel went far beyond that allowed elsewhere.[84] Large numbers of readily available disciplined patients made ideal subjects for controlled and prolonged medical and scientific experimentation. Far from 'the edge of utility', soldiers were increasingly acknowledged as a central source of medical exploration and innovative practice.[85] Numerous medical trials, from smallpox inoculation and venereal therapeutics, to wound management and amputation, were performed on soldiers.[86] Much of the experimentation was carried out with the absolute complicity and general encouragement of a military regime eager to reduce manpower wastage by all means available.

Manpower was one of the most valued possessions of an eighteenth-century army.[87] Numerous articles and publications have stressed the recruitment shortages and manpower problems that plagued the British armed forces throughout the eighteenth and nineteenth centuries.[88] Henry Marshall has spoken of the difficulties of recruiting, and more recently V. E. Neuberg and Linda Colley have discussed the increasingly sophisticated methods that governments employed to raise new corps throughout the eighteenth century.[89] Certainly, there is evidence to suggest that in times of hasty mass recruitment there were indeed temporary shortfalls in the army.[90] This manpower problem has usually been explained in terms of an 'inelastic labour supply schedule' created by self-imposed health and height restrictions, and the disamenities of service. However, a recent anthropometric study has challenged this traditional assumption, by suggesting that the gap between establishment and 'effectives' was rarely large – signifying, in other words, that the Army was actually able to sustain recruitment requirements.[91] But, whereas Roderick Floud, Kenneth Wachter and Annabel Gregory have emphasised the role of an unstable Georgian labour market in making 'a large fraction of the British working class' available for service, the most prized and valued personnel were experienced and trained servicemen.[92]

It was the loss of this scarce veteran manpower, crucial to the fighting efficiency of all military formations, which alarmed line officers rather than an absence of raw recruits.[93] Not only were seasoned troops hardened and disciplined in the rigours of military life, the longer they served the more cost-effective they became. As Alan Guy has so rightly pointed out, senior officers often perceived eighteenth-century soldiers as commodities.[94] The economic characteristics of the army were fundamental to a regimental organisation based on 'propriety command'. Within this commercial enterprise, proprietary ranks of captain and colonel pocketed dividends from the management of the regimental finances at their disposal, and the extent of regimental funds depended upon the number of soldiers under their command.[95] Enlisting and training raw recruits were expensive and the loss of trained soldiers was sorely felt. Thus, efficacious hernia treatments had financial incentives as well as practical martial benefits for recruitment and service longevity.

One manifestation of this determination to retain the service of experienced troops was the fervent military patronage and substantial War Office funding for two medical trials for the cure of hernias, running almost uninterrupted from 1721 to 1770. In December 1721, Thomas Renton, acting Physician-Extraordinary to George II, approached the Board of Commissioners, at the Royal Hospital, Chelsea, and offered to treat pensioners with hernia. Supported in his claim by numerous witnesses including the militarily experienced Surgeon-General and Royal Hospital surgeon, Alexander Inglis, and crucially endorsed with royal patronage, Renton was admitted as a supernumerary hospital surgeon and paid fifty pounds per annum in order to 'trial' and 'perfect his secret remedy'.[96] Although the particulars of the experimentation were not recorded, details of his 'secret remedy' became public knowledge in the course of a widely publicised scandal. Five years after beginning his experiments at Chelsea, Renton secured a knighthood, doctorate by royal decree, £5,000 bounty and £500 annual gratuity in exchange for his 'Art, Skill and Mystery in curing of Ruptures'.[97]

On publication, the 'secret' was revealed to be a simple caustic compound familiar to continental European herniotomists since the fourteenth century.[98] In a self-proclaimed 'polemic doggerel attack against Quackery in general', and Renton in particular, Robert Houston proclaimed the 'mighty Arcanum' nothing less than a financial and medical fraud. Houston wrote a two-hundred-and-fifty-page tirade, defaming Renton as an uneducated charlatan who had sold nothing more than a well-known and much mistrusted rupture 'cure' as a unique and efficacious 'secret remedy'.[99] How many ex-soldiers were treated in this way and with what success is unknown, although it was later noted that the 'method proved upon trial ineffectual'.[100] Despite damaged creditability, and tarnished reputation, Renton retained his powerful royal patronage, and with it the hospital appointment, until his death in 1740.

Ten years later another secret cure for ruptures made an appearance at Chelsea. Apprenticed son of a surgeon and member of the Corporation of Surgeons, Samuel Lee acquired notoriety as a 'rupture doctor'. As friend and associate of William Mitchell, surgeon to the prestigious Horse Guards regiment of Royal Blues, Lee gained the confidence of General John Ligonier – the then Regimental Colonel and soon to be Commander-in-Chief of the British Army.[101] Lee's acquaintance with Ligonier proved extremely important for the remainder of his military medical career. Under the patronage of Ligonier and Admiral George Anson, Lee acquired the right to 'trial' his cure at both Chelsea and Greenwich hospitals.[102]

Unlike Renton's experimentation of thirty years earlier, the early-1750s trials were intended to validate rather than facilitate the cure. In effect, the function of 'trial' had changed from one of experiment to one of assessment. Wary of secret remedies and under the guidance of the hospital medical staff, both sets of hospital commissioners ordered Lee to provide evidence of cure before he could be appointed. The negotiation for the appropriate measures of proving the efficacy of a 'secret remedy', became the focus of a bitter and drawn-out dispute. What originated as a simple request for 'ocular proofs', concluded in several public court cases and the controversial dismissal of Lee. At its height, some of the most prestigious surgeons and physicians in England were drawn into the heart of a controversy. The medical authority of such notable figures as William Cheselden, William and John Hunter, Percivall Pott, and Caesar Hawkins was marshalled behind the first Master of the newly formed Company of Surgeons, Serjeant-Surgeon, Master Surgeon to the Royal Hospital at Chelsea and chief protagonist, John Ranby. Ranby insisted that Lee subject his 'secret remedy' to methodical and public testing that would disclose, as a 'matter of fact', whether it was an efficacious cure for hernia, or merely another fraudulent claim. Lee, on the other hand preferred to hide his 'secret remedy' behind patient testimony and the affidavits of the social élite, and the inherent credibility he possessed as a gentleman.[103] But this is another story.[104] What is important, for the purposes of this paper, is the significant role servicemen and pensioners played in these medical trials.

The Board selected ten of the thirty-six ruptured Chelsea in-pensioners for the medical trials.[105] Lee isolated his patients in a separate ward and jealously guarded them from the attentions of the hospital surgeons. This was necessary, in the opinion of Lee, to prevent accidental, or intentional, exposure of his much-valued secret. After six weeks, Lee presented the complimentary affidavits of four 'cured' pensioners to the board. When Ranby challenged the validity of such evidence, Lee retorted with the disingenuous remark that it was 'no contradiction to suppose, that – The *Oath* of a *poor Pensioner* may POSSIBLY be as true as the *Word* of a *Serjeant Surgeon*'.[106] But, as Ranby had the ear of the Hospital Board, Lee reluctantly agreed to a publicly witnessed physical examination of the pensioners. One examination, however, was not enough. The Board rejected this evidence on the grounds that:

> The Proof of Cure [resting] wholly on [soldiers'] Declarations and Affidavits, and upon such Inspection and Examination, as, at the most, could only produce a Declaration that their Ruptures were not down at that Time.[107]

According to Ranby at least two or three months were needed to assess the efficacy of a rupture cure:

> [I]n which Time [the practitioner] ought to make various Trials with different Kinds and Degrees of Exercise, before he could, upon any just Foundation, conclude that his Cure was really compleat [*sic*] and perfect.[108]

It was the last time that the obstinate and increasingly disconsolate Lee co-operated with his medical counterparts at the hospitals. The patience of the hospital boards gradually eroded over the next two years until they seized absolute control over the experimental patients and imposed a draconian regime of enforced multiple-examinations. Over several weeks the pensioners were repeatedly examined, with or without their consent. Stripped from the waist down, they were marched and paraded before a mixed board of surgeons and house officers. Partially dressed, the ruptured men were prodded, probed, examined and 'exercised with Coughing, Jumping, etc.' until signs of hernia were evident.[109] Considering the sensitive nature of the disorder, these actions were unusual. Physical examination was occasional and far from routine, even for surgeons whose terrain comprised the externals of the body.[110] Perhaps, this legacy of a polite culture that stigmatised even the most superficial physical examination as manual work did not apply to handling servicemen.[111] In dealing with poor pensioners, at least, Ranby showed no obvious qualms about violating accepted social etiquette. At times, Ranby went a good deal further. Lee complained to the Sick and Hurt Board of the Admiralty about the 'ungentlemanly' methods

165

and practices employed by Ranby in the course of the trials. When examining pensioner George Dix, for example, Ranby 'squeezed his testicles so much that the poor man was in great pain for four days after'.[112] Nevertheless, the pressure of physical truth overcame the objections and protestations of gentlemanly trust and on 2 April 1752:

> The Board having taken the whole into Consideration, and finding no Cures performed, but many Mal-Practices carried on by Mr Lee, have judged him no Ways intitled [*sic*] to any Reward for one Year's Experiments... and do forbid him all attendance upon the Hospital for the future.[113]

The rupture hospital

As outlined above, military imperatives and patronage were central to the rupture trials at Greenwich and Chelsea. They were perhaps even more important in the establishment of a military hospital for ruptured soldiers in 1758. The facility began life in 1756 as a voluntary hospital for the relief of 'poor indigent sick persons of either sex'.[114] As sources of civic pride and private prestige, hospitals were increasingly recognised for their practical merit.[115] Not surprising then, the hospital subscription list included local merchants as well as some prominent military and political figures, from whom an impressive committee was formed, headed by Lord Halifax as President and George Dodington as Vice President.[116] It was located near the 'Westminster Bridge-foot, in Lambeth' – in a prominent position and only about twenty minutes stroll from Lee's private residence on Arundel Street.[117]

The precise size and character of the building are unknown. But as Adrian Wilson has indicated, specialist facilities were notably small institutions,[118] and the rupture hospital was unlikely to be any different. Since Lee never mentioned treating more than a dozen patients at any one moment, it is reasonable to assume that the hospital contained some ten to fifteen beds. It was certainly residential, as the 'eminent council and Serjeant-at-Law', John Glynn confirmed when he noted in 1764 that Lee had 'provided a house and proper accommodations for ruptured persons'.[119] Quite possibly the 'hospital' was little more than a rented floor in one of the numerous riverside warehouses found in that area. Whatever the size and nature, Lee probably found it a considerable advantage in his private practice to call himself 'Surgeon to the Hospital'.

The fact that the hospital treated a specific disorder was not particularly remarkable, as the founding of specialist facilities was far from unique in Georgian London. This hospital was simply one more specialist institution, alongside bladder stone and eye clinics, and venereal hospitals that appeared in the 1740s and 50s.[120] The principal difference about the rupture hospital was that not long after opening to the public, it became a military establishment. After an initial period of public service, Ligonier suggested that the hospital deal exclusively with ruptured soldiers. When the members of the hospital committee were acquainted with these proposed developments:

[T]hey declared their intention was to support an hospital for the relief of indigent persons, and not for the army, so capable of providing for themselves; in consequence of which, the soldiers being admitted, all meetings of the subscribers dropped.[121]

In April 1758, a royal warrant defined the hospital as a military post.[122] Appointed permanent hospital director, Lee also assumed the rank of Surgeon General to the Army.[123]

As a military establishment, the rupture hospital was regulated under standard military hospital instructions first instigated during the latter stages of the War of Austrian Succession.[124] To aid the implementation of military discipline and medical policy, the hospital was assigned a guard of regular soldiers. Ligonier ordered that a sergeant of the Guards daily attended:

Mr Lee, from whom he is to receive a list of the patients, with the places of their abode; and when any of them neglect attending, he is to go to them to know the cause of such neglect; and if they can give no sufficient reason for it, he is to confine them in the Savoy.... And if any of the patients are guilty of any irregular or indecent behaviour, he is likewise to confine them.[125]

Patients without passes were prevented from leaving the premises and those who broke hospital rules were subject to punishment. The guards were also intended to supervise patient–civilian interaction. Local 'tippling houses' were patrolled 'to prevent any men from Drinking & quarrelling with the inhabitants'.[126]

There were strict admittance policies and procedures. Regimental officers were commanded by general order to send ruptured soldiers for treatment to the hospital. Arrivals were required to present a letter of recommendation, signed by the regimental surgeon and a company officer: 'Sir, Please to admit the bearer [blank space] into your hospital, for the cure of a rupture, with which he is afflicted, and thereby rendered incapable of duty'.[127] This presented Lee with a theoretical medical monopoly over ruptured soldiers. It remained only theoretical, because archival evidence indicates that field surgeons continued to treat and pension ruptured soldiers during this same period without reference to a rupture hospital.[128] Besides which, Lee had no practical means of enforcing his prerogative. The fact that the only patients known to have attended the hospital were all stationed in and around London at the time of treatment[129] implies that the hospital was, at best, restricted to serving the regiments and garrisons stationed in the south east of England.

Unfortunately, little known documentation remains of the hospital's medical regime. One nineteenth-century commentator was certain that Lee had performed herniotomies, 'not to relieve strangulated hernia, but to cure the rupture of every patient who placed himself in his care'.[130] However, according to Sheldrake, after several fatal operations, Lee changed his methods and 'instead of committing murder, was contented to be guilty of fraud, for the rest of his life he pretended to cure ruptures by application of astringent washes, bandages, &c'.[131] One soldier testified in court that Lee did 'anoint the groin' with some secret curative lotion as part of a six-week intensive therapy he had received.[132]

In all probability, Lee practised a near-conventional course of treatment consistent with contemporary palliative methods. During the Greenwich experiments, Lee 'employed [two bosuns and two mates] to prevent those People of strolling about or eating or drinking to excess' and insisted that his patients were fed an adjusted oil and fat-free diet consisting of 'milk potage' and 'hasty pudding' in place of beef.[133] Having then reduced the hernia by regular means, Lee then applied an astringent lotion, over which he fitted a specially designed truss. In public court, Private John Oxlade stated that having had a rupture for sixteen months Lee had cured him in less than four weeks. When asked how, Oxlade stated that before treatment he 'only wore a Truss of the common form; but Mr Lee's is an ingenious Invention'.[134] After several weeks of treatment, Lee sent the cured soldiers back to their regiments with a precautionary bandage for support. If the disorder returned, Lee would claim, as he often did at Chelsea and Greenwich, that it was an entirely new rupture.[135]

Whichever therapeutic methods were employed, expertise and hospitalisation were relatively expensive ventures. Lee's annual salary was an impressive £300 per annum for his limited and specialised services. This was a sum that matched the retainer of the extremely prestigious position of master surgeon at the Royal Hospital, Chelsea.[136] In addition, there were, amongst numerable sundries, the wages of the other hospital personnel and military guard to consider, as well as the expenses incurred transporting soldiers to and from the hospital. Regimental surgeons and staff surgeons, in comparison, were paid 4s per day (or £73 a year), and 10s per day (or £184 10s a year) respectively, for treating the whole spectrum of ailments and injuries *in situ*, and without incurring extra costs.

If patronage fathered the rupture hospital, war nurtured and peace smothered it. The hospital received War Office funding for eight consecutive years, before the conjunction of three events conspired to bring about its closure in 1765. The first came with the close of the Seven Years War. Having stood at an impressive paper-strength of 120,000 troops in 1763, the British army shrank to a little over 30,000 by the end of the following year. Along with this general demobilisation came a habitual reduction in the military budget.[137] Thus, parliamentary measures had the dual effect of diminishing the actual number of ruptured soldiers and, just as importantly, drastically curtailing military expenditure. Under the influence of intensive financial constraints, the rupture hospital was just one of many military institutions to disappear at this time. Second, Lord Barrington was re-instated as Secretary-at-War. This appointment could have hardly been worse for Lee and the hospital. Barrington had been specifically re-appointed to implement the economic restrictions that the Government had imposed on the armed forces after the signing of peace, and was therefore unlikely to fund a contentious and expensive hospital.[138] Perhaps more importantly, Barrington had little regard or respect for either Lee or Ligonier. Having experienced several disagreeable encounters with them both in his first term of office, it must have given him considerable personal satisfaction to foreclose on the project of two men with whom he had so often quarrelled over issues of authority.[139] Finally, the health and political power of the aged Ligonier were fading. Removed from office at the same moment that his army was being dismantled, and suffering a debilitating disease, Ligonier was to all intents and purposes powerless to help Lee or the hospital, and with the death of Ligonier in 1770 the fate of the rupture hospital and the specific treatment of ruptured soldiers were sealed.

Conclusion

The exact number and rate of hernia occurrence in the Georgian British Army are beyond the reach of the historian. That an image of obese, periodically malnourished, diseased and constipated, occasionally physically overworked, and perpetually unfit British troops manning camps and barracks, ringing with hacking smoker's coughs and the distinctive short consumptive bark, may be a gross characterisation should not detract from the fact that the underlying causes of hernia were endemic characteristics of eighteenth-century soldiers and soldiering. That hernia was a significant cause of manpower wastage should not be doubted. To counter this debilitating disorder, the army required an efficacious cure that conventional therapeutics could not deliver. This inability to find a cure conflicts with the ever-present military imperative of maintaining as many men as possible in the field at all times. It also strained relations between medicine and the Army. Indeed, it has been the claim of this paper that the military reaction to the medical inability to cure hernias tells us a great deal about the Army, medicine, and their awkward relationship.

Both the Army and military hospitals were environments extremely congenial to the performance clinical trials. Nowhere else in society were disciplined patients readily available in such numbers. Nor did any other institution have the infrastructure and financial collateral that could, and did, support large-scale medical endeavours of this kind. But the Army was not an homogeneous organisation. Much depended upon the personal interests and powers of individual commanders. Patronage, as we have seen above, went far beyond the recruitment of individuals. It had the power to create military vacancies and initiate medical careers as well as end them. It could also support or resist particular therapeutic practices. But, as in the case of hernia treatment, even though patronage was directly responsible for the establishment of a preferred treatment in a military hospital, it was unable to resist the implications of war and peace.

It was not mere coincidence that Lee sought and was given military support to treat ex-servicemen during the peace of 1749–55, and serving soldiers during the Seven Years War (1756–63). The demise of the hospital and Lee's military career were explicitly linked to the social and economic changes that were set in motion after the signing of the peace treaty. The demobilisation that followed over the next two years eroded the self-professed *raison d'être* of a hospital specifically maintained for the cure of ruptured servicemen. Besides which, in times of peace, the expenditure upon and concern for the health and fitness of soldiers lessened proportionally to their estimated use. Indeed, it has been suggested that any enthusiasm for the armed forces acquired after even the most victorious campaigns quickly evaporated on the cessation of war.[140] Consequently, when the powerful patronage of Ligonier ended with his death, Lee and the treatment of ruptured soldiers slipped back into the margins of military and medical consciousness.

Acknowledgement

I would like to thank Chris Lawrence, the late Roy Porter, Mark Jenner, Michael McVaugh, Caroline Essex, and Geoff Hudson, from whose comments this paper has greatly benefited.

Notes

1. G. Carlisle, 'An Account of an Uncommon Large Hernia, in a Letter from Dr George Carlisle, to the Right Rev. The Lord Bishop of Carlisle, FRS', in *The Royal Society of London Philosophical Transactions* [*RSLPT*], 55 (1766), 133-41.

2. R. Porter, 'Gout: Framing and Fantasising Disease', *Bulletin of the History of Medicine*, 68 (1994), 1-28; R. Porter and G.S. Rousseau, *Gout: The Patrician Malady* (New Haven and London: Yale University Press, 1998).

3. Calculated from fourteen separate surveys published between 1900 and the 1940s and tabulated in L.M. Zimmerman and B.J. Anson, *Anatomy and Surgery of Hernia* (Baltimore: Williams & Wilkins, 1953), 21.

4. H.A.L. Howell, 'The Story of the Army Surgeon and the Care of the Sick and Wounded in the British Army, from 1715–1748', part I and II, *Journal of Royal Army Medical Corps*, 22 (1914), 320–34 and 455–71; G. Gask, 'John Hunter in the Campaign in Portugal, 1762–3', *idem, Essays in the History of Medicine* (London: Butterworth, 1950), 116-44; P.E. Kopperman, 'Medical Services in the British Army, 1742–1783', *Journal of the History of Medicine and Allied Sciences*, 34 (1979), 428-55; and relevant chapters in N. Cantlie, *A History of the Army Medical Department*, 2 vols (London: Churchill Livingstone, 1974); R.C. Engelman and R.J.T. Joy, *Two Hundred Years of Military Medicine* (Fort Detrick: Maryland, 1975); R.A. Gabriel and K.S. Metz, *A History of Military Medicine, Vol. 2: From the Renaissance through Modern Times* (New York: Greenwood Press, 1992); F.H. Garrison, *Notes on the History of Military Medicine* (Washington: Association of Military Surgeons, 1922); M.H. Kaufman, *Surgeons at War: Medical Arrangements for the Treatment of the Sick and Wounded in the British Army During the Late Eighteenth and Nineteenth Centuries* (London: Greenwood Press, 2001); M. Howard, *Wellington's Doctors: The British Army Medical Services in the Napoleonic Wars* (Staplehurst: Spellmount, 2002).

5. L. Colley, *Britons: Forging the Nation, 1707–1837* (London: Pimlico, 1992); J. Brewer, *The Sinews of Power: War, Money and the English State, 1688–1783* (London: Routledge, 1994).

6. M. Harrison, 'Medicine and the Management of Modern Warfare', *History of Science*, 34 (1996), 379–410; *idem*, 'Medicine and the Management of Modern Warfare: an Introduction', in R. Cooter, M. Harrison and S. Sturdy (eds), *Medicine and Modern Warfare* (Amsterdam: Rodopi, 1999), 1-27; M. Harrison, *Medicine and Victory: British Military Medicine in the Second World War* (Oxford: Oxford University Press, 2004), 1–7, *passim*; R.N. Buckley, *The British Army in the West Indies: Society and the Military in the Revolutionary Age* (Gainsville: University Press of Florida, 1998) 272–324.

7. M. Foucault, 'The Politics of Health in the Eighteenth Century', in C. Gordon (ed.), *Power/Knowledge: Selected Interviews and other Writings by Michel Foucault* (Worcester: Harvest Press, 1988), 166–82; *idem, Discipline and Punish: The Birth of the Prison*, trans. A. Sheridan (Harmondsworth: Penguin, 1977); *idem*, 'La Politique de la Santé au 18e Siècle' in his *Les Machines à Guérir: Aux Origines de l'Hôpital Moderne* (Bruxelles: Pierre Mardaga 1979), 7–18.

8. C. Lawrence, 'Disciplining Disease: Scurvy, the Navy and Imperial Expansion' in D. Miller and P. Reill (eds), *Visions of Empire* (Cambridge:

Cambridge University Press, 1994), 80–106.

9. H.J. Cook, 'Practical Medicine and the British Armed Forces after the "Glorious Revolution", *Medical History*, 34 (1990), 1–26, 3; P. Mathias, 'Swords and Ploughshares: The Armed Forces, Medicine and Public Health in the Late Eighteenth Century', in J.M. Winter (ed.), *War and Economic Development: Essays in Memory of David Joslin* (Cambridge: Cambridge University Press, 1975), 73–90.

10. For an overview of the role of military experience in the development of French medicine in the eighteenth century see C. Jones, 'The Welfare of the French Foot-Soldier from Richleau to Napoleon', in his *The Charitable Imperative: Hospitals and Nursing in Ancien Regime and Revolutionary France* (London: Routledge, 1989), 80–106; *idem*, 'The Construction of the Hospital Patient in Early Modern France', in N. Finzch and R. Jutte (eds), *Institutions of Confinement: Hospitals, Asylums and Prisons in Western Europe and North America, 1500–1950* (Cambridge: Cambridge University Press, 1998), 55–74.

11. R. Cooter, 'War and Modern Medicine', in W.F. Bynum and R. Porter (eds), *Companion Encyclopaedia of the History of Medicine* (London: Routledge, 1994), 1536–73; for examples of the role of military medicine as a medical career, see M. Ackroyd, *et al.*, *Advancing with the Army: Medicine, the Professions, and Social Mobility in the British Isles, 1790–1850* (Oxford: Oxford University Press, 2006); M.H. Kaufman, *The Regius Chair of Military Surgery in the University of Edinburgh, 1806–55* (Amsterdam: Rodopi, 2003).

12. S. Blancard, *The Physical Dictionary Wherein the Terms of Anatomy, the Names and Causes of Diseases, Chyrurgical Instruments, and their Use, are Accurately Described* (London, 1708), 153.

13. J. Quincy, *Lexicon Physico-Medicum: Or a New Medicinal Dictionary; Explaining the Different Terms used in the Several Branches of the Profession, and in such Parts of Natural Philosophy as are Introductionary [sic] Thereto: with an Account of the Things Signified by such Terms; Collected from the Most Eminent Authors; and Particularly those who have Wrote upon Mechanical Principles*, 3rd edn (London, 1726), 210.

14. According to L.M. Nymus and H.N. Harkins less than ten per cent of hernias are caused exclusively by acquired defects, *idem*, *Hernia* (London: Pitman Medical Publishing, 1964).

15. T. Brand, *Chirurigical Essays, on the Causes and Symptoms of Rupture; their Natural Consequences, if Neglected, and the Various Dangers in Applying Trusses with Cases to Illustrate the Success of an Improved Method of Treatment and Cure: To which are Added, the Opinions of the Late Sir Edward Barry; John Hunter esq.; Surgeon Extraordinary to the King, Confirming the Peculiar Efficiency of the Elastic Bandages Applied by the Author* (London, 1782), 2.

16. I would like to thank surgeon and historian Piers Mitchell for taking the time to explain the current understanding of the anatomical and causal characteristics of hernia. Any inaccuracies in interpretation, of course, are entirely my own. S. Eubanks, 'Hernias', in D.C. Sabiston and H.K. Lyerly (eds), *Textbook of Surgery: The Biological Basis of Modern Surgical Practice*, 15th edn (Philadelphia: W.B. Saunders Company, 1997), 1215–33.

17. R.C. Read, 'Collagen synthesis and direct inguinal herniation', in M.E. Arregui and R.F. Nagan (eds), *Inguinal Hernia: Advances or Controversies?* (Oxford: Radcliff Medical Press, 1994); *idem*, 'The Role of Protease–Antiprotease in the Pathogenesis of Herniation and Abdominal Aortic Aneurysm in Certain Smokers', *Postgraduate General Surgery*, 14 (1992), 161; J.I. Weitz, *et al.*, 'Increased Neutrophil Elastase Activity in Cigarette Smokers', *Ann. Intern. Med.*, 107 (1987), 686; K. Bielecki and R. Puawski, 'Is Cigarette Smoking a Causative Factor in the Development of Inguinal Hernia?', *Pol. Tyg. Lek.*, 43 (1988), 974.

18. G.L Apperson, *The Social History of Smoking* (London: Martin Secker, 1914), 174; J. Goodman, *Tobacco in History: The Cultures of Dependence* (London: Routledge, 1993), 59–89; J. Walvin, *Fruits of Empire: Exotic Produce and British Taste, 1660–1800* (London: Macmillan, 1997), 66–88.

19. G. Cleghorn, *Observations on the Epidemical Diseases in Minorca: From the Year 1744 to 1749: To Which is Prefixed, A Short Account of the Climate, Productions, Inhabitants, and Endemical Distempers of that Island* (London: Wilson, 1751), 56–7.

20. See, for example, C. Amyand, 'Of an Inguinal Rupture, with a Pin in the Appendix Coeci, incrusted with Stone; Some Observations on Wounds in the Guts', in *RSLPT*, 39 (1735–6), 329–42; J. Buchanan, *Regimental Practice or Short History of Diseases Common to His Majesties own Royale Regiment of Horse Guards, Commonly Called the Blews, when Abroard*, (*c.*1746–1750), Wellcome Library [hereafter WL], RAMC 1037, 216; and the letters from John Huxham, in *RSLPT*, 41 (1741), 640–5.

21. J. Ranby, 'An Account of What Appeared Most Remarkable on Opening the Body of Ann Edwards, Who Died January 5th 1730 [ns] Having a Large Umbilical Rupture', in *RSLPT*, Vol. 37 (1731–2), 221–2.

22. A. Stuart, *New Discoveries and Improvements in the Most Considerable Branches of Anatomy and Surgery* (London, 1738), 19–23.

23. See, for example, A. Monro, 'Surgery', Vol. II (1790), WL, MS. 3618; J. Parkinson, Hints for the Improvement of Trusses; Intended to Render Their use Less Inconvenient, and to Prevent the Necessity of an Understrap (London: H.D. Symonds, 1802), note on 13; note also that as James Sharpe has pointed out, growing anxiety about the large numbers of disabled labourers stimulated the founding of a number of friendly societies intended to distribute free trusses amongst the ruptured poor: J.A. Sharpe, *Early*

Modern England: A Social History, 1550–1750 (London: Edward Arnold, 1987), 208.

24. The dominant explanation of congenital causes, established in P. Pott, *A Treatise on Ruptures* (London: C. Hitch and L. Hawes, 1756), 11–21, remained unchanged until the publication of A. Cooper's *The Anatomy and Surgical Treatment of Abdominal Hernia* (London, 1804) almost fifty years later.

25. R.C. Read, 'The Development of Inguinal Herniorrhaphy', *Surgical Clinics of North America*, 64 (1984), 185–96.

26. *Ibid.*, 189.

27. T. Sheldrake, *Useful Hints to Those Who are Afflicted with Ruptures: Nature, Cure and Consequences of the Disease and of the Empirical Practices of the Present Day* (London, 1803), 6–8.

28. Pott, *op. cit.* (note 24), 11, my emphasis.

29. With the exception of S.R. Frey, *The British Soldier in America: A Social History of Military Life in the Revolutionary Period* (Austin: University of Texas Press, 1981), 3–52; M. Sikora, *Disziplin und Desertion: Strukturprobleme militärischer Organisation im 18 Jahrhundert* (Berlin: Duncker and Humblot, 1996); M. Lorenz, *Kriminelle Körper – Gestörte Gemöter: Die Normierung des Individuums in Gerichtsmedizin und Psychiatrie der* Aufklörung (Hamburg: Hamburger Edition, 1999), esp. 189–254.

30. J. Black, *Britain as a Military Power, 1688–1815* (London: UCL, 1999).

31. J. Keegan, *The Face of Battle: A Study of Agincourt, Waterloo and the Somme* (London: Pimlico, 1976); A. Brett-James, *Life in Wellington's Army* (London: Allen and Unwin, 1972).

32. J.M. Tanner, *A History of the Study of Human Growth* (Cambridge: Cambridge University Press, 1981), 98–100; A.N. Gilbert, 'An Analysis of Some Eighteenth Century Army Recruiting Records', *Journal of the Society for Army Historical Research*, 54 (1976), 38–47; A.J. Guy, 'Reinforcements for Portugal 1762: Recruiting for Rank at the End of the Seven Years' War', *Annual Report of the National Army Museum*, (1978–9), 30–43; B. Harris, 'Health, Height and History: An Overview of Recent Developments in Anthropometric History', *Social History of Medicine*, 7 (1993), 343–66.

33. Despite popular opinion, gentlemen rankers and career soldiers were a rarity in the eighteenth-century British Army, even amongst the militia. See J.R. Western, *The English Militia in the Eighteenth Century: The Story of a Political Issue, 1660–1802* (London: Routledge, 1965), 255-72; G.A. Steppler, *Britons To Arm! The Story of the British Volunteer Soldier and Volunteer Tradition in Leicestershire and Rutland* (London: Alan Stroud, 1992).

34. G.A. Steppler, 'The Common Soldier in the Reign of George III, 1760–1793' (unpublished University of Oxford PhD thesis, 1984); S. Brumwell, 'The British Soldier in North America, 1755–63' (unpublished

PhD thesis, University of Leeds, 1998).

35. Cantlie, *op. cit.* (note 4), 104.

36. Particular significance was given to the age and height of potential recruits. Article seven of regimental 'Recruiting Instructions' insisted that: 'None to be Inlisted [*sic*] between twenty & thirty five years of age under five feet six inches, & from Sixteen to twenty years of Age under five feet five inches in their Stocking feet, & care to be taken that the Standard be just, & none under sixteen or upwards of thirty five to be Inlisted for the Regiment'. Tall soldiers were regarded as preferable to short ones. Not only were they considered to be generally healthier and stronger; they covered more ground on the march because of a greater length of stride and handled the long-barrelled muskets more easily. See A. Guy, *Colonel Samuel Bageshawe and the Army of George II, 1731–1762* (London: Bodley Head, 1990), 211; Tanner, *op. cit.* (note 32), 98–100.

37. The National Archives [hereafter NA], WO 34/73, contained in a letter from General Jeffery Amherst, New York, to the War Office in London, 16 February 1758.

38. Guy, *op. cit.* (note 36), 260.

39. NA, SP 37/8, S. Lee, 'Memorial and Petition to the King's most excellent Majesty, on the Principles of Public Faith, common Justice and His own Royal Promise, 16th Jan. 1771', f.4 [hereafter 1771a]; *idem, A Memorial and Petition to the King's most Excellent Majesty, On the Principles of Public Faith, Common Justice and His Own Royal Promise, Delivered to the King at St James's, On Wednesday the 23rd January, 1771* (London: J. Williams, 1771), 5 [hereafter 1771b]; *idem, A Narrative of some Proceedings in the Management of Chelsea Hospital: As far as relates to the Appointment and Dismission [sic] of Samuel Lee, Surgeon* (London: W. Owen, 1753); *idem,* A *Proper Reply to the Serjeant Surgeons Defence of their Conduct at Chelsea Hospital* (London: W. Owen, 1754).

40. Quoted in C. Duffy, *The Military Experience in the Age of Reason* (London: Routledge and Kegan Paul, 1987), 147.

41. Much more research into army food and supplies is needed. But for a comparative study on naval victuals see Patricia Crimmin in this publication. For discussion on the use and abuse of alcohol in the army see P.E. Kopperman, 'The Cheapest Pay: Alcohol Abuse in the Eighteenth-Century British Army' *The Journal of Military History*, 60 (1996), 445–70.

42. See, for example, NA, WO 34/63, f. 231.

43. N.A.M. Rodger, *The Wooden World: An Anatomy of the Georgian Navy* (London: Fontana Press, 1986), 82–112.

44. For a detailed discussion on the problem of food supply see R.A. Bowler, *Logistics and the Failure of the British Army in America, 1775–1783* (Princeton: Princeton University Press, 1975), 41–91.

45. For the experiences encountered by the British Army in the Caribbean see R.N. Buckley, 'The Destruction of the British Army in the West Indies, 1793–1815: A Medical History', *JSAHR*, 56 (1978), 79–92; *idem, The British Army in the West Indies: Society and the Military in the Revolutionary Age* (Gainesville: University Press of Florida, 1998); and for a brief, but useful, overview of the British Army experience in North America, see N. St. John Williams, *Redcoats Along the Hudson: The Struggle for North America, 1754–63* (London: Brassey's Classics, 1997).

46. Eubanks, *op. cit.* (note 16), 1219.

47. J. Pringle, 'Medical Annotations', 10 vols (*c.*1752–77), held at the Royal College of Physicians of Edinburgh, Vol. 5, f. 239. All the Pringle MSS held at the College are handwritten. Under the terms of his last will and testament, 'they are never to be lent out on any pretence whatsoever, and... are never to be published.'

48. Buchanan, *op. cit.* (note 20), 143.

49. Cleghorn, *op. cit.* (note 19), 54–7.

50. *Ibid.*, 71.

51. For an introduction to the extent that tuberculosis affected early modern society see W.D. Johnston, 'Tuberculosis', in K.F. Kiple (ed.), *The Cambridge World History of Human Disease* (Cambridge: Cambridge University Press, 1993), 1059–68; and for wider medical and social significance see, G. Palfi, *et al.* (eds), *Tuberculosis: Past and Present* (Szeged: Golden Book Publishers, 1999).

52. See for example, J. Pringle, *Observations on the Diseases of the Army, in Camp and Garrison: In Three Parts. With an Appendix Containing Some Papers of Experiments, Read at Several Meetings of the Royal Society* (London: Millar & Wilson, 1752); R. Hamilton, *The Duties of a Regimental Surgeon Considered: with Observations on his General Qualifications; and Hints Relative to a More Respectable Practice, and Better Regulation of that Department. Wherein are Interpreted many Medical Anecdotes [sic], and Subjects Discussed, Equally Interesting to Every Practitioner,* 2 vols (London: Johnson, 1787); R. Brocklesby, *Oeconomical and Medical Observations, In Two Parts: From the Year 1758 to the Year 1763, inclusive. Tending to The Improvement of Military Hospitals, and to The Cure of Camp Diseases, incident to Soldiers. To which is Subjoined, An Appendix, containing a curious Account of the Climate and Diseases in Africa, upon the Great River Senegal, and farther up than the Island of Senegal. In a letter from Mr. Boone, Practitioner in Physic to that Garrison for three Years, to Dr. Brocklesby* (London: Becket and De Hondt, 1764); D. Monro, *An Account of the Diseases which were most Frequent in the British Military Hospitals in Germany, From January 1761 to the Return of the Troops to England in March 1763. To which is added, An Essay on the Means of Preserving the Health of Soldiers, and conducting Military Hospitals* (London:

Millar, Wilson, Durham, Payne, 1764), who refer to the commonality of coughs amongst the troops, especially in overcrowded winter quarters.

53. Brocklesby, *ibid.*, 109–11.
54. For a detailed analysis of soldier fatigue after sustained periods of rest see Duffy, *op. cit.* (note 40), 157–73.
55. Lee, *A Proper Reply, op. cit.* (note 39), 8.
56. R. Whitworth, *Field Marshal Lord Ligonier: A Story of the British Army, 1702–1770* (Oxford: Clarendon Press, 1958), 385.
57. These figures are calculated from the available data found in the Royal Hospital Chelsea Admissions Books, NA, WO 116/1–3, from 3 October 1715 to 14 February 1746.
58. Quoted in L.G. Stevenson, 'John Hunter, Surgeon-General 1790–1793', *History of Medicine*, 19 (1964), 239–66: 245.
59. Carlisle, *op. cit.* (note 1), 134.
60. Pott, *op. cit.* (note 24), Preface, vii–ix, xii.
61. For details of these procedures see L.M. Zimmerman and B.J. Anson, 'Hernia Through the Ages', in *idem, op. cit.* (note 3), 1–15; P.D. Olch and H.N. Harkins, 'Historical Survey of the Treatment of Inguinal Hernia', in Nymus and Harkins, *op. cit.* (note 14), 1–13.
62. A. Monro (Primus), 'A Tratise [*sic*] on the Operations of Chirurgery', WL, WMS.934 (1734), 119.
63. J. Hunter, 'Lectures on Surgery', WL, WMS.2959 (1779), 277.
64. For an interesting insight into the psychological and sociological implications of male castration see G. Taylor, *Castration: An Abbreviated History of Western Manhood* (New York and London: Routledge, 2000).
65. See Edmund Andrews, 'A History of the Development of the Technique of Herniotomy', *Annals of Medical History*, 7 (1935), 451–66: 461.
66. J. Geyer-Kordesch and F. Macdonald, *Physicians and Surgeons in Glasgow: The History of the Royal College of Physicians of Glasgow, 1599–1858* (London: The Hambledon Press, 1999), 65–6.
67. Andrews, *op. cit.* (note 65); and J.E. Raaf, 'Hernia Healers', *Annals of Medical History*, 4 (1932), 377–89: 377.
68. Pott, *op. cit.* (note 24), 173.
69. A. Monro (secundus), 'Lectures on Surgery', Vol. 1, WL, WMS.3619, 337–40.
70. See, for example, Sheldrake, *op. cit.* (note 27); M.W. Hilles, *Treatise on Hernia: Comprising the Surgical Anatomy, Operative Surgery, and Treatment of that Important Disease in All its Forms* (London: Henry Renshaw, 1838).
71. See, for example, John Clerk's letter of advice to his uncle suffering from an 'Hernia incompleta' in H.M. Dingwall, *Physicians, Surgeons and Apothecaries: Medicine in Seventeenth-Century Edinburgh* (East Heriton: Tuckwell Press, 1995), 141–2.

72. W. Hunter, 'Lectures on Anatomy' (1755), WL, WMS.2965, 276.

73. G.S. Acret, *A Treatise on Hernia, Explaining its Varieties, Situation, Symptoms, and Causes: To which is Added a Full Description of the Construction and Application of the most Approved Mechanical Remedies* (London: Houlston & Son, 1835), 59.

74. G. Arnaud, *A Dissertation on Hernia* (London: A. Millar, 1748), preface, n.p.

75. R. Brand, *The Method of Applying of Trusses* (London, 1771), 19–27.

76. I am much indebted to Patricia Crimmin for this and many more references to the treatment of hernias in Admiralty papers kept at the National Maritime Museum [NMM]. NMM/F/11, 3 April 1752.

77. For examples, see: D. Lysons, *Collectanea: Or, a Collection of Advertisements and Paragraphs from the Newspapers, Relating to Various Subjects* [dated 1660–1825] (London, no publication date).

78. S. Mihles, *The Elements of Surgery: In which are Contained All the Essential and Necessary Principles of the ART; With an Account of the Nature and Treatment of Chirurgical Disorders, and a Description of the Operations, Bandages, Instruments, and Dressings, According to the Modern and most Approved Practice: Adapted to the Use of the Camp and Navy, as well as the Domestic Surgeon,* 2nd edn ['altered and considerably augmented with several of the latest improvements in Practice and Operations. By Alexander Reid, assistant surgeon to Chelsea Hospital'] (London: Robert Horsfield, 1764).

79. Hamilton, *op. cit.* (note 52), Vol. 1, 326.

80. For an overview of medical duties of the Naval Sick and Hurt Board, see P. Crimmin in this volume.

81. NMM ADM/E/11.

82. For an example of soldiers concealing hernias behind tight fitting clothing see J. Ranby and C. Hawkins, *The True Account of All the Transactions Before the Right Honourable the Lords, and Others the Commissioners for the Affairs of Chelsea Hospital; As Far as Relates to the Admission and Dismission [sic] of Samuel Lee, Surgeon: To which is Prefixed, A Short Account of the Nature of a Rupture* (London, 1754), 42.

83. For an assessment on the quantity of experimentation on patients in late-eighteenth-century hospital wards see G.B. Risse, *Hospital Life in Enlightenment Scotland: Care and Teaching at the Royal Infirmary of Edinburgh* (Cambridge: Cambridge University Press, 1986); and L. Rosner, *Medical Education in the Age of Improvement: Edinburgh Students and Apprentices, 1760–1826* (Edinburgh: Edinburgh University Press, 1991).

84. Slaves may be the other exception, see: L. Stewart, 'The Edge of Utility: Slaves and Smallpox in the Early Eighteenth Century", *Medical History*, 29 (1985), 54–70.

85. In an open letter to a friend and benefactor in Scotland, John Pringle informed Andrew Mitchell that a physician or surgeon could learn more in a

month of active service than a year of university education, Pringle to Mitchell, 15 October 1742, British Library [hereafter BL], AMS 6861, f. 178.

86. For an example of medical innovation and experimentation with medicines, drugs and soldiers see Mark Harrison's article in this volume.

87. See, for example, J. Black, 'Introduction', in *idem* (ed.), *European Warfare, 1453–1815* (London: Macmillan Press, 1999), 1–22; S. Brumwell, *White Devil: An Epic Story of Revenge from the Savage War that Inspired the Last of the Mohicans* (London: Phoenix, 2004), 173–4; S. Brumwell, *Redcoats: The British Soldier and the War in the Americas, 1755–1763* (London: Phoenix, 2001), 55–137; N.A.M. Rodger, *The Wooden World: An Anatomy of the Georgian Navy* (London: Fontana Press, 1986) 98–105.

88. See, for example, J.A. Houlding, *Fit for Service: The Training of the British Army, 1715–1795* (London: Clarenden Press, 1981); J.W. Fortescue, *A History of the British Army*, Vols 1–3 (London: Macmillan, 1899–1906); H. De Watteville, *The British Soldier* (London, 1954); E.M. Spiers, *The Army and Society, 1815–1914* (London: Longman, 1980); A.R. Skelley, *The Victorian Army at Home* (London: Croom Helm, 1977).

89. H. Marshall, *Military Miscellany* (London, 1846); V.E. Neuburg, 'The British Army in the Eighteenth Century', *Journal of the Society for Army Historical Research*, 61 (1983), 39–47; Colley, *op. cit.* (note 5), 283–319.

90. M. Mann, *The Veterans* (Norwich: Michael Russell, 1997); C.G.T. Dean, 'The Corps of Invalids', *Journal of the Royal United Service Institution* (hereafter *JRUSI*), 89 (1944), 281–7; and 'The Corps of Invalids, part II', *JRUSI*, 91 (1946), 584–9.

91. R. Floud, K. Wachter and A. Gregory, *Height, Health and History: Nutritional Status in the United Kingdom, 1750–1980* (Cambridge: Cambridge University Press, 1990).

92. Houlding, *op. cit.* (note 88), 116–37.

93. J. Keegan and R. Holmes, *Soldiers: A History of Men in Battle* (London: Hamilton, 1985); R. Holmes, *Firing Line* (London: Cape, 1985).

94. See Guy, *op. cit.* (note 36), 15–16; R. Holmes, *Redcoat: The British Soldier in the Age of Horse and Musket* (London: Harper Collins, 2001).

95. For a detailed exposition of the regimental finance, see: A. Guy, *Oeconomy and Discipline: Officership and Administration in the British Army, 1714–63* (Manchester: Manchester University Press, 1985).

96. NA, WO 250/459, 'Royal Hospital Chelsea Journal, 1715–1749 [hereafter *RHCJ*], 67.

97. BL, Add. MS. 34327, f. 6. When assessing the potential rewards for 'discovering' and disclosing useful medical 'cures' it is interesting to note that in 1726, £5,000 was approximately the equivalent of £250,000 in today's money.

98. See M. McVaugh, 'Treatment of Hernia in the Later Middle Ages: Surgical Correction and Social Construction', in R. French, *et al.* (eds), *Medicine from the Black Death to the French Disease* (Aldershot: Ashgate, 1998), 131–55.

99. R[obert] H[ouston], *The History of Ruptures and Rupture-Curers: Wherein Both are Thoroughly and Impartially Considered. Occasioned by a Letter from a Physician of Paris, to a Physician at London, Concerning a New, and Never Failing Way of Curing all Sorts of Ruptures in Men, Women, and Children, by an Infallible Remedy, a Secret: With a Genuine Receipt of the whole Secret, Part of which was Lately Sold for an Immense Sum of Money, As also of a Famous Stiptick* [*sic*], *Both Laid Open for the Satisfaction of the Curious, and Benefit of the Publick* (London, 1726), 43.

100. Ranby and Hawkins, *op. cit.* (note 82), 10–1.

101. I have not found a commission or warrant to support this proposition, but Lee certainly possessed both the devoted patronage of Ligonier and the medical support of Mitchell throughout the controversy.

102. C.G.T. Dean, *The Royal Hospital, Chelsea* (London: Hutchingson, 1950); C. Lloyd and J.L.S. Coulter, *Medicine and the Navy, 1220–1900, Vol. III, 1714–1815* (Edinburgh and London: Livingstone, 1961), 208; see also NA, ADM 67/10, 25 May 1752.

103. For an excellent exploration of trust, truth and scientific knowledge see S. Shapin, *A Social History of Truth: Civility and Science in Seventeenth-Century England* (Chicago: University of Chicago Press, 1995); and for an interpretation of how Boylean scientific methodology was intended for medical practice see B. Beigun Kaplan, *Divulging of Useful Truths in Physick: The Medical Agenda of Robert Boyle* (Baltimore: Johns Hopkins University Press, 1993).

104. See P.R. Mills, 'The Nature of a Rupture: Concepts of Truth and Trust during a Medical Dispute in the Treatment of Hernia in Eighteenth-Century London', in submission.

105. NA, WO 250/460, *Chelsea Hospital Journal, 1749–1771* [*CHJ*], f. 8.

106. Lee, *A Proper Reply, op. cit.* (note 39), 30–1.

107. Ranby and Hawkins, *op. cit.* (note 82), 12.

108. *Ibid.*, 13.

109. Lee, *Appointment and Dismission, op. cit.* (note 39), 17.

110. R. Porter, 'The Rise of the Physical Examination', in W.F. Bynum and R. Porter (eds), *Medicine and the Five Senses* (Cambridge: Cambridge University Press, 1993), 179–97.

111. See M. Nicolson, 'Giovanni Battista Morgani and Eighteenth-Century Physical Examination', in C. Lawrence (ed.), *Medical Theory, Surgical Practice: Studies in the History of Surgery* (London: Routledge, 1992), 101–33.

112. NMM ADM/F/11.

113. *CHJ, op. cit.* (note 105), f.50.

114. Lee, *Memorial and Petition* [1771b], *op. cit.* (note 39), 3.

115. M.E. Fissell, *Patients, Power, and the Poor in Eighteenth-Century Bristol* (Cambridge: Cambridge University Press, 1991), esp. 74–94.

116. Lee, *Memorial and Petition* [1771b], *op. cit.* (note 39), 3.

117. *Ibid.,* 4.

118. A. Wilson, 'The Politics of Medical Improvement in Early Hanoverian London', in A. Cunningham and R. French, *The Medical Enlightenment of the Eighteenth Century* (Cambridge: Cambridge University Press, 1990), 4–39: 10–24.

119. Lee, *Memorial and Petition* [1771b], *op. cit.* (note 39), 22.

120. D. Andrew, 'Two Medical Charities in Eighteenth-Century London: The Lock Hospital and the Lying-In Charity for Married Women', in J. Barry and C. Jones (eds), *Medicine and Charity Before the Welfare State* (London: Routledge, 1991), 82–97; L. Granshaw, '"Fame and Fortune by Means of Bricks and Mortar": The Medical Profession and Specialist Hospitals in Britain, 1800–1948', in L. Granshaw and R. Porter (eds), *The Hospital in History* (London: Routledge, 1989), 199–220.

121. Lee, *Memorial and Petition* [1771b], *op. cit.* (note 39), 6.

122. NA, WO 248/63, f. 124.

123. On the title page of the memorial of 1771, Lee described himself as 'Surgeon-General to the Army by the Appointment of his late and present Majesty'; Lee, *Memorial and Petition, op. cit.* (note 39).

124. For examples of these instructions see NA, WO 1/5, f. 50; NA, WO 26/19, f. 450; RADCP 2/5.

125. Lee, *Memorial and Petition, op. cit.* (note 39), 9.

126. Royal College of Surgeons, Loudoun Papers, Vol. 1, letter 27.

127. Lee, *Memorial and Petition, op. cit.* (note 39), 11.

128. See, for example, the admittance details in NA, WO 116/4–8, February 1746–September 1775.

129. Lee, *Memorial and Petition* [1771b], *op. cit.* (note 39), 5.

130. Sheldrake included a short footnote biography of Lee, *op. cit.* (note 27), 14–15.

131. *Ibid.,* 14–15, 19, 147.

132. Lee, *Appointment and Dismission, op. cit.* (note 39), 60–1; see also *idem, A Proper Reply, op. cit.* (note 39).

133. NMM ADM/F/11, 3 July 1752 and 5 March 1752.

134. Lee, *Appointment and Dismission, op. cit.* (note 39), 53–4.

135. Lee, *A Proper Reply, op. cit.* (note 39), 59–61.

136. Dean, *op. cit.* (note 102).

137. See Brewer, *op. cit.* (note 5).

138. T. Hayter, *An Eighteenth-Century Secretary at War: The Papers of William,*

Viscount Barrington (London: Bodley Head, 1988), 3–18.

139. For a brief overview of the relationship between Barrington and Ligonier see relevant papers in Hayter, *ibid.*, and Whitworth, *op. cit.* (note 56).

140. See Guy, *op. cit.* (note 95); *idem, op. cit.* (note 36), esp. 1–20; Houlding, *op. cit.* (note 88), 99–136.

7

British Naval Health, 1700–1800:
Improvement over Time?

Patricia Kathleen Crimmin

Did British naval health improve over the course of the eighteenth century? The Sick and Hurt Board sought cures for common ailments such as scurvy by encouraging experimentation, and the development of cheap universal treatments. It also strove to provide a healthful environment and diet. Overall, prevention rather than the development of cures was very much the focus. This chapter also argues that too much emphasis has been placed on the authoritarian nature of the British Navy in the eighteenth century.

If one considers Admiral Hosier's expedition to the West Indies in 1726, when 'in two years a squadron of 4,750 men lost over 4,000 dead, including the admiral and his successor, seven captains and fifty lieutenants' and compares it with Admiral Lord St Vincent's return to Plymouth, from the blockade of Brest in November 1800, with a fleet of 28,000 men, of which only sixteen needed hospital treatment after a cruise of eight months, it seems obvious that naval health had improved during the course of the eighteenth century.[1] Earlier in that century it was impossible to conduct operations for a prolonged period without losing large numbers of men to sickness and death. Only in the 1790s could Nelson, then in the Mediterranean, declare a cruise of six weeks nothing extraordinary and this was, in great part, because he was an officer careful of his men's health, serving under an admiral, Sir John Jervis, later Earl St Vincent, who took the greatest care of everything connected with it.

The Royal Navy was not indifferent to the health of seamen: far from it. Manning the service was a continual and insoluble problem throughout the century, and the illnesses of seamen and their deaths from disease were important contributory factors. Naval health was thus often a high priority for the Admiralty and for its subordinate department, the Commission for the Taking Care of Sick and Wounded Seamen and for the Care and Treatment of Prisoners of War, more commonly known as the Sick and Hurt

Board. The very existence of such an organisation argues the Navy's concern with seamen's health, but the office only became permanent from the 1740s, during a period of prolonged warfare. The Sick and Hurt Board was an administrative body, working through its appointed agents and surgeons, making contracts for the supply of hospitals, sick quarters, medical care, and food, in the earlier period, later undertaking these functions itself, but always aiming to contain, and if possible cure, sickness and return men to duty. The early commissioners were civil servants who had often worked in other branches of naval bureaucracy. This provided them with ample administrative experience but they had no medical knowledge.

In the 1740s and for some years thereafter, the Board had no physician among its members. Though Dr Maxwell served as one of the commissioners from 1757 until 1771, the balance in favour of doctors as commissioners only tipped in their favour in 1795, when Drs Blaine, Blair and Sir William Gibbons formed the London board with Dr Johnston as a resident commissioner at the Royal Naval Hospital, Haslar. This medical predominance remained thereafter until the Board's abolition in 1806. Before that shift, the commissioners relied for necessary medical advice on external experts. In 1740, they consulted Dr Mead on the prevention of scurvy, taking additional advice from Doctors Monrow and Cockburn; and in March 1754, faced with proposals by Dr James Lind, their surgeon at Haslar hospital, Gosport, on better ways of improving seamen's health on long voyages, they consulted Drs Schomberg and James, as acknowledged experts.[2]

Yet in the 1740s, the Admiralty was increasingly asking the Board for more and more detailed information on the numbers of men sick ashore at home and abroad, the greatest number sick ashore at various ports since July 1739 to August 1740, and for monthly accounts of the sick. The bureaucratic difficulties of compiling such statistics produced only partial answers, but those statistics that were produced in 1740 were sufficiently sobering, and perhaps for the first time the Admiralty glimpsed the scale of the war-time health problem. There were 9,775 men sick ashore, over 3,000 at Plymouth, the remainder at Gosport, over 3,500 were ashore at the eastern ports of Woolwich, Rochester Sheerness and Deal. The Board could produce no figures from abroad for comparison in this period, though figures for earlier in 1739, eight hundred sick at Gibraltar in February, one thousand at Port Mahon in April, were sufficiently alarming.[3] The Admiralty requested such figures because of a crisis in manning the fleet. War with Spain, begun in 1739, called for a greater effort in raising men but the lists of newly raised men were being outstripped by the sick lists, thanks to an epidemic of typhus. In 1744, when war with France developed, the problem was one of desertion. The Admiralty, insisting on better and more frequent reports on numbers of men raised, wished to discover how greatly sickness and desertion eroded these numbers.[4] It was one thing to quantify this problem; quite another to solve it. In May 1744, the Admiralty wished to know the reason for 'so extraordinary a sickness' at Gosport contract hospital and on the *Blenheim* hospital ship there, what the diseases were, their cause, and the possibility of the seamen's recovery. The Sick and Hurt Board were unable to answer these questions. They did not consider that anything 'extraordinary or epidemic' had occurred. While certain ships were more sickly than others, only those on board knew the reasons for this, the Commissioners did not pretend to know why. The sickness was already declining and of 1,337 men sick ashore, only 391 were very ill.[5]

From the 1730s, but increasingly in the next two decades, the logic of establishing large hospitals run by the Navy, and producing answers to such questions, therefore grew stronger. Sick seamen ashore were traditionally housed in sick quarters, hired by the Board through their local agents. These quarters were often in unsuitable private houses or inns, where drink prevented cures and from where men easily deserted, or in buildings run by a contractor who supplied the furniture, medicines, nurses, and food for an agreed price. Many complaints concerning these quarters: of ill treatment, dirt, over-crowding, the lack of medical care and of provision of a suitable invalid diet, and the mixing together of men with different complaints – swell the correspondence of the Board. The bulk of such complaints was chiefly from naval officers who objected to these abuses and the wastage of seamen as a result, and thought the civilians who ran the system corrupt and inefficient. Those working in the system saw it differently. Sir James Barclay, one of the doctors at Gosport, censured for his lack of care of seamen in 1740, declared in his defence, that the Dockyard Commissioner and all the captains at Portsmouth wanted a naval hospital and for this reason they painted as black a picture as possible of the sick quarters there.[6] But complaints were too often justified, and flaws in the existing system, notably inadequate space in hired quarters, often hampered recovery.[7] The major barrier to building naval hospitals was cost – a powerful one in the Walpole era – and the fact that a permanent naval hospital would be permanently more expensive than temporary lodgings for the sick. There was no major war between 1714 and 1744 and both the Treasury and the Admiralty hoped these temporary structures and organisations would suffice to deal with emergencies. Continued war eventually dispelled that hope but it died hard. The epidemic of 1739–41 overwhelmed the existing services and encouraged the Admiralty to question whether the contract system could provide proper care. By April 1740, it was considering building its own hospitals and the Sick and Hurt Board confirmed this would be cheaper than dealing with contractors. Nothing was done until 1745, when Parliament granted an initial £12,000 to build a naval hospital at Portsmouth and Haslar hospital was begun. Baugh has called Haslar 'a monument to the disasters of 1740 and 1741' and the beginning of the era of permanent naval hospitals.[8] So it was. Partly occupied in 1754, by 1760 it was already holding 1,300 men and although annual salary costs were then approximately £1500, an enlargement of staff numbers was being sought. When it was finished in 1761 it was, and remained for some years, the largest brick building in Europe and had cost over £100,000, enough to build three battleships.[9] This is convincing proof of the Navy's commitment to providing better health care, but there was also a considerable hospital building programme in the next two decades. A new hospital was begun at Stonehouse, near Plymouth, in 1758, built on a pavilion system, the first of its kind in Britain, which encouraged the free circulation of air and allowed wards to be isolated. Temporary accommodation for one hundred sick seamen was ready two years later, and the total number planned for was 1,200. In 1761, there were proposals for a new hospital at Antigua, an upgrading of the existing hospital at Jamaica and additional medical establishments were proposed for Barbadoes, Halifax, Minorca and Gibraltar.[10] All these facilities witness to the successful growth of empire and its cost in health as much as to advances in health care. Since the building and maintenance of naval hospitals abroad was often difficult and expensive, the system of contract hospitals was continued to supplement naval hospitals there. Sick quarters at home and overseas were also not totally abandoned, for this was a gradual process both administratively and in terms of how the naval authorities saw health care. The earlier system's prime function had been to remove sick men from ships (where they could not be properly cared for) before they could infect others. The system implicit in the building of naval hospitals was to preserve lives and restore health, while controlling desertion through greater security.

The commitment to naval hospitals, even the complaints they provoked, reveals a desire to achieve the best possible health care for seamen and some idea of a standard to which to aspire. Again and again, phrases urging that seamen are 'carefully and diligently looked after' and 'all caution be taken for using them well... for effecting their speedy recovery', or 'the doing right to the seamen and preventing such hardships to them and clamours and trouble upon the service', can be found in official letters. This seems to me more than a trite formula, parroted by officials who had no intention of implementing it.[11] The Admiralty and the Sick and Hurt Board always responded to complaints about the lack of medical care, ill treatment or deliberate neglect of sick seamen and poor or inadequate food, partly in the spirit of the age of benevolence, increasingly apparent as the century progressed, but also as a matter of enlightened self-interest, as throughout the century the Navy required more and more men to man more and larger ships worldwide.

The Sick and Hurt Board was not a research institute. Yet the commissioners and their agents speculated on causes of sickness and discussed and sometimes initiated experiments to improve health. So far, I have discovered twenty-five offers of cures for or alleviations of conditions or disease; thirteen cures for scurvy were offered between 1771 and 1782 alone. These numbers do not include suggestions for improvements in preserving food or obtaining fresh food, which might lead to improvements in health. A selection of some of these cures and alleviations, offered to the Sick and Hurt Board, will illustrate their range, and the Board's response.[12] Thus, in 1752, when the Admiralty ordered an experiment to be made in ships on the efficacy of Dr James's powders to cure inflammatory fevers, 'to make a rational judgement' if they were for the good of the service, the Board suggested testing them instead in naval hospitals at home. Reports from surgeons abroad were uncertain and the regular monthly accounts from the home-based surgeons could be more accurately monitored.[13] They permitted Mr Lee's experiments involving different types of trusses on ten Greenwich pensioners with severe cases of rupture, in 1751. Lee's method of tight bandaging led to disputes between him and the hospital medical staff. The Board considered a cure very difficult, even for a young man who had been ruptured, especially 'if he is obliged to labour, as all foremast men are on board, particularly either in spreading a yard, getting anchors up, tacks on board or sheets aft'.[14] Since the majority of ruptured seamen would have been unable to perform the necessary heavy work of a ship and were at least partially disabled, the Board were anxious to find some alleviation of a serious problem. Between 1746 and 1748, 1366 trusses had been supplied to seamen at a cost of £303.[15] In 1782, Mr Brand, a surgeon at Greenwich Hospital, proposed the introduction of elastic trusses and was supported by Admiral Rodney; John Hunter, the famous surgeon; and the surgeon and physician at the hospital, John Hossack and William Taylor; who had all found them efficacious.[16] But the Surgeons Company, whom the Board consulted after seeking advice from the surgeons of St Thomas's, Guy's and St Bartholemew's hospitals, thought traditional steel trusses best. In 1772, the Board, under Admiralty direction, ordered trials of carrot marmalade as a cure for scurvy on *HMS Resolution* and *Adventure*, commanded by Captain James Cook on his second voyage to the southern seas. On Cook's return, a report of the trials was to be sent to the Admiralty.[17] In 1747, Mr Neeler had offered medicinal belts, rolls of canvas stuffed with a dried herbal mixture, which he claimed would cure scurvy and the itch and prevent vermin. The Board ordered a trial, perhaps with memories of recent fever epidemics in mind, but the belts proved useless against scurvy and only partially effective against the itch and vermin. Men wearing them caught colds when they discarded them and sometimes became entangled in the rigging, so trials were stopped the following year. Fifty years later, in December 1796, Dr Wilkinson suggested servicemen in the West Indies should wear his herbal stomacher, a canvas belt inter-lined with tobacco, rue and camphor, to prevent and cure infectious diseases, particularly yellow fever, then decimating men in the West Indian campaigns of 1795–6. Wilkinson claimed that those wearing the stomacher would breathe in an anti-pestilential vapour and that medicinal effluvia would be absorbed through the skin. But the Board rejected Wilkinson's offer as impractical and refused a trial.[18] In 1782, James Rymer, a naval surgeon, concerned by the lack of tourniquets in battle, which caused many men to bleed to death, offered a new type he had invented which, when applied, did not slip or slacken, and the Admiralty asked the Board to investigate these claims.[19] In 1795 John Robertson offered, as a cure for flux, a mixture of soap, sugar and rum, which the Admiralty directed the Board to try on patients at Haslar hospital in February. Two weeks later, trials were extended to the hospitals at Forton and Portchester Castle in the Portsmouth area, containing prisoners-of-war. The results were almost uniformly fatal and the trials were discontinued in April.[20]

But in general. the Board was concerned with dealing with the common illnesses and diseases which afflicted seamen. What were these? Apart from battle wounds, generally handled with skill and speed, seamen suffered from scurvy, dysentery, gravel, rheumatism, rupture, ulcers, fevers such as typhus, malaria and yellow fever, smallpox, depression, madness, and venereal disease. Some of these were the consequences of diet, of working conditions and lifestyle; some, the foreign fevers particularly, of place of work and the extension of empire. Apart from battle wounds, many of these complaints were not so different from those which afflicted their contemporaries ashore. The alleviation or prevention of these diseases could be secured by better ventilation; an avoidance of over-crowding; better, and better-preserved, food; clean, warm clothing; and a warm, dry atmosphere. None of these requirements were medical solutions in themselves. All were quite difficult to achieve in the eighteenth-century navy.

The Royal Navy practised preventive medicine, often successfully and frequently founded on careful observation by its surgeons and physicians. The emphasis on cleanliness rightly identified dirt with disease, without always discovering specific carriers or reasons for it. The contemporary belief in foul air as a cause of disease made cleanliness and ventilation of first importance and British ships were kept as clean as possible. The upper decks were washed daily; the lower decks where men lived, regularly. In many ships the external sides were washed regularly too. Specific orders forbad men to use the hold or cable tiers as lavatories, though lavatory accommodation – the heads, in the bows of the ship, floored with gratings so that the sea could help to cleanse them – was cold, wet, and insufficient, especially when dysentery attacked a crew.[21] Adequate ventilation, another problem in ships, was partially solved by Dr Hales' pump, a hand-powered pump which forced air through tubes to the lowest decks. It was first introduced in 1747 by Admiral Boscawen, whose wife was a family connection of Hales, and more widely introduced in 1756.[22] Fumigation to destroy contagion and purify the air was another pre-occupation of naval officers, achieved by washing decks, with vinegar, carefully lighting fires in the hold and between decks and placing pots of burning sulphur between decks. In 1796, the Sick and Hurt Board tried Dr Carmichael Smyth's methods of fumigation, unfortunately not clearly described but containing nitrous acid, at the naval hospital at Deal and in the *Union* hospital ship at Sheerness, which was suffering from an outbreak of typhus, with some success.[23]

While all this had some effect, especially in larger ships of seventy-four guns and upwards and with complements ranging from 650 to 950 men, over-crowding was a fact of life. Sailors were allowed 14 inches of sleeping room. At sea, thanks to the watch system, when part of the crew was on duty at given times, this became twenty-eight inches, but it was not spacious.

> On the same deck with me, when the crew was complete, slept between five and six hundred men; and the ports being necessarily closed from evening to morning, the heat in this cavern of only six feet high, and so entirely filled with human bodies, was overpowering.[24]

Robert Wilson's description of life between decks in a warship in 1800 clearly illustrates the need for cleanliness, ventilation, and fumigation when hundreds of 'frowsty carnivores' were sleeping together in a sealed box, a potential breeding ground for contagious diseases. Little or nothing could be done about this. That was how ships were designed and how seamen lived in them.

For much of the century, sick seamen were confined in a sick-berth, which was often part of the lower deck, curtained off but not otherwise segregated, difficult to access, and with little air. Sometimes they were placed near the galley because it was thought the smoke was helpful for some diseases, but this belief was discredited by 1793. Admiralty regulations only recommended the most airy part of the ship in accordance with current views on the beneficial effects of pure air. The major change came in the late 1790s, when Captain Markham, later one of the Admiralty commissioners, introduced a new type of sick-berth on his ship *HMS Centaur*, moving it from the lower to the upper deck on the starboard side, under the forecastle, and partitioned it off to isolate the sick men. This gave more light and air and access to the roundhouse or lavatory. In 1798 Admiral Lord St Vincent ordered this type of sick-berth to be adopted throughout the Mediterranean fleet and extended it to the Channel fleet in 1800, when he commanded there. Yet no Admiralty regulations enforced this in the navy as a whole.[25]

Personal hygiene for sailors was always difficult. Some captains insisted on men changing their linen as regularly as possible, others did not. There was always a shortage of fresh water, and though seamen did wash their clothes in salt water, this was unsatisfactory. The crew of *HMS Reunion* complained that:

> Captain Baynham also obliges us to wash our linen twice a week in salt water and to put two shirts on every week and if they do not look as clean as if they were washed in fresh water he stops the person's grog.[26]

Soap was not a standard issue until the end of the century when Admiral Lord St Vincent introduced it into the Mediterranean fleet in February 1796, for sick-berths, and more generally in September.

Common seamen had no official uniform until the nineteenth century and most naval officers and surgeons agreed that the clothes new recruits came in, often dirty and louse-ridden, were a source of infection. If men had been pressed, they had spent some time, perhaps weeks, crammed with others in a receiving ship. After William Pitt's Quota Acts of 1795, many men came from jails. All carried with them any infection contracted in these places. Once entered on a particular ship's books and actually on board, men were clothed, but not before, for fear they would desert and sell their new clothes. The problem of manning, of holding onto men, even if infected, thus had its impact on naval health. Men were also provided with a hammock and mattress. For most of the century flock mattresses were used, often stuffed with old rags or re-used flock, frequently mouldy. In 1743, the Sick and Hurt Board suggested the use of hair mattresses as more healthy, but there was a problem over the supply and cost of suitable animal hair, which came from abroad, so hair mattresses were not introduced until the 1790s, and were not standard issue to all ships until St Vincent became first Lord of the Admiralty in 1801.[27]

Most authorities agreed that warm, dry clothing preserved seamen from many ailments and advocated the use of flannel. Both Admiral St Vincent, Commander-in-Chief of the Channel fleet in 1800, and Dr Thomas Trotter, physician to that fleet, strongly supported seamen wearing flannel, though since both were stubborn and self-opinionated men, they quarrelled about the method of use. St Vincent ordered flannel worn next to the skin. Trotter insisted that cotton or linen should be worn next the skin for cleanliness.

Advocates of good practice could disagree but in such disagreements, and in all that concerned the life and health of the crew, the views of the naval officer generally prevailed. One reason for this was the low status of ships' surgeons. They were not commissioned but warrant officers. That is, they did not hold the King's commission, issued by the Admiralty, which conferred gentility, but a warrant, issued by the subordinate Navy Board, which classed them with masters, carpenters, boatswains and gunners, who, for much of the century, were more highly paid and frequently more highly regarded as being essential to the ship. Surgeons could not walk the quarter deck with other officers and gentlemen; until 1805 they had no distinguishing uniform.[28] The surgeon of *HMS Prince George*, Admiral Digby's flagship, on passage to North America in 1781, was never invited to dine with the admiral during the voyage, though all the lieutenants, midshipmen, master's mates, and other officers were. These distinctive marks of gentility were important in the intensely hierarchical naval society in which ships' surgeons lived.[29]

A surgeon's pay, often in arrears, was low; £5 a month at the beginning of the century and only a few shillings more in 1780, when surgeons petitioned, unsuccessfully, for an increase. A half pay system was introduced in 1729 but only for two hundred senior naval surgeons. Before receiving his warrant, a surgeon was orally examined by the Company of Barber Surgeons, or, after 1745 by the Surgeons' Company at Surgeons' Hall, but only in surgery, not in physic, though as a ship's doctor he had to practice both.[30] The comments of the Sick and Hurt Board's surgeon and agent at Bristol in June 1740 illustrate the difficulties that could result from this division. Edward French had been dealing with an outbreak of typhus amongst the crew of *HMS Bristol*, then in the port of Bristol, caring for 180 of the sick put ashore, twenty of whom had died of the infection. French thought it fortunate for the crew that he had the advantage:

> [W]hich very few of my profession have; for being a City Physician here, frequent opportunities have occurr'd to me of seeing the same Sickness in our Prisons which not only gave me more Courage in venturing among the Men, but also made me much less at a loss how to manage the Distemper, for it was in all its Symptoms the Gaol Fever.[31]

Every surgeon also had to provide a chest containing medicines at his own expense. This was examined at Apothecaries' Hall and sealed before the surgeon came on board. From 1796, some drugs were provided free by government and from 1804, all drugs were so provided, but the surgeon still had to provide his own instruments.[32] The result of this niggardly financial provision, the lack of status and the hazards of the job meant that there were never enough surgeons for all ships to carry one, with inevitable consequences for seamen's health. The quality of surgeons undoubtedly varied throughout the century. Some were brutal, uncaring, and unqualified, like that of *HMS Pompée*, according to Admiral Lord St Vincent 'a butcher of men and I impute the deaths of all who have been lost to the King's service in the *Pompée* to him'.[33] But there were also men of ability and concern. James Anthony Gardner, a naval officer serving between 1783 and 1814, recalled many of the surgeons he had known. Though some were 'mad with drink' or 'crabbed as the devil', he noted others as 'highly respected' and 'the first to relieve those in distress'. Gardner served with Thomas Trotter and considered him 'a most excellent fellow with first rate abilities' so his judgement may be taken as sound.[34]

One important factor in preserving the health of seamen was the supply of sufficient good food. The Navy recognised this and produced a diet, which though monotonous, was better than most working people ate ashore. Sailors were supplied weekly with seven pounds of bread, seven gallons of beer, four pounds of beef and two of pork, six ounces of butter and six of cheese, three pints of oatmeal and two pints of peas. Of necessity, much of this food was preserved, but when possible fresh food was introduced for variety and health. An order of 1703 to victual ships returning from the West Indies with fresh provisions in lieu of salt for ten days, for the health of seamen and to provide fresh food to all ships in port for a stated number of weekdays for the same purpose, illustrates the connection had been made between feeding men too long on salt provisions and illness. But the economic and logistic implications, and problems of such orders were considerable. In 1704, the Victualling Board, the subordinate naval department responsible for supplying the navy with food and drink, was contemplating having to provide supplies regularly for forty thousand men and their anxious response to Admiralty orders reveal the complexity of the problems they faced. Seamen were quick to complain about poor or inadequate provisions and complaints about bad beer and poorly baked bread, provided by private contractors, which gave rise to sickness amongst seamen in 1706, resulted in the establishment of naval bake, and brew-houses at Portsmouth and Plymouth, at an estimated cost of £20,000, 'to set the Contractors a standard for the goodness of the provisions'.[35] The Sick and Hurt Board introduced portable soup, beef stock dried into cakes or slabs and reconstituted with water, in the middle of the century, at first for sick seamen only. Fresh vegetables were often added to it to make a nourishing and popular broth, and its use was extended in the 1750s to seamen going abroad. In 1773, the Board was ordered to supply it to healthy seamen when no fresh provisions were available in the East Indies; finally it was issued to all seamen. Whenever possible fresh vegetables were issued, though regular supply proved difficult and logistical problems remained throughout the century. Attempts were made to preserve vegetables without using salt, to retain their essence and health-giving properties. In 1777, the Victualling Board was offered a scheme to make a preserve of turnips, similar to the preserved cabbage or sauerkraut used against scurvy. Ten tons were made as an experiment, tasted by the Board and found good and put on victualling transports for New York to see if it kept and whether it was as useful as the preserved cabbage.[36] Admiral Lord Howe recommended, in 1782, an invention of John Grafen, dried and preserved kale, to the Admiralty. Experiments had been made in the Channel fleet when he was Commander-in-Chief, by which small quantities of the kale, added with barley and shallots to portable soup made 'a grateful and nourishing food for convalescents'.[37] Not all preparations were so harmless. In 1774, Henry Phillips proposed a varnish of cinnabar, a compound of mercury and sulphur, with which to paint ships' bread rooms, casks, and bread bags, which would destroy vermin and preserve bread. But the Victualling Board were not sure how safe this compound was and as it cost seven shillings per pound, they thought the expense too great and declined the offer.[38]

It was not merely the difficulty of preserving food; indeed, given the amounts handled, food storage was quite successful.[39] Nor were the considerable problems of actually finding and buying fresh meat, lemons or cabbages in foreign countries, where the British contractor often faced an unfavourable exchange rate, the only difficulties.[40] There remained the task of getting such supplies to the fleets in all seasons and weathers and against other hazards. In December 1804, *HMS Tribune* pressed two men out of a naval victualling transport, bringing provisions for the Mediterranean fleet, and refused to give them up. The crews of such transports were, theoretically, exempt from pressing, but *Tribune* was short of men and her captain's necessity knew no law. Yet if this practice went unchecked, crews would not be found for transports and the whole provisioning system would grind to a halt and food supplies would run short with consequent effects on the health of seamen. In this case the Commander-in-Chief, Admiral Nelson, was asked to intervene. Even he was not always able to command success. Captain Boyle of *HMS Seahorse*, who pressed the second mate of the *Berwick* transport at Gibraltar in January 1804, was still finding excuses not to give up such a useful seaman in March 1805.[41]

Much then, depended on the attitudes of captains of ships and commanders of fleets. Most officers were concerned with the health of their men and some made suggestions or tried experiments to improve or preserve it. Captain Robert Harland had asked to be supplied with Neeler's medicinal belts when these were first tried, 'being glad to use every expedient to preserve the health of my people.'[42] As the century progressed, many captains reported the beneficial effect of citrus fruits on the health of seamen. Some were more actively concerned, like Captain Roger Curtis, who in 1794 published a pamphlet on the eradication of fever from *HMS Brunswick* in 1791. Captain Francs Austen, Jane Austen's brother, recommended the whitewashing of cheeses, to preserve them from insects and waste, to the Victualling Board in November 1801. Vice-Admiral Gambier had suggested this method of preservation and Austen decided to try an experiment. He ordered a number of cheeses for his ship, *HMS Neptune*, from Plymouth. After drying them well in the sun he had them whitewashed and put on racks in the bread room or repacked in casks and stowed in the afterhold. The results were excellent. Every whitewashed cheese remained perfectly dry and free from insects. Those cheeses not so treated, though also placed on racks, became moist, rotten and full of vermin, lost weight and were less wholesome and nutritious.

Though the various boards received these suggestions, they did not always adopt them. Admiral Sir Charles Hardy's suggestion of December 1780, to the governing council of Haslar hospital, that rows of lime and elm trees should be planted around the hospital to provide shelter from the high winds and 'to meliorate the air' the better to cure 'those diseases which originate from the sea' was declined; the Sick and Hurt Board thought of no particular benefit and that trees would not survive on such an exposed site.[43] Officers could also delay improvements. In 1760, the Sick and Hurt Board confessed to the Admiralty that they had long thought the sick were deprived of the benefits of portable soup by the disinclination of pursers and others to issue and keep an account of it. The reason pursers did not demand 'what they themselves allow to be the best thing introduced aboard ship for the use of the sick' was the long-winded process of passing the accounts and the affidavits required. So the pursers often urged their captains, successfully, not to demand the soup, and the Board begged the Admiralty to enforce the orders to commanders of ships to ask for portable soup when fitting for sea. The Admiralty promptly complied, directing the Board to report to them who did and who did not ask for the soup.[44]

Conclusion

Naval health and health care had improved by the end of this period. Sick rates amongst serving seamen had fallen, from one man in 2.45 in 1779 to 1 in 10.75 by 1813 and death rates for the same years from 1 man in 42, to 1 man in 143.[45] Advances in medicine had not played much part in this. Though scurvy had been largely eliminated through dietary improvements, smallpox could be contained by vaccination, and there was some success against malaria through the issue of quinine mixed with wine, the causes and thus the cures of most seamen's illnesses and diseases, particularly the fevers, were still unknown at the end of the period. The real advances had been in hygiene, improved diet, and the more regular provision of clean, warm clothing.

Peter Mathias has attributed the success of measures to promote health and curb disease to the authoritarian regimes to which enforced them, found uniquely in the late-eighteenth-century British Army and Royal Navy. But the eighteenth-century Navy was not a single authoritarian structure. What may be considered 'local regimes' in the Navy behaved in a somewhat comparable way to those contemporary civilian authorities Mathias describes as resisting 'centralising forces and the authoritarian pressure of professional opinion' so making 'the gap between knowledge and effective compulsory action... very wide'.[46] With regard to seamen's health, much was left to the individual initiative of admirals or captains, particularly on distant stations where central naval bureaucratic control was weak, especially at the beginning of the period. Only as that control increased, as Admiralty power grew and the individual power of naval officers over their crews and squadrons correspondingly lessened, did it become possible to impose greater uniformity in health care, as in matters of discipline and manning. The slow growth in the professional status of the surgeon within the naval hierarchy also helped this shift in power and attitude. But admirals were in overall command and physicians and surgeons, however distinguished, were subordinate to them. As yet, it is difficult to say how considerable and significant was the role of individual naval officers in the promotion of seamen's health. The part played by Admirals Rodney, Howe, and St Vincent in introducing and implementing reforms affecting health are well documented. The papers of other officers may reveal a similar story.

There was plenty of opportunity for experiment in an authoritarian community like the navy. Such experiments, often in the controlled conditions of hospitals and ships, were driven by a desire to achieve the essential result of an improvement in health, which would solve the manning problem.[47] Though the experiments of surgeons and physicians – such as Lind, Blane and Trotter – were based on a belief in the efficacy of the scientific method, this was never predominant in the calculations of the Sick and Hurt Board, particularly during the first half of the eighteenth century when it was dominated by non-medical administrators. Even when doctors formed a majority on the Board, that Board was still subject to Admiralty authority, which was moved by a number of competing considerations, not merely those of health. The pre-eminent imperative of manning the Navy drove the Sick and Hurt Board to preventive medicine rather than to discovering the causes of disease. There was no time for such research in the imminence of ensuring national defence, planning campaigns or dealing with everyday war-time emergencies which pressed relentlessly upon the naval authorities. Thus, time lags between invention or discovery and implementation were, necessarily, often considerable, and Mathias illustrates how 'medical ignorance... blunted the edge of preventive measures as well as preventing cures' quoting Lind's advocacy of boiling citrus fruit down to a 'rob' as a cure for scurvy and by that process destroying most of the fruit's vitamin content.[48] Moreover captains and others could be careless or indifferent about obeying regulations. Some thought better health care 'spoiled' the men, perhaps particularly after the mutinies of 1797 which shook the mutual trust between officers and men. Nor was it always possible under war conditions to get supplies of lemon juice or soap or adequate clothing, to avoid fever-ridden conditions, to find a source of clean drinking water or to avoid running out of all medical supplies before deliveries arrived from home.

Much then, remained to be done. At times the balance between success and failure was precarious and the warship of *c.*1800 was still, potentially, the engine of disease it had been in 1700. Yet overall, the health of seamen had improved throughout the century, and while advances in medicine may not have had much to do with this improvement, those advances that had been made, based on observations and experience, had begun to form a sound basis for nineteenth-century progress in public as well as in naval health.

Notes

1. N.A.M. Rodger, *The Wooden World: An Anatomy of the Georgian Navy* (London: Collins, 1986), 98; J.S. Tucker, *Memoirs of Admiral the Right Honourable the Earl of St. Vincent*, 2 vols (London: R. Bentley, 1844), Vol. 2, 31.

2. The National Archives [hereafter NA], ADM1/3528, *Sick and Hurt Board to Admiralty*, 25 September 1740; National Maritime Museum [hereafter NMM], ADM/F/11, *Sick and Hurt Board to Admiralty*, 6 March 1754 enclosing reports by Schomberg and James.

3. NA, ADM1/3528, *Sick and Hurt Board to Admiralty*, 10 October 1740, enclosures 1, 3, 6; NMM, ADM/E/11, *Admiralty to Sick and Hurt Board*, for similar queries in November 1744.

4. D.A. Baugh, *British Naval Administration in the Age of Walpole* (Princeton: Princeton University Press, 1965), 179, 206 *et seq.*

5. NMM, ADM/E/11, *Admiralty to Sick and Hurt Board*, 19 May 1744; ADM/F/4, *Sick and Hurt Board to Admiralty*, 20 June 1744.

6 . NA, ADM1/3528, *Sick and Hurt Board to Admiralty*, 1 May 1740 enclosing Barclay's letter to the Board of 28 April. Complaints were speedily investigated in Britain by personal visits from the Sick and Hurt commissioners. This was impossible abroad and here the Board relied on the inspections and reports of naval officers, not always in sympathy with shore

based civilian bureaucrats and their problems.

7. A large house in Plymouth, bought in 1694 as a prison, later served as a hospital for sick seamen ashore but could only accommodate 165 men. NA, ADM1/3528, *Sick and Hurt Board to Admiralty*, 26 October 1733.

8. Baugh, *op. cit.* (note 4), 51.

9. NMM, ADM/F/20, *Sick and Hurt to Admiralty*, 7 February 1760; Rodger, *op. cit.* (note 1), 110.

10. NMM, ADM/F/21, *Sick and Hurt Board to Admiralty*, 7 March 1761; ADM/F/22, *Sick and Hurt Board to Admiralty*, 'An Account of Officers and Employments existing... in the Department of the Office for Sick and Wounded Seamen... also the Names and Salaries of Officers in that Department as they stood on the 5 January 1779'.

11. NMM, ADM/E/1, *Admiralty to Sick and Hurt Board*, f. 175, 9 January, f. 295, 3 June 1703. There are many similar expressions throughout the correspondence.

12. I hope to examine these offers in a later article. Major gaps in the Sick and Hurt Board's records at the National Maritime Museum prevent me tracing the results of some of these trials at present. It will be possible to follow them through the Board's minutes and letters, held at the National Archive and not yet consulted.

13. NMM, ADM/F/11, *Sick and Hurt Board to Admiralty*, 8 December 1752. An Admiralty minute of 22 December on the reverse of the letter agrees.

14. *Ibid.*, *Sick and Hurt Board to Admiralty*, 9 March and 3 July 1752, 5 March 1753.

15. *Ibid.*, 3 April 1752. The authorities provided steel trusses at the inadequate rate of five per one hundred men. In March 1744, although one truss was issued free to men already ruptured, if a second truss was required it was charged, at half a guinea, against the man's wages. The Board urged that when men were wearing trusses they should not 'be obliged to hand or reef because the pressure they must meet with in that service would be very apt to force the intestines into the scrotum notwithstanding the trusses'. ANM/E/11, *Sick and Hurt Board to Admiralty*, 1 March 1744.

16. NMM, ADM/E/43, *Admiralty to Sick and Hurt Board*, 9 January 1782, enclosing the letters of Rodney, Hunter, Hosack, and Taylor, 4–7 December 1781. Rodney also wrote a long memorandum to the Admiralty, one of many on seamen's health, on the difficulties caused by rupture. He was preparing to take command in the West Indies and was taking Dr Gilbert Blane with him as his personal physician and physician to his squadron. D. Spinney, *Rodney* (London: George Allen and Unwin, 1969), 384.

17. The recipe had been sent to the Society for the Encouragement of Arts, Manufacture and Commerce by their corresponding member in Berlin, Baron Stosch, who had tried it, successfully, on the peasants of his estates.

They forwarded it to the Admiralty who sent copies to the Victualling and Sick and Hurt Boards. NMM, ADM/G/785, *Admiralty to Victualling Board,* 25 November 1771, ADM/E/41, *Admiralty to Sick and Hurt Board,* 20 January 1772.

18. NMM, ADM/E/12, *Admiralty to Sick and Hurt Board,* 15 October, 11 December 1747, 24 May, 27 December 1748, ADM/E/45, *Admiralty to Sick and Hurt Board,* 8 December 1796, enclosing Wilkinson to Admiralty of 21 September 1796. Wilkinson argued that in the Great Plague of London, 1665, it was well known that the houses of druggists and tobacconists had all escaped infection.

19. NMM, ADM/E/43, *Admiralty to Sick and Hurt Board,* 14 October 1782 containing Rymer's letter to the Admiralty of 11 October.

20. NMM, ADM/E/45, *Admiralty to Sick and Hurt Board,* 16 and 27 February; 2 April 1795.

21. B. Lavery, *Nelson's Navy: The Ships, Men and Organisation 1793–1815* (London: Conway, 1989), 200–1, 203, 207.

22. Rodger, *op. cit.* (note 1), 106–7.

23. NMM, ADM/E/45, *Admiralty to Sick and Hurt Board,* 16 February, 14 March 1796. See the letter of Mr Bassan, surgeon of the *Union* to Dr Smyth, 'The dejection and melancholy occasioned by the dread of the disease prior to the trying the experiment was evident in every countenance and really affecting and distressing, but the circumstance of its being stopped at present has diffused joy and cheerfulness and all look forward with hopes and expectation of soon becoming a wholesome ship.' ADM/E/45, 7 December 1795 enclosed in *Admiralty to Sick and Hurt Board,* 10 December.

24. Lavery, *op. cit.* (note 21), 207.

25. *Ibid.,* 213–14.

26. *Ibid.,* 204.

27. NMM, ADM/F/3, *Sick and Hurt Board to Admiralty,* 24 March 1743.

28. J.J. Keevil, C. Lloyd and J.L.S. Coulter, *Medicine and the Navy 1200–1900,* 4 vols (Edinburgh and London: E and S Livingstone, 1961), Vol. 3, 10–11. The right to appoint surgeons was transferred from the Navy to the Sick and Hurt Board in July 1796; ADM/E/45, *Admiralty to Sick and Hurt Board,* 29 July 1796.

29. B. Lavery (ed.), *Shipboard Life and Organisation, 1731–1815,* Navy Records Society, Vol. 138 (Aldershot: Ashgate, 1998), 613.

30. Keevil, *et al., op. cit.* (note 28), Vol. 2, 278–81.

31. NA, ADM1/3528, *Sick and Hurt Board to Admiralty,* 2 July 1740 enclosing French's letter to Board of 18 June.

32. Keevil, *et al., op. cit.* (note 28), Vol. 3, 10–16.

33. St Vincent to Dr Blane, 24 July 1800, in Tucker, *op. cit.* (note 1), Vol. 2, 84–5.

34. R. Vesey Hamilton and J.K. Laughton (eds), *Recollections of James Anthony Gardner, R.N* (London: Navy Records Society, 1906), Vol. 31, 63, 53, 39, 248, 91.

35. NMM, ADM/G/773, *Admiralty to Victualling Board*, fo.126r-v, 27 October 1703; fo.131r-v, 22 December 1703; fo.132r-v, 6 January 1704; ADM/D/2, *Victualling Board to Admiralty*, 23 December 1703; ADM/D/5, *Victualling Board to Admiralty*, 20 December 1706, 17 January, 8 February 1707.

36. NMM, ADM/DP/109, *Victualling Board to Admiralty*, 7 July 1777; ADM/G/787, *Admiralty to Victualling Board*, 14 July 1777.

37. NMM, ADM/E/43, *Admiralty to Sick and Hurt Board*, 16 August 1782 enclosing Howe's letter of 22 July 1782.

38. NMM, ADM/DP/106, *Victualling Board to Admiralty*, 2 February 1774.

39. Rodger, *op. cit.* (note 1), 85.

40. An outbreak of scurvy in the winter of 1804/5, affecting 260 men in the Mediterranean fleet by April 1805, was caused by the closure of the Spanish provision market upon Spain's entry into the war as France's ally in December 1804. For several months it proved difficult to find alternative sources of fresh food, particularly lemon and orange juice. This illustrates how quickly the disease could establish itself if anti-scorbutics were absent. P. K. Crimmin, 'Letters and Documents Relating to the Service of Nelson's Ships, 1780–1805: A Critical Report', *Historical Research*, 70 (1997), 59.

41. *Ibid.*, 55.

42. NMM, ADM/E/12, *Harland to Admiralty*, 7 July 1746; I am grateful to Dr Margarette Lincoln for the Curtis reference.

43. NMM, AUS/7, *Letter Book of Captain Francis Austen 1801–1806, Austen to Victualling Board*, 18 November 1801; ADM/E/42, *Admiralty to Sick and Hurt Board*, 13 January 1780, *Sick and Hurt to Admiralty*, 8 December 1779.

44. NMM, ADM/F/21, *Sick and Hurt Board to Admiralty*, 3 December 1760, Admiralty minute 5 February 1761.

45. P. Mathias (ed.), 'Swords and Ploughshares: The Armed Forces, Medicine and Public Health in the Late Eighteenth Century,' *The Transformation of England: Essays in the Economic and Social History of England in the Eighteenth Century* (London: Methuen, 1979), 280.

46. *Ibid.*, 280-1.

47. Even in the controlled environment of the hospital, attempts at uniformity were subject to human nature. Hospital staff did not always obey regulations or were difficult to work with. Complaints against Mr Lott, Sick and Hurt Board agent at Plymouth in 1774, reveal a disruptive personality, quarrels, disobeyed orders, a constant source of animosities and arguments, with whom no-one would willingly work and who threatened to bring the work of the hospital to a halt, a serious matter if large numbers of men were

admitted. Lott was suspended by Admiralty order on 20 July and his deputy appointed in his place. NMM, ADM/FP/17, *Sick and Hurt Board to Admiralty*, 8 July 1774.

48. Mathias, *op. cit.* (note 45), 272.

8

The Medical Profession and Representations of the Navy, 1750–1815

Margarette Lincoln

This chapter focuses on the interrelationship between naval medicine and broader society, discussing medical representations of the Navy in the late-eighteenth century, and arguing that naval medicine was a matter of keen debate, perceived as important for the country. Navy servicemen were represented in contradictory ways: as a tool of empire, heroes deserving care for their service to their country, and a source of contagion and ill discipline in need of paternal attention from officers and medics.

Naval doctors and the public

Few authors writing about medicine and the sea in the eighteenth and early-nineteenth centuries have considered how medical discourses construct the objects of their enquiry in social terms. Such terms play little or no part in the seminal account of the development of naval medicine provided by C. Lloyd and J.S. Coulter; or in the detailed accounts by K.J. Carpenter, and others of the development of a cure for scurvy. The same might be said of discussions outlining the beginnings of institutional care during this period, although such studies do show how civilian hospitals played an important role in projecting images of civic well-being, philanthropy and medical 'progress'.[1] But it can be argued that medical discourse is always shaped by social assumptions – for example, about gender, or race, or class – which it tends to naturalise. I argue that discourses of naval medicine naturalised, and so helped to promote, particular assumptions about the Navy, which are supplementary to their immediate medical concerns. During the period 1750–1815, Britain was often at war and the Navy was high on the public agenda. The Navy was represented in a wide range of media, including paintings, ceramics, ballads, newspapers, sermons, and government propaganda. In these forms, an image of the Navy was constructed, often by different elements of society, to help shape public opinion. This study focuses on one strand of a much larger picture during a critical period of

201

national expansion, and concentrates on works of naval medicine and examples of public interest in the health of the Navy.

In the second half of the eighteenth century, doctors and men of science increasingly influenced public opinion by publishing their work in books and essays aimed at the polite reader.[2] The Navy offered excellent opportunities for medical observation – in wartime, on voyages of discovery or in experiments on crews. Medical writings helped to complicate the public image of the Navy, although those by naval surgeons were also products of their own desire for higher status. All warships carried surgeons.[3] These men had first-hand experience of both life at sea and the Navy as an institution, but in the eighteenth century they were often poorly trained and their status was low. As one handbook for naval surgeons made clear, they were expected to acquire much of their skill on the job, and were apt to view ships' crews as a testing ground. 'For common and general Parts of Surgery', wrote John Atkins in 1737, 'I know no better School to improve in, than the NAVY, especially in time of War. Accidents are frequent, and the Industrious illustrate Practice by their Cures.'[4] Later, they were better trained, but he status of naval surgeons was lower than that of army surgeons. They were often dissatisfied with the lack of respect shown them on board ship and with the class of men, with whom their assistants were forced to associate, below deck. Naval surgeons did not obtain officer status and a uniform until January 1805, and even afterwards they were still subordinate to lieutenants on the ships in which they served. Not surprisingly, naval surgeons were keen to improve their status and publication was one means to this end. Until surgeons' rank and salary improved in 1805, they were badly paid and subject to dismissal at the end of a war; some later achieved success in civilian practice but on the whole, their skills were lightly regarded ashore, partly because they had lacked opportunities to network.[5] In this period, works concerning naval medicine often reveal signs of tension between physicians and naval surgeons. In 1798, a well-trained doctor could still write dismissively of a surgeon's ability. 'It is a notorious truth, that at sea they amputate like the barbarians of Abyssinia; only with this difference, they use a knife instead of a hatchet.'[6] As late as 1808, a former naval surgeon was still complaining about the practice in the Army or Navy of accepting raw apothecaries' boys as hospital mates or assistant surgeons, 'whose whole education has been acquired, in the course of a year or two, behind the counter of some obscure apothecary or barber-surgeon'. Worse still, he thought some naval surgeons still performed operations 'in a way that would disgrace a farrier of any repute'.[7]

In the first half of the eighteenth century, there were several well-known treatises and guides for ship surgeons. It was recognised that crews on long voyages generally became ill, whether or not individuals met with accidents or were wounded in battle. The various causes of sickness were not well understood – there was no conception of vitamin deficiency or of germ theory – and in the course of the century, as Britain worked to achieve and maintain naval supremacy, shipboard diseases became a more pressing problem. It was the circumstances of Anson's expedition against Spain and circumnavigation in the 1740s, that drew particular attention to seamen's health.[8] Anson did manage to capture a Spanish treasure ship but during the course of his arduous commission, he lost over eighty per cent of his ships' company: four men from enemy action and over 1,300 from disease. After this tragedy, doctors scrutinised accounts of the voyage, searching for clues that would explain the level of sickness. The Admiralty considered fitting all warships with Samuel Sutton's machine for extracting foul air out of ships, but balked at the expense. The published account of Sutton's invention included a supporting 'Discourse on the Scurvy' by the King's own physician, the suave Dr Richard Mead, who maintained that foul air contributed to scurvy. He conceded that humanity alone might not prompt greater care for seamen's health but argued that considerations of policy, military success, and professional honour made such care advisable[9]. Mead's intervention itself suggests an element of self-interest; here was an opportunity for a prominent clinician to increase his standing by aligning himself and his profession with wider national aims.[10] A steady flow of publications on naval medicine followed the Anson episode, by doctors whose writing often suggests a comparable awareness of both their own and their readers' self-interest. In general handbooks and in essays on specific diseases or epidemics, they helped to bring the health of the Navy to the public's attention.

Of course, it is difficult to determine precisely who read these medical books, other than doctors themselves who regularly quoted each other; but clearly these works did not fall dead from the press. Of the contemporary books footnoted here, fifty per cent enjoyed a second edition and over thirty per cent three or more editions. Roy Porter and others have shown that in the eighteenth century, sufferers played an active role in managing their own state of health and turned to a variety of books, magazines and pamphlets for medical advice. Public-spirited, well-informed, responsible people were expected to have a general familiarity with medicine. For example, the surviving record of borrowings from the Bristol subscription library, 1773–84, shows that works of medicine and anatomy were provided for general readers. Popular publications instructed in medical self-help and played an important role in the diffusion of medical initiatives. This was the case with the *Gentleman's Magazine*, at least until 1810, or so when it began to report on the medical profession in a way that implied that the lay public would have little involvement in its activities. At its peak, the magazine had a circulation possibly of over 10,000 copies and far more readers. In its pages, medical books were both listed and reviewed, and readers shared information about specific ailments or wrote in to ask for particular advice. In 1767, for example, one correspondent described a home-made bandage as 'a method to cure, or at least prevent, the increase of any naval rupture', indicating the commonplace nature of such injuries at sea and the spirit of self-help that enabled sufferers to cope with such chronic ailments.[11] Editors of the magazine certainly felt that the health of seamen was of sufficiently broad interest to carry articles on the subject and also to justify the expense of including prints of Royal Naval Hospital, Haslar, Portsmouth.[12]

Naval health and the image of the seaman

A detailed examination of references to naval medicine in the *Gentleman's Magazine* during this period helps us to judge the extent of public interest in keeping crews healthy. In the mid-1750s there was substantial curiosity in the ventilation of ships. The Rev. Dr Hales, Clerk of the Closet to the Princess of Wales, suggested various means of introducing fresh air into the lower decks, which were reported with recommendations by ship's captains. Hales also published proposals for fumigating ships to rid them of infection. These proposals applied to merchant ships as well as naval vessels but vividly communicated to readers the claustrophobic, airless conditions below deck on warships and the importance of cleanliness to reduce disease.[13] The *Gentleman's Magazine* soon became a favoured means by which naval officers communicated to a wider public the useful health tips gleaned on longer voyages. A letter from the captain of the *Tyger* in 1755 'containing some few Observations that may be of public Service' was sent to the editor because it was felt these observations could not be better communicated 'than thro' the Channel of the Gentleman's Magazine'.[14] He wrote from St Augustin's Bay, Madagascar, and congratulated himself on keeping the ship's crew healthy. 'I have had about three fevers in the ship since I left *England*, which were occasioned by drinking great quantities of spirits at *Plymouth*, but Dr *James's* Powder soon removed these.'[15] The letter shows how, in passing on medical advice, a particular image of hard-drinking seamen could be reinforced. It also confirms that naval officers were often aware of recent works on naval medicine. The correspondent had ordered his ship's doctor to treat a severe case of scurvy according to the recommendations of Dr Antony Addington who wrote an essay on sea scurvy in 1753. He also expected his men to drink and bathe in sea water every day, leading by example himself, and believed that this had kept scurvy at bay. In 1760, the captain of the *Torbay* wrote to the *Gentleman's Magazine* from Plymouth Sound explaining that he had kept his ship healthy by enforcing cleanliness. He shamed men who were found to be dirty or to have sold their clothes for drink, fumigated the decks, and treated the few scorbutic cases on board with lemon juice.[16]

Issues related to naval medicine and the image of British seamen were actually debated in the *Gentleman's Magazine*. At the time of great public debate about the state of the Navy, following Admiral Byng's court martial for alleged cowardice and neglect of duty, one correspondent saw a link between scurvy and idleness in the Navy. He pointed out that scurvy was more prevalent in the Navy than in the merchantmen, even though warships were better ventilated from having gunports, and suggested that merchant seamen were fortunately obliged to keep up a healthy sweat necessary because their ships were less well manned. He wrote, 'it is well known in the navy, especially on board large ships, what numbers continually sculk [*sic*] below, and there indulge themselves in sleep and inactivity,' adding 'It is a doctrine, 'tis true, that will be in no ways agreeable to unthinking tars.'[17] The Editor was moved to disagree, pointing out the extent to which sailors suffered on Anson's circumnavigation and noting that the late Dr Richard Mead who had read accounts of the voyage and talked with Anson never mentioned inactivity as the cause. The Editor also referred to Mr Pascoe Thomas's account of the Anson voyage, which described how sailors suffering from scurvy, were falsely accused of idleness, and kicked and punched to do their duty when utterly incapable of it. This gives an insight into naval discipline of the time and the desperate situation that could result on board if the numbers of sick rose to the extent that there were too few seamen to work the ship.

In 1758, when the fleets were fitting out for long voyages, the *Gentleman's Magazine* printed Thomas Reynolds's proposals for the management of the sick in the Navy on the grounds that they had never been published before and might help to save lives. Reynolds, a former naval surgeon, recommended good food, warm clothes, and the paternal care of officers. In doing so, he conveyed an image of a navy prone to drunkenness – seamen, he argued, must be mustered regularly and forced to display their clothes to prevent them from selling them for drink. Reynolds also throws light on the kind of men who served in the Navy at that time and what drove them to sea. He commented that when seamen were dangerously ill:

[M]any of them reflect with great severity on their own misdoings, which brought them first to sea, and consequently into their present calamitous condition, being now under the fullest conviction that if they had regarded the admonitions of their parents and friends, and in obedience to their advice would have submitted to get their bread by honest judicious means, they might have lived a less hazardous as well as a more easy life in the midst of peace and plenty.[18]

In the 1760s and 1770s, while Britain was engaged in no major war, the *Gentleman's Magazine* carried less information about naval medicine, although general medicine was still a popular topic and, in particular, methods of smallpox inoculation attracted attention. By 1779, when the war with the American colonies was going badly, medical correspondents to the *Gentleman's Magazine* were advising general inoculation of the poor and citing the advantage to Britain's army and navy. 'The soldier and sailor [would] do service to their country without fear of being cut off in prime of life to the great loss and disappointment of the public.'[19] Military medicine features more strongly in the *Gentleman's Magazine* once more from the onset of the French Revolutionary Wars. In 1793, Dr Moseley's new edition of his *Treatise on Tropical Diseases* was welcomed as useful and important. 'Our distant colonies, our militia, our fleets, and armies, are under great obligation to this writer.'[20] In 1794, a correspondent warned readers against using any substitute for Dr James's Powders in the Tropics. The correspondent explained that when the Sick and Hurt Board had asked the College of Physicians in 1789 whether or not to supply warships with the less expensive *puvis antimonialis,* the College could only report that no trials had been conducted that allowed them to say it was any better.[21] While his prime purpose was to defend an established remedy against rival substances, the correspondent raises the public profile of naval health in the context of the cost of national defence and the progress of medicine. At this time, scurvy at sea once more becomes a matter for public debate. An inhabitant of Lincoln recommended the juice of goose-grass; earlier letters were cited blaming scurvy on putrid air and salt provisions. A 'Friend to the Navy' proposed that the Admiralty supply the root of the garden carrot, which was easily casked and less liable to spoil than lemon juice; another recommended instead 'small spirit of vitriol'.[22]

Medical findings, as they related to the Navy, were also frequently reported in *The Times*. On 1 December 1796, for example, readers were informed, 'Dr. CARMICHAEL SMITH's mode of stopping contagion, by nitrous fumigation, is now very properly adopted through the whole of the British Navy, and will certainly be productive of the most salutary consequences.' This piece refers to James Carmichael Smyth's book, published earlier that year, describing an experiment to reduce infection on board the *Union* hospital ship, which had docked at Sheerness with about 200 sick on board.[23] Such notices kept naval medicine firmly in the public eye – as did public disputes between doctors themselves. On 26 December 1807, for example, 'an Old Navy Surgeon' wrote to *The Times* refuting Dr Harness's claims to be responsible for the prevention of scurvy in the Navy by introducing lemon juice into men's rations. As the correspondent pointed out, it had first been necessary to discover how to preserve lemon juice – and

Figure 8.1

'Midshipman Blockhead, fitting out Mastr Willm Blockhead, HM Ship Hellfire, West India Station.' Produced by George Cruikshank (engraver) and Thomas McLean (Publisher), 1 August 1835.
© National Maritime Museum.

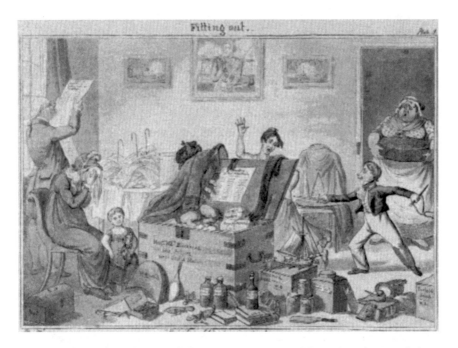

Dr Gilbert Blane discovered this as commissioner of the Sick and Wounded Board.

Seamen, their families, and all those who travelled by sea, naturally had a keen interest in finding out how to stay healthy on long voyages or in tropical climates. An appeal printed in five issues of *The Times* during 1794 illustrates the quality of this common interest and shows how patent medicines and the writing of naval surgeons were recommended to a wider reading public. The appeal is addressed 'particularly to the officers of the army and navy serving in the West Indies and other hot climates.' The writer explains that violent fevers in the West Indies have been fatal to many officers in the previous year and given serious alarm to the friends of those destined to serve there. He claims that doctors who have practised in that climate recommend James's Powders, and continues:

[F]or more positive proofs of its efficacy, reference may be had to Dr James's 'Dissertation on Fevers'; in which accounts are published from Surgeons of our ships, both in the *East* and *West Indies,* where the crews had been seized with violent malignant Fevers, and cured after other means had failed, by taking this medicine.[24]

The first print in George Cruickshank's series called 'The Progress of a Midshipman Exemplified in the Career of Master Blockhead', which was produced from sketches by Captain Frederick Marryat, suggests that naval families took this advice to heart or at least that it was well known. The print, shown in Figure 8.1, shows the fitting out of young Blockhead before he goes to sea. He is destined for the West Indies and his parents have remembered to put James's Powders into his sea chest. Clearly, medical works were relevant to the imperial enterprise, although after Trafalgar, the lack of references to the health of the Navy in the *Gentleman's Magazine* suggests that public interest in the topic slowly waned.

The scale of the Navy's health problem

The perspective of doctors writing about naval medicine changed and developed in the course of the eighteenth century, and successive publications helped to shape public understanding of this aspect of life at sea. Earlier books on naval medicine published in the 1750s may have been partly written to counteract the damning publicity given to naval surgeons in Tobias Smollett's *Roderick Random.*[25] The novel, which appeared in 1748, was a great success and remained popular for decades. Smollett's account of Admiral Vernon's disastrous attack on Cartagena and the death of thousands in the British fleet from yellow fever, was based on his own experience as a surgeon's mate and eye witness. A patriotic Scot with perhaps little sympathy for Britain's imperial mission, Smollett denounced Vernon's ability to lead, to carry out combined operations, and even to take proper responsibility for his men. Life on board was depicted as a stinking ordeal with little chance of survival if this depended on the ship's surgeon. It was the worst possible propaganda for the Navy and naval medicine. No wonder if doctors attempted publicly to re-affirm the primacy of medical discourse over Smollett's racy and colourful descriptions.

But in the 1750s, doctors themselves displayed marked anxiety over the scale of the naval health care problem. Whenever it manifested itself in home waters, it was frequently in excess of any resources that port towns could muster. When a fleet returned, many hundreds of men could be put ashore with scurvy. Dr John Huxham was so appalled by the numbers he saw suffering from scurvy in Plymouth that he drew up proposals for preventing the disease and distributed copies to the captains of warships:

I have known many a Ship's Company set out on a Cruize [*sic*] in high Health, and yet in two or three months return vastly sickly, and eaten out with the Scurvy, a third Part of them being half rotten, and utterly unfit for the Service. – About four or five weeks after they have been out, they begin to drop down one after another, and at length by Dozens, till at last scarce half the *Complement* can stand to their Duty.[26]

John Huxham's account implies that scurvy was unavoidable on longer voyages. Certainly, the sailors had no control over the sequence of events. Yet Huxham understood that scurvy was linked to poor diet and that 'Apples, Oranges, and Lemons, alone, have been often known to do surprising Things in the Cure of very deplorable scorbutic Cases'. He recommends the use of vinegar to purify water on board and the addition of 'inferior wines' to the seaman's diet. In justifying the additional cost of these rations, he alludes to Britain's dependence on the Navy for defence and imperial ambition, drawing a parallel between Rome and Britain: Rome issued its soldiers with vinegar and wine, and if Rome thought such lives worth the expense, why shouldn't Britain have as much regard for its sailors, 'altogether as brave and useful to the Commonwealth?'[27] John Huxham contributes to the growing public image of the Navy as an essential tool of empire but suggests that seamen were undervalued and, given current medical provision, almost certain to become ill in the service.

Doctors continued to use John Huxham's patriotic arguments when lobbying the public. Others, to the very end of the period under review, emphasised the economic case for better healthcare at sea: Parliament expended vast sums on hospitals and medical supplies; it was expensive to replace men and support invalids; savings could be made if crews could be kept healthy. Also, seamen, by the very nature of their calling, represented a considerable investment. Dr Thomas Trotter reiterated the accepted view in 1819:

The soldier can be perfected in his exercise in a few days; and it little avails what kind of trade he has been employed in; but no person will have the hardihood to contend, that a seaman's duty can be learned in less than seven years, or after twenty-one years of age. He must be accustomed to it from boyhood; for no adult being can ever be brought to endure the privations, dangers, and hardships, which are inseparable from a sea-life.[28]

Doctors throughout this period reinforced a perception of the Navy as a demanding profession requiring both skill and endurance.

Manning the Navy was a persistent problem and Government had taken some steps to encourage volunteers.[29] But in the mid-eighteenth century, the need to attract men to the service and preserve them in it did not immediately win ministers' support for improved health measures, although medical provision in the Royal Navy still exceeded that in the merchant service. In 1757, James Lind, a dedicated naval doctor, could refer to this with national pride (after all, in the French navy seamen had their pay stopped when ill). On occasion, therefore, doctors represented the Navy as honourable employment with some degree of security:

> Nor is it a small additional Pleasure, to a Seamen in the Royal Navy to reflect, that whatever Misfortunes, incident to his Way of Life, may befall him, in the Service of his country, he will be honourably rewarded, and, under many Circumstances of but small Accident, obtain a Pension for Life.[30]

Large naval hospitals – Haslar in Portsmouth, begun in 1745, and Stonehouse, near Plymouth, begun in 1758 – were visible reminders that Government ostensibly took great care of the health of its seamen and, by association, that the Navy was acknowledged to be of vital importance to the nation. For example, Dr George Pinckard, Deputy Inspector-General of Hospitals to his Majesty's Forces, was particularly impressed by Haslar:

> Connected with our country's greatness, it called up a similar train of ideas, and I felt it an honor [*sic*] to England that so noble an institution should offer, to our brave tars, the comforts required in sickness. Too much cannot be done for our navy, nor can the provision for our sick and wounded defenders be too liberal; they merit all their country can bestow.[31]

George Pinckard was writing during the Napoleonic Wars when there was general consensus about the debt that the country owed to the Navy but Haslar was a remarkable building. Completed in 1761, it was for many years the largest brick building in Europe. Built at great expense, the hospitals provided valuable statistics on the frequency of diseases and helped to spread good practice formerly confined to isolated ships. Together with Greenwich Hospital for retired seamen, they were often reproduced in prints. Greenwich Hospital early became a tourist attraction.[32] In 1789, its two chaplains wrote a history of the Hospital which invited readers to regard the building as a work of national grandeur as well as a monument to wisdom and benevolence. The history was used as a guidebook, which, adapted or augmented, saw eight English and two French editions by 1820.

Doctors of the mid-eighteenth century, commenting on naval health, were able to position themselves as reformers. They depict the Navy as an institution bound by tradition, in which sickness was fostered by 'too strict an Attachment to Old Regulations and Customs'.[33] If the role of reformer offered opportunities to increase their status in some quarters, their role as servants of the state helpfully seeking to point out economies, offered opportunities in others. Yet, their writings were probably compromised in the eyes of the authorities since surgeons, throughout the period, were also clearly writing in the hope of improving their own pay and conditions of service.[34] They were seemingly caught between two imperatives – between wanting to do good and wanting to do well. Doctors reiterated similar arguments over decades until the beginning of the nineteenth century, which suggests that when they tried to improve the treatment of sailors, they did not easily win support until the exigencies of the Napoleonic Wars made the conservation of men imperative.

Improvements in naval medicine

In this period, important developments in medical care came to affect the way in which doctors represented the Navy. From the mid-eighteenth century, doctors placed greater emphasis on observation and on recording both the symptoms of illness and the effect of medicines in order to categorise results and produce statistics.[35] Military hospitals and, from 1770, newly-founded dispensaries, added impetus to this trend by providing opportunities for the study of disease.[36] When Dr John Pringle, Physician-General of the British Army from 1744 to 1752, found that military diseases had been neglected by earlier writers, typically, he began to collect factual observations about different diseases and to compile his own statistics. In this area, medical works had the potential to impress on the reader uncomfortable truths that patriotic discourse about the armed forces tended to conceal, and medical writings attest to the human cost of victories glorified in the public media. Pringle's case histories of men dying in agony, in sordid circumstances, owe their power to his clinical descriptions of horrific symptoms, and must have offered a contemporary counterpoint to campaign accounts of a more heroic nature. Pringle opened their bodies subsequently to see what he could record. In illness and in death the body was a field for observation.

Dr James Lind, in 1757, similarly represented the Navy as an excellent subject for medical observation. Warship crews, being both disciplined and confined to a small area, lent themselves to this practice:

> All the ships, which compose a squadron, are under the same influence of diet and of climate, the circumstances of the men being likewise in other respects for the most part similar. Hence an infection may often spread itself unsuspected over a town or village, while in a fleet of ships its influence becomes more apparent, from its confinement to one or more ships.[37]

When Gilbert Blane was appointed Physician to the Fleet in 1780, he determined to make the best use he could of 'the advantages, which this field of observation afforded'.[38] The fleet had sailed to the West Indies – a notoriously unhealthy location for British seamen where the death rate was one in seven. Blane collected and arranged into tables all the available facts concerning the causes of disease. The Commander-in-Chief ordered every surgeon in the fleet to send Blane a monthly return stating the prevalence of sickness, mortality figures, and other circumstances relating to the health of their ships. This allowed Blane to regulate hospital admissions, to keep the Commander-in-Chief informed and also to collect a body of facts relating to the causes and course of disease.

Statistical evidence helped doctors like Gilbert Blane to promote a better image of the Navy, particularly at the end of the century when healthcare at sea had improved – mostly due to advances in preventative medicine. Following improvements in hygiene, ventilation, and diet, mortality in the Navy decreased substantially. Lemon juice was finally included in seamen's rations in 1795, cleanliness was strictly enforced and actually mentioned in instructions to naval commanders from 1806, and the sick-bay on warships was improved and better equipped. Using tables of mortality, at the end of the Napoleonic Wars, Blane was able to calculate that if the Navy had been as subject to disease in 1813 as it had been in 1779, the number of deaths in 1813 would have been 6,674 higher. He concluded triumphantly, 'Under such an annual waste of life, the national stock of mariners must have been exhausted.' Clearly, medicine had helped to win the war. Blane was able to depict a much more caring, more effective navy but he had to admit that though his statistics proved that mortality in the Navy has decreased, the death rate was still high compared to that of men 'of the same age, in other situations of life'.[39]

From the 1780s, the weight of numerical evidence added validity to doctors' published findings but such writing also confirmed the impression that military forces, subject to orders anyway, could be used as the basis of experiment.[40] In general, people at this time were still apt to challenge their doctors. If they did not like the treatment, and could afford to do so, they sought second and third opinions. When Lind experimented on seamen to find a cure for scurvy, the men presumably had no choice as to whether they took vinegar or citrus juice for their complaint.

Voyages of exploration had also allowed various remedies to be tested on seamen and observations to be made, for example, bark (quinine) was administered for fever on Captain James Cook's *Resolution* voyage and proved more effective than the usual copious bleedings.[41] This result was verified by Dr William Robertson, naval surgeon on board *Juno* and *Edgar* from 4 April 1776 to 30 November 1781. The two ships served in American waters, the Mediterranean and the Channel. During the voyage, Robertson compiled accurate tables detailing the success of different methods of treating fevers on board, and showed the great efficacy of using Peruvian bark (quinine).[42] Cook had been celebrated for keeping his crews healthy and free from scurvy. Medical and dietary details were carefully recorded in published accounts of his voyages and were influential in promoting the role of paternalistic commander.[43] Joseph Adams, physician at a London smallpox hospital, shows how records of Cook's *Endeavour* voyage were still being used in the early-nineteenth century. Adams wrote a paper on the elusive 'itch insect'. He suspected that there might be a connection between such insects and stubborn eye infections. As evidence, he quoted a letter from Sir Joseph Banks describing how a Tahitian woman had used splinters of bamboo to extract minute lice from the eye when Cook's seamen were troubled with a tormenting itch around the eyelids.[44] Even if naval doctors applied what proved to be mistaken theories and administered ineffective medicines in their treatment of illness, the observations they recorded were extremely important to the investigations of later doctors attempting to define diseases. Seamen were often in the front line in more ways than one.

Historians have tried to use Michel Foucault's discussion of French Enlightenment medicine, his *The Birth of the Clinic*, for example, as a model for interpreting developments in British medicine at this time, with variable success. At another level, though, Foucault's analysis does afford a model by which to understand some of the ways in which medical men in Britain came to exercise greater control over their patients. Certainly, this control is evident in naval medicine. Sailors were institutionalised and although doubtless they learned to work the system, their commanders had a high degree of control over their bodies and actions. Mary E. Fissell has analysed the way in which, towards the end of the eighteenth century when doctors were trained more in hospitals, the diagnostic process altered in two ways. Firstly, doctors took more notice of the signs of disease in the body – rather than of what patients wanted to tell them about their symptoms. Secondly, they favoured anatomic enquiry after death. Fissell argues that the essays published by doctors helped to reconstruct the meaning of illness in ways that shifted the authority from patient to medical man. She also notes that many surgeons given this new hospital-based training subsequently made their career in the Navy but, as we can see, their influence there would have reinforced an existing trend.[45]

Naval medicine and the ethos of command

The writings of naval doctors influenced the ethos of command operating on board the King's ships and helped to publicise this development. Gilbert Blane, in particular, encouraged a paternalistic relationship between officers and men. He deduced that the health of a ship depended principally on the power of officers – even more than on doctors. Different ships in the same fleet had varying numbers of sick even when they had been at sea the same length of time and the men had been fed on the same food. As a result, the prevention of illness depended chiefly on order and discipline, which officers alone could enforce.[46] Professional standards and peer group pressure had created a code of behaviour based on strong leadership. Doctors helped to modify this by publicly emphasising the parent-like responsibilities of naval officers to their men. In 1794, Sir Roger Curtis, captain of the *Brunswick,* wrote 'It has been wisely said, that the fatherly care of a commander is the *Seaman's best Physician.*' The crew were 'entitled to kindness in return for obedience'.[47] It has been argued that Curtis's remark indicates that officers resented the influence that preventative medicine brought naval surgeons and wished to return to an older paternalism.[48] It is true that by the end of the century, order was enforced by strict discipline in large warships that were likely to have significant quotas of landmen and pressed men.[49] However, most key works of naval medicine from the 1780s to the end of the Napoleonic Wars continue to promote the concept of fatherly care that Curtis has internalised.[50] Curtis continues by saying that commanders should have in their libraries the works of medical men like Gilbert Blane and James Lind to enable them to carry out their duties. This persistent medical theme should be viewed in the context of increasing support in society, from the mid-eighteenth century, for what had traditionally been considered softer, 'feminine' values.[51] Once again, medical works help to promote a vivid image of naval life, though individual commanders would have determined the degree to which it matched reality.

Increasingly, naval doctors largely complied with and helped to bolster the stereotypical view of a navy comprised of honest Jack Tars. Since impressed men were so apt to desert, this image of the British seaman may have been widely publicised in the hope that men would live up to it. Certainly, it complemented the support naval doctors generally gave to a paternalistic bond between officers and men. Thomas Trotter displays a subtle difference in attitude when he writes in 1797 that 'to relieve effectually the distresses of a particular class of men, as the British seamen, we must associate with the character, and keep aloof from none of their frailties'.[52] Trotter attributed the 'striking singularities' in the character of the British seaman to sea life itself and the little communication it afforded with the common manners of society. The courage of such men, partly innate, was increased by their habits of life. They associated with others who were accustomed to danger and who, 'from national prowess, consider themselves at sea, as rulers by birthright'. Trotter's balanced description of the character of a seaman, has often been quoted:

The mind, by custom and example, is thus trained to brave the fury of the elements, in their different forms, with a degree of contempt, at danger and death, that is to be met with no where else, and which has become proverbial. Excluded, by the employment which they have chosen, from all society, but people of similar dispositions, the deficiencies of education are not felt, and information on general affairs is seldom courted. Their pride consists in being reputed a thorough bred seaman; and they look upon all landmen, as beings of inferior order.... Having little intercourse with the world, they are easily defrauded, and dupes to the deceitful, wherever they go: their money is lavished with the most thoughtless profusion.... With minds uncultivated and uninformed, they are equally credulous and superstitious.... The true-bred seaman, is seldom a profligate character; his vices, if he had any, rarely partake of premeditated villainy, or turpitude of conduct; but rather originate from want of reflection, and a narrow understanding.... In his pleasures he is coarse, and in his person slovenly: he acquires no experience from past misfortunes, and is heedless of futurity.[53]

Thomas Trotter was writing during the Revolutionary and Napoleonic Wars when victories at sea were celebrated above all others. He recognised, for example, that newspaper accounts of sea-battles portraying the Navy as the chief means of securing the independence of a free people helped to win it great patriotic support until 'the names of our great admirals are therefore revered as so many tutelatory deities of our island'.[54] By 1798, it was possible to complain that 'it is the fashion to extol our sailors and overlook our soldiers, as of little or no consequence.'[55] The physician George Pinckard, visiting Haslar in 1795, was moved to exclaim that however difficult it was to describe the character of seamen 'yet it may be given in one short sentence, for – *they are a race of heroes!*'[56]

Yet, seamen were also notoriously intemperate, often accused of recruiting their strength for work by getting drunk. Doctors did little to efface this image despite elsewhere helping to promulgate the image of the likeable Jack Tar. Throughout the period, they sternly warned seamen against the dangers of intoxication, as was common in contemporary writings addressed to the poor.[57] Additionally, stray comments in medical publications reveal another, harsher side to life in the Navy. Gilbert Blane, for example, notes that 'nothing tends more to shorten life than excessive bodily labour and watching' and consequently seamen are, in general, short-lived: 'their countenance and general appearance make them appear older that they really are by several years.' Thomas Trotter alludes to the destructive effects of mercury treatment for venereal disease on seamen's constitutions already weakened by scurvy and hard labour, 'hence... that rotten old age so early to be found among them'.[58] Dr C. Fletcher, advocated the appointment of chaplains to warships, claiming that deprived of the benefits of public devotion, seamen were activated only by fear and when discipline was relaxed, as when ashore, they broke all bounds of restraint.[59] Caricatures of the time allude to the damage sailors inflict on their health by excessive drinking, but make both the seaman and his doctor figures of fun, perhaps reflecting a popular desire for a more transparent medical discourse that allowed ordinary people to understand their ailments and take effective action. For example, 'Jack hove down with a Grog Blossom Fever' (Figure 8.2) shows Jack rejecting treatment from an incompetent doctor: 'You may batter my Hull as long as you like, but I'll be d – 'nd if ever you board me with your Glyster pipe.' That sailors drank excessively was nothing new but only naval doctors claimed that such intoxication was a disease. This print is further evidence that the readership for medical works was wider than the profession itself. It indicates too, how certain details relating to the image of the Navy, being of wider public interest, might be promulgated to a less literate audience.

Contagion and amputation

The writings of naval doctors also confirmed what the public had long apprehended, namely that seamen were a source of contagion in ports and coastal towns, and a threat to the local population. Wharves, the chief resort of sailors for business and pleasure were understood to be desperately unhealthy places. The *Gentleman's Magazine* for June 1782 printed an extract from the Post Letter from Plymouth, which replicated the contents of almost all the letters from the sea ports apparently suffering from an outbreak of influenza. 'The present epidemical disorder rages violently here, and at Dock; also on board the men-of-war lying here. The troops in town too, and in barracks, are affected with it, more or less; scarce a family, but has some person ill in it.'[60] The great outbreak of yellow fever in Philadelphia in 1797 was traced to seamen arriving from the West Indies. The American physician, Benjamin Rush, believed that every ship should be obliged by law to carry a ventilator 'calculated to prevent not only the decay of ships and cargoes, but a very frequent source of pestilential diseases of all kinds, in commercial cities'.[61] Naval hospitals took stringent measures to prevent infection escaping into neighbouring areas – and deserters escaping anywhere. Ordinary seamen might have been admired but their company was best avoided.

However, those who had never left the land could hardly appreciate life at sea. To some extent, the writings of doctors helped to create an appreciation of the space on board ship and a sense of what it was like to be in the Navy. Doctors observed that a species of distemper broke out in crowded, ill-ventilated ships similar to jail-fever on land.[62] Indeed, men at sea

Figure 8.2

'Jack Hove Down with a Grog Blossom Fever.' Published 12 August 1811 by X.Y. [sic] and Thomas Tegg (publisher). © National Maritime Museum.

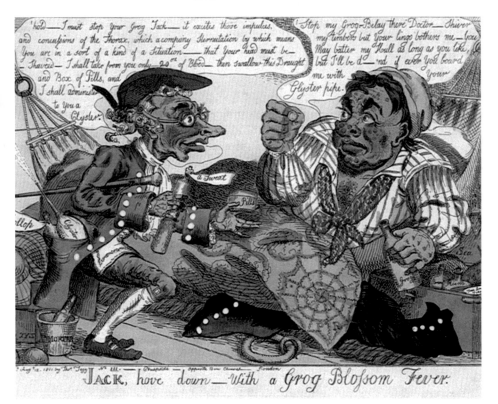

were confined to a species of jail, forced to breathe poisonous air and associate with carriers of disease. It was natural, then, that naval doctors came to insist on strict procedures of hygiene and cleanliness.

James Lind, regarded as the founder of naval hygiene in England, strongly advocated preventative medicine, which he considered often more effective than any attempt to cure illness. His observations concerning probable sources of contagion on ships had earlier presented a baleful picture of the constitution of the Navy in wartime:

> In the Equipment of a Fleet there are two Sorts of Men from whome the
> Sickness may be apprehended, *viz.* Sailors imprest after a long Voyage from

the *East* or *West Indies,* or the Coast of *Guinea,* and such idle Fellows as are picked from the Streets or the Prisons.[63]

As Lind's work gained acceptance, and we have seen that by the 1790s commanders were advised to buy his books for their own use, his advice came to change administrative procedures on board ship. For example, he advised that the captain regulating impressed men should record the details of a seaman's last voyage, ordering him fresh provisions if the voyage had been sickly. Similarly, he was to record the last place of residence of all landmen and enquire of their state of health.

Ironically, though it may be considered a basic human right to be allowed the self-management of one's own health, preventative medicine had to be strictly enforced to be effective. In 1780, Gilbert Blane wrote, that since pressing men was unavoidable, and since it was the greatest means of generating and spreading disease, it was necessary to prevent the effects of contagion on newly pressed men: 'This is done by stripping and washing their bodies; by cutting off their hair; and destroying all their clothes, before they are allowed to mix with the ship's company in which they are going to enter.'[64] This procedure amounts to an initiation ceremony, encouraging a loss of identity. Some critics, referring to the work of Foucault, consider that 'the conceptualisation of the body as property owned and operated by an individual is a relatively recent phenomenon of bourgeois culture.'[65] Certainly, self-management was effectively denied to the seaman. Lind considered that any man found remiss in keeping his clothes and bedding aired and dry 'should be compelled to become more cleanly'.[66] In a short time, doctors were legitimately able to represent British warships as more disciplined and better run than those of the French, which were dirty and badly ventilated.

Mutilation was common in the Navy and the loss of a limb was to be born with equanimity. Amputations are portrayed as opportunities to display personal courage, and here doctors contribute to popular conceptions of heroism. For example, the surgeon Edward Ives relates how a sixteen-year-old boy, almost as a matter of personal honour, endured the amputation of his leg without a groan that could be heard a yard away.[67] In contrast, protracted deaths from fever, dysentery or scurvy do not lend themselves to this treatment and are described according to their symptoms, not as individual acts of bravery that can be used to encourage others. Amputation was one instance, perhaps, when patients could be asked to exercise great self-control. In other cases, once they had consented to place themselves in the hands of a doctor, the severity of the treatment – vomits, purges, and blisters – meant that effectively patients had limited control over the consequences. This emphasis is reflected in popular prints.

Figure 8.3

'Droll Doings No 29: Shiver my Timbers, Jack.' Produced by F.C. [sic] (artist) and William Spooner, (publisher). © National Maritime Museum.

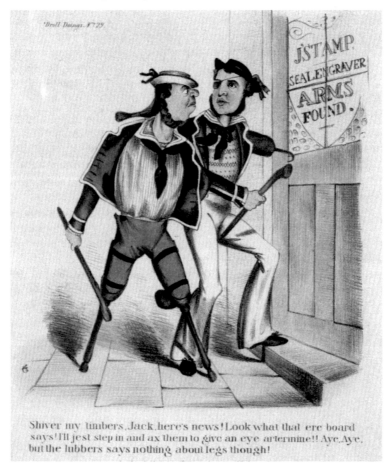

Shiver my timbers, Jack, here's news! Look what that ere board says! I'll jest step in and ax them to give an eye arternine!! Aye, Aye, but the lubbers says nothing about legs though!

Caricatures like 'Shiver my timbers, Jack...' (Figure 8.3) show a pragmatic attitude to dismemberment while humourously playing on seamen's supposed naivety. In military circles at this period, death from disease seems to have been considered somehow ignoble, a death for cowards and common men. Wounds, on the other hand were badges of bravery.

In the 1790s, doctors who were politically active diagnosed widespread ill-health in Britain as symptomatic of the rottenness of the *ancien régime* body politic.[68] Parliament, after all, had taken little interest in organising healthcare provision. In doing so, they embraced the idiom of natural human rights, which included the right to be healthy. People, they contended, were entitled to competent advice about their health and its self-management. Opinion thereafter was divided. Should ordinary people, given basic information about healthcare, be left to treat themselves? Or should they always be encouraged to seek trained help? The problem was that people rarely acted in their best interests, were absurdly credulous when it came to health matters, and often had to be compelled to follow doctors' orders. Ironically, the example of the Navy indicated that oligarchy was far from inimical to the health of the people: once cleanliness was enforced, health improved. The fleet was inoculated against smallpox long before there was widespread inoculation in Britain's cities, or even in the army – sailors had little choice.[69] Naval doctors, by celebrating these advances and representing the Navy as a successful experiment in controlled healthcare, lent support to the Government. In this instance, an apparent denial of basic rights produced better propaganda for the ruling classes.

On the other hand, doctors were broadly united in their condemnation of impressment. The most sustained criticism of the Navy was focused on this one issue. Impressment was in direct opposition to propaganda celebrating the liberty of the British people and it was hard to lessen the negative effect this had on the Navy's image. Impressment clearly had a detrimental effect upon the health of crews. John Huxham wrote:

> The usual Method of impressing Seamen on their Return from long and tedious Voyages, void of Necessaries, chagrined at not seeing their Friends and Families, and most commonly in a bad state of Health, and not allowed Time and Opportunity to recover it, hath been the Bane of thousands: And I could wish, for the Honour of the Nation, a Method of manning our fleet could be found out more consistent with common Humanity and *British* Liberty.[70]

Thomas Trotter observed that a newly impressed seaman had 'a sulkiness of disposition' which was only gradually overcome and which caused problems for both the commander and the doctor. The seaman watched 'every opportunity for effecting his escape'. He was also liable to try to deceive the doctor, assuming diseases in order to be 'an object for invaliding'.[71] After the Napoleonic Wars, when there was less pressure for all good patriots to support the Navy as an institution, Trotter wrote a vigorously argued paper against impressment. Holding up the spectre of the 1797 naval mutinies and making a case for creating a more contented body of men, he dismissed the argument that pressing was sanctioned by custom.

He contended that the popular celebration of British seamen was both hollow and cynical:

> The seaman is like the victim in sacrifice, that is gilded and decked out to be consumed; for his valour is blazoned with triumphal songs and feats, while himself is dragged from his home and his endearments, and ultimately consigned to neglect.[72]

Yet, as I have indicated, there is a sense in which doctors helped to create the type that the public loved to extol 'the plain and honest, though unthinking seaman', who was nevertheless a great lover of his country.[73] The paternalistic relationship between officers and men, that doctors helped to foster, can only have encouraged a lack of responsibility in sailors. The emphasis doctors came to place on enforced cleanliness and preventative medicine helped to deprive the men of individual identity.

Unremarkably, perhaps, in these medical writings there seems to be a tension between the general and the particular. Doctors observed individual symptoms and individual cases and then tried to generalise in order to deduce common causes and cures – which would help them to advance in their careers. A similar tension in attitudes to the Navy existed in the country at large: the public had a keen sense of the debt society owed to the Navy but a distaste for individual sailors whom they tried to efface from their conscience. The difference, of course, is that the more committed doctors also cared for the individual. This is evident in Thomas Trotter's conclusion to his paper on impressment, when he makes a sad plea for the seaman. He writes:

> I am afraid there has been too often a want of sympathy for his condition, by seeing him in his idle hours of dissipation and low pleasure. His slovenly appearance and awkward gait have to the beholder's eye, too frequently obliterated all the remembrance of his naval glory; and the honours of... the battle of the Nile, Camperdown, Trafalgar, etc, have been at once forgotten, on seeing him stagger from the bar of a tavern.[74]

This was an age of great public interest in health matters and growing medical consumerism.[75] As we have seen, by 1815, progress in preventative medicine had brought about real improvements to healthcare in the Navy. In many ways doctors continued to promulgate stereotypical views of the Navy favoured by ballad and print makers, the popular theatre, and some government propagandists, but their published works helped to convey to a wider public both improvements in conditions of service and associated developments in the ethos of naval command. Medical writings made a significant contribution to the public image of the Navy as an institution.

Acknowledgements

I am grateful to the John Carter Brown Library for awarding me the Alexander O. Vietor Fellowship to research this article. This essay was first published in M. Lincoln, *Representing the Royal Navy. British Sea Power, 1750–1815* (Aldershot: Ashgate, 2003).

Notes

1. See C. Lloyd and J.L.S. Coulter, *Medicine and the Navy 1200–1900,* Vol. III (Edinburgh: Livingstone, 1961). For scurvy in particular, see K.J. Carpenter, *The History of Scurvy and Vitamin C* (Cambridge: Cambridge University Press, 1986). Useful works on institutional care of the period include: M. Ignatieff, *A Just Measure of Pain: The Penitentiary in the Industrial Revolution, 1750–1850* (London: Macmillan Press, 1978); C. Hamlin, 'Predisposing Causes and Public Health in Early-Nineteeth-Century Medical Thought', *Social History of Medicine*, V (1992), 43–70; C. Lawrence, *Medicine and the Making of Modern Britain, 1700–1920* (London: William Collins, 1994).

2. Throughout 'doctors' is used to denote all medical practitioners, including surgeons, although strictly only physicians were MDs.

3. There were few physicians in the Navy. Larger overseas squadrons carried one. See N.A.M. Rodger, *The Wooden World: An Anatomy of the Georgian Navy* (London: William Collins, 1986), 20.

4. J. Atkins, *The Navy-Surgeon: Or a Practical System of Surgery,* 2nd edn (London, 1737), x.

5. Even towards the end of the period, when their status had improved, since their numbers had increased they still found it difficult to gain positions ashore in peacetime. See *Gentleman's Magazine,* LXXIII (1803), 5.

6. J. Ring, *Reflections on the Surgeons' Bill: In Answer to Three Pamphlets in Defence of that Bill* (London, 1798), 36. Ring (1752–1821) was trained at Winchester College and published tracts on vaccination.

7. C. Dunne, *The Chirurgical Candidate; Or, Reflections on Education: indispensable to complete Naval, Military, and Other Surgeons* (London, 1801), 20, 83.

8. Eg. see *Gentleman's Magazine,* XXVIII (1758), 160.

9. S. Sutton, *An Historical Account of a New Method for extracting the foul Air out of Ships etc., To Which are Annexed... A Discourse on the Scurvy by Dr Mead,* 2nd. edn (London, 1749), 73. First edn 1745. Thanks to Mead's influence, Sutton's ventilators were installed in warships ten years after their invention. See *Gentleman's Magazine,* XXXIV (1764), 275.

10. C. Lawrence confirms that scurvy was a key area in which doctors advanced their claims for higher social status. See his 'Disciplining Disease: Scurvy, the Navy, and Imperial Expansion, 1750–1825' in D. Miller and P. Reill, *Visions of Empire: Voyages, Botany and Representations of Nature* (Cambridge: Cambridge University Press, 1996), 81 and 85.

11. See R. Porter, 'Lay Medical Knowledge in the Eighteenth Century: the Evidence of the *Gentleman's Magazine*', *Medical History*, XXIX (1985), 138–68; 149. For reviews, see *Gentleman's Magazine*, XXXIII (1763), 602 and XXXIX (1769), 156.

12. See *Gentleman's Magazine*, XVII (1747), 467–69; XXI (1751), 408; LX (1790), 493.

13. *Gentleman's Magazine*, XXIV (1754), 114–15, 543–4.

14. *Gentleman's Magazine*, XXV (1755), 175. The latest medical publications were also advertised in the *Gentleman's Magazine*, see XXV (1755) 478.

15. *Ibid.*, 175. Cf. *Gentleman's Magazine*, XXVIII (1758), 160.

16. *Gentleman's Magazine*, XXX (1760), 557.

17. *Gentleman's Magazine*, XXVI (1756), 418–20.

18. *Gentleman's Magazine*, XXVIII (1758), 105. See also *Ibid.*, 61–3.

19. *Gentleman's Magazine*, XLIX (1779), 193.

20. *Gentleman's Magazine*, LXIII (1793), 291. Cf. LXXIII (1803), 897.

21. *Gentleman's Magazine*, LXIV (1794), 422.

22. *Gentleman's Magazine*, LXII (1792), 604; LXIV (1794), 690; LXVIII (1798), 823, 945, 1029.

23. See J.C. Smyth, *An Account of the Experiment made at the Desire of the Lords Commissioners of the Admiralty, on Board the Union Hospital Ship* (London, 1796).

24. *The Times*, 24 April, 16 May, 15 August, 5 September, and 29 September 1794.

25. See W. Turnbull, *The Naval Surgeon* (London, 1806), vii.

26. J. Huxham, *An Essay on Fevers* (London, 1750), 47–8.

27. *Ibid.*, 26, 264. See also J. Lind, A*n Essay on the Most Effectual Means of Preserving the Health of Seamen in the Royal Navy* (London, 1757), xiv–xv.

28. T. Trotter, *A Practicable Plan for Manning the Royal Navy and Preserving our Maritime Ascendancy without Impressment* (Newcastle, 1819), 37–8. Cf. G. Blane, *A Short Account of the Most Effectual Means of Preserving the Health of Seamen, particularly in the Royal Navy* (London, 1780), 2.

29. Eg. The 1758 Navy Act enforced more frequent paying of ships. It also introduced a new mechanism by which men might send money home, free, by government channels.

30. Lind, *op. cit.* (note 27), 109–10.

31. G. Pinckard, *Notes on the West Indies Written during the Expedition under the Command of the late General Sir Ralph Abercomby*, 3 vols (London, 1806),

42. Greenwich Hospital was supported by a tax on seamen.

32. See S. Monks, 'National Heterotopia: Greenwich as Spectacle, 1694–1869', *Rising East: The Journal of East London Studies*, 2, 1 (1998), 156–66.

33. This is true of three of the four prominent doctors publishing between 1745 and 1760. See Lind, *op. cit.* (note 27), xvi; R. Mead, *A Discourse on Scurvy*, 75; T. Reynolds, *The Gentleman's Magazine*, XXVIII (1758), 210.

34. For example, see T. Trotter, *Medicina Nautica* (London, 1797), 18.

35. See U. Tröhler, 'Quantification in British Medicine and Surgery 1750–1830; with Special Reference to its Introduction into Therapeutics' (PhD thesis, University of London, 1978). Also, O. Keel, 'The Politics of Health and the Institutionalisation of Clinical Practices in Europe in the Second Half of the Eighteenth Century', in W.F. Bynum and R. Porter (eds), *William Hunter and the Eighteenth-Century Medical World* (Cambridge: Cambridge University Press, 1985), 231.

36. I.S.L. Loudon, 'The Origins and Growth of the Dispensary Movement in England' *Bulletin of the History of Medicine*, LV (1981), 322–42.

37. Lind, *op. cit.* (note 27), 36. Army surgeons advised the same for doctors in the colonies, see G. Cleghorn, *Observations on the Epidemical Diseases in Minorca, from the year 1744–1749* (London, 1751), v.

38. G. Blane, *Observations on the Diseases Incident to Seamen* (London, 1785), v.

39. G. Blane, *Select Dissertations on Several Subjects of Medical Science* (London, 1822), 2–3 and 22. See also L. Brockliss, J. Cardwell and M. Moss, *Nelson's Surgeon: William Beatty, Naval Medicine, and the Battle of Trafalgar* (Oxford: Oxford University Press, 2005).

40. The Sick and Hurt Board conducted 17 experiments on ships' crews between 1740 and 1782. See P.K. Crimmin, 'The Sick and Hurt Board and the Health of Seamen, *c*.1700–1806', *Journal for Maritime Research* (December 1999), http://www.jmr.nmm.ac.uk/server/show/ conJmrArticle.12. The lessons of naval medicine were understood to be of potential public benefit. See *Gentleman's Magazine*, XXVIII (1758), 209.

41. J. Millar, *Observations on the Management of the Prevailing Diseases in Great Britain, particularly in the Army and Navy* (London, 1779), 204.

42. J. Millar, *Observations on the Change of Public Opinion in Religion, Politics, and Medicine on the Conduct of the War; on the Prevailing Diseases in Great Britain; and on Medical Arrangements in the Army and Navy*, 2 vols (London, 1805), II, 38.

43. See *Gentleman's Magazine*, XLVII (1777), 179.

44. J. Adams, *On Morbid Poisons*, 2nd edn (London, 1807), 307.

45. M.E. Fissell, *Patients, Power, and the Poor in Eighteenth-Century Bristol* (Cambridge: Cambridge University Press, 1991), 145, 148–9.

46. G. Blane, *op. cit.* (note 39), 4.

47. R. Curtis, *The Means to Eradicate a Malignant Fever which raged on board his*

Majesty's Ship Brunswick at Spithead in the Spring of the Year 1791 (London, 1794), 24.

48. See Lawrence, *op. cit.* (note 10).

49. See Rodger, *op. cit.* (note 3), 346.

50. See Blane, *op. cit.* (note 28), 4 and *op. cit.* (note 39), 71; Millar, *op. cit.* (note 42), cxvi; W. Turnbull, *op. cit.* (note 25), 49; A. C. Hutchison, *Practical Observations in Surgery: More Particularly as Regards the Naval and Military Service*, 2nd edn (London, 1826), 192, 1st ed. 1816.

51. For example, see T. Eagleton, *The Rape of Clarissa* (Minneapolis: University of Minnesota Press, 1982), 15–16.

52. Trotter, *op. cit.* (note 34), 4.

53. *Ibid.*, 38–9.

54. *Ibid.*, 37.

55. Ring, *op. cit.* (note 6), 39.

56. Pinckard, *op. cit.* (note 31), I, 42–3.

57. Atkins, *op. cit.* (note 4), 8. Also, T.M. Winterbottom, *Medical Directions for the Navigators and Settlers in Hot Climates*, 2nd edn (London, 1803), 9; T. Trotter, *An Essay, Medical, Philosophical, and Chemical on Drunkenness* (London, 1804); Turnbull, *op. cit.* (note 25), 112.

58. Blane, *op. cit.* (note 38), 323 and J. Trotter, *Observations on the Scurvy* (London, 1786), 89. Cf. Trotter, *op. cit.* (note 52), 41.

59. C. Fletcher, *The Naval Guardian*, 2nd edn, 2 vols (London, 1805), I, 169.

60. *Gentleman's Magazine*, LII (1782), 306.

61. B. Rush, *Medical Inquiries and Observations: Containing an Account of the Yellow Fever, as it Appeared in Philadelphia in 1797*, Vol. V (Philadelphia, 1798), 55.

62. For example, see J. Pringle, *Observations on the Diseases of the Army, in Camp and Garrison* (London, 1752), 291.

63. Lind, *op. cit.* (note 27), 1.

64. Blane, *op. cit.* (note 28), 8–9.

65. V. Kelly, and D.E. Von Mücke, *Body & Text in the Eighteenth Century* (California: Stanford University Press, 1994), 6.

66. Blane, *op. cit.* (note 38), 109. Men were forced to wash their clothes and air their bedding.

67. E. Ives, *A Voyage from England to India in the Year MDCCLIV* (London, 1773), 133.

68. R. Porter, *Doctor of Society: Thomas Beddoes and the Sick Trade in Late-Enlightenment England* (London and New York: Routledge, 1992), 158.

69. G. Blane states that enforced inoculation against smallpox in the Navy and Army 'has by no means been followed among the civil population of England' in *op. cit.* (note 39), 354. Cf. *Gentleman's Magazine*, LXXI (1801), 318; LXXIII (1803), 520.

70. Huxham, *op. cit.* (note 26), 264–5.
71. Trotter, *op. cit.* (note 34), 40. Cf. Hutchison, *op. cit.* (note 50), 142, 184.
72. T. Trotter, *A Practicable Plan for Manning the Royal Navy and Preserving our Maritime Ascendancy without Impressment* (Newcastle, 1819), viii, 30.
73. Blane, *op. cit.* (note 38), 97.
74. Trotter, *op. cit.* (note 72), 31–2.
75. D. Porter and R. Porter, *Patient's Progress: Doctors and Doctoring in Eighteenth-Century England* (Oxford: Polity, 1989), 214.

9

From Palace to Hut:
The Architecture of Military and Naval Medicine

Christine Stevenson

The walls separating medicine from society break down in this examination of early-British hospital architecture, which stresses the similarities and continuities between the civilian and the military. The hospitals examined include those for sick and wounded in the Empire, and later at home and those built for long-term chronic cases. Stevenson considers how matters of state, as well as medical theory and its changes, affected architecture.

The illustrations of the hut, Figures 9.1 and 9.2 overleaf, were published in 1813, by James Tilton (1745–1822), a former 'Physician and Surgeon in the Revolutionary Army of the United States'. Tilton's *Observations on Military Hospitals* includes some vivid recollections of the Revolutionary War, and more than thirty years later what he most remembered were the cold and the excrement. The latter was all over the camp at King's Bridge, New York in 1776, and with it a 'disagreeable smell'. 'A putrid diarrhoea was the consequence.... Many died, melting as it were and running off by the bowels.' When the enemy shifted, so did the Americans, who left their 'infectious camp and the attendant diseases behind them'. It was remarkable, Tilton wrote, how the officers and men were 'always more healthy in motion, than in fixed camps' before they were 'reduced to strict discipline and order'.[1]

A very old understanding of disease underpins this account of the King's Bridge 'infection'. Even a smell that is merely disagreeable might also be deadly; it caused the putridity, which then killed the 'melting' men. Discipline, burying the faeces to be precise, had averted the threat and permitted stasis, the camp that could stay put.

Even so, the best accommodation for sick soldiers was always transient, in the sense of ephemeral. Tilton preferred tents, but they could not be used during the hard winter of 1779–80, so he had his cabin-hospital built of unhewn logs. The middle ward, just over thirty feet long, housed feverish

Figure 9.1

"Log military hospital" from J. Tilton's Observations on Military Hospitals *(1813). Courtesy: Wellcome Library, London.*

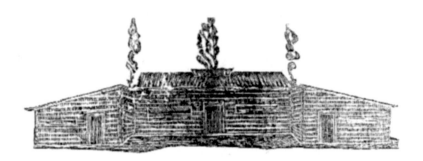

Figure 9.2

Plan of hospital" from J. Tilton's Observations on Military Hospitals *(1813). Courtesy: Wellcome Library, London.*

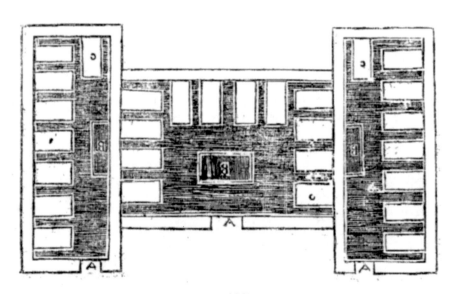

patients, and the cross-wards were for the wounded and 'other cases of topical affection'. The earthen floor was a 'neutralising' or 'correcting' influence, and smoke from open fires escaped through holes in the roof, combating infection on the way. Tilton explained that this was all 'upon the plan of an Indian hut', and that in it he could safely accommodate many more sick than could normally be kept in a space this size, that is, in a less primitive house.[2]

This survey of military and naval hospital architecture begins with the 'palaces', the great veterans' hospitals begun in the late-seventeenth century. Chelsea and Greenwich were not clinical hospitals, but the distinction was not maintained in the period, at least not in the latter's case, and in some ways these large and expensive complexes do not differ as much from Tilton's hut as we might assume. My major examples of clinical hospitals will be those built by the Navy on the Haslar peninsula near Portsmouth in Hampshire (1746–61) and at Plymouth, Devon (1758–62), for they were the century's major examples. The Army did not build general hospitals, as opposed to relatively small, regimental establishments, until the end of the century,[3] but it produced the writers, whose influence extended well beyond their professional sphere. The British Army physicians, or former physicians, John Pringle, Richard Brocklesby, and Donald Monro were Tilton's acknowledged inspirations, and their writings will, at the end of this essay, bring us back to the virtues of transience.

The palaces

Though it had forerunners – in 1641 the young John Evelyn (1620–1705) greatly admired Amsterdam's Soldatengasthuis, a 'Hospitall for... lame and decrepid souldiers'[4] – the Hôtel des Invalides in Paris, founded in 1670, effectively inaugurated the veterans' hospital as a building type. A very concrete manifestation of the 'military revolution', it was an idea whose time had come.[5] Yet the Invalides' importance as a model also owed much to the skill with which it was publicised as a direct manifestation of Louis XIV's loving charity and martial valour.[6] The combination probably intrigued Charles II, and the architecture certainly did. The Duke of Monmouth twice viewed the great work in progress on his father's behalf, and William Robinson (1645–1712), Surveyor-General to the Army in Ireland, was in 1677 very likely sent to inspect the Invalides too.[7] Three years later work began, to Robinson's designs, on the Royal Hospital at Kilmainham near Dublin, in effect, the first of the English veterans' hospitals.

Kilmainham adhered more closely to the French prototype than the Chelsea and Greenwich hospitals would. It was – and, as the Irish Museum of Modern Art, still is – a quadrangle formed by wings consisting of rows of rooms, with two beds to a room, and two men to a bed, fronted at ground level by an open arcade and above by a closed gallery, or corridor. This arrangement is like that of some of the Invalides' wings, though the latter has many quadrangles, and the resemblance between the two extends to some ornamental details.[8]

Veterans' hospitals had a particular meaning in a reign that had begun with a regicide; not for nothing was Kilmainham's chapel dedicated to King Charles the Martyr. In scouting for funds for the next, at Chelsea, Charles II explained that he had often and 'with great grief observed that many of our loyal subjects, who formerly took up arms for us, our royal father of blessed memory, to resist that torrent of prosperous rebellion, which at last overturned this monarchy, & Church', were now reduced to such 'extreme poverty' that some were forced to beg for their bread.[9] In this way, the King explained in-pensioning as his patriarchal duty. The hospitals were, in this specific sense, palaces; regal houses offering charitable hospitality to poor and loyal dependents.

Palatialness was not only metaphorical or symbolic. At Chelsea, begun in 1682, Christopher Wren (1632–1723) opened up the Invalides' and Kilmainham's quadrangles to make a U-shape facing the Thames, with ward wings at right angles to, but narrowly separated from, the central range with its chapel and hall. The display was entirely appropriate to what King Charles called 'so pious, & charitable a work' stemming from 'our own royal bounty'.[10] The river provided both convenient transport and the position from which the Royal Hospital appears to best advantage, and for the same reasons this is how London's royal palaces were then planned, although they were not built. It was a dim era for real palaces, but a brilliant one for these surrogates.

At the same time, Chelsea's shape allows more light and air to reach the men's galleries than a quadrangular arrangement would, and we can infer that this was part of Wren's reasoning.[11] The inference is in no way anachronistic. Like his friend Robert Hooke (1635–1703), another scientist–architect, Wren had keenly investigated the effects of air, and of the lack of air, on the human body. More generally, sunlight and clean air in gentle motion were central to the early modern understanding of a healthy environment, in part because of a fear of pathogenic smells, which James Tilton shared.[12] In one respect, Wren's hospitals' accommodation resembled that of the best clinical hospitals of their day: they provided 'cabins' or bed-cubicles, as Kilmainham and the Invalides did not. Compare, for example, a civil hospital in Rotterdam, where Wren's future acquaintance the naval surgeon James Yonge (1647–1721) found himself a prisoner-of-war in the mid-1660s. Yonge admired this 'fair house' with its long high wards, where the 'beds were enclosed like cabins... each having a window in it'.[13] The cabins offered privacy and warmth as required. A similar type was used at a garrison hospital built in Portsmouth in the early 1680s, where each bed formed its own enclosure, '4 foot wide by 6 foot 3 inches long.... In front of each curtain rods with two hooks and a corni[ce] at the top of each bedstead', which was eight feet high.[14] These beds were narrower but a little longer than Chelsea's cabins, designed a year or so later, which line each side of the ward-ranges' partition walls. Most comparable to Chelsea was the recent example of Hooke's rebuilding (1674–6) of London's Bethlem Hospital for the Insane, the other great hospital-construction project of Charles II's reign. Nearly six hundred feet long, Bethlem comprised rows of individual 'cells', a word also used for Chelsea's cabins. These were fronted by galleries serving as day-rooms, an institutional innovation that Wren adopted for his hospitals.

The construction of the Royal Hospital for sailors began in 1694, appropriately enough with Wren's conversion of the building designed by John Webb (1611–72) for a new Greenwich Palace, although this project was abandoned in 1670. What is now called the King Charles Building comprises Webb's original range, whose long thin rooms lent themselves nicely to their new purpose, and the new 'Base Block', lying parallel across a narrow court.[15] Wren's intention was always to balance the King Charles Building with another, named for Queen Anne, but on paper he experimented with different arrangements for the rest of the complex. One would have had twelve detached ward blocks – plus another pair for the chapel and the dining halls – in two parallel rows behind the Charles and Anne buildings; and the Greenwich Directors took another, smaller scheme, with a total of six blocks, seriously enough to have it engraved for subscribers in 1699.[16] Though for unknown reasons free-standing blocks were rejected soon afterwards, in favour of the three-sided King William and Queen Mary buildings which stand today, this project remained in circulation because pirated copies of the 1699 engraving were published until the early-1730s (Figure 9.3, overleaf). This was long after the hospital's final form was fixed, though two decades before it was finished.

These unexecuted designs are interesting because with them Wren departed from the palatial model.[17] Chelsea's planning struck a balance of sorts between the regal and the utilitarian, and as it was built, Greenwich did too. Even so, its 'parts' might be called, as Samuel Johnson did, 'too much detached to make one great whole',[18] and the early projects look frankly institutional to modern eyes. They have even been heralded as an anticipation of the 'pavilion' plan, which began to dominate hospital construction in the 1860s and remained the norm until well into the twentieth century.[19] They are not, however, in as much as pavilion wards are large open wards, and for healthy pensioners Wren planned a more complex arrangement of open-topped cabins in six-cabin rooms, which was retained

Figure 9.3

*Greenwich as engraved by Sutton Nicholls in 1728, even though the
arrangement of rear blocks in parallel had long been abandoned.
Courtesy: Wellcome Library, London.*

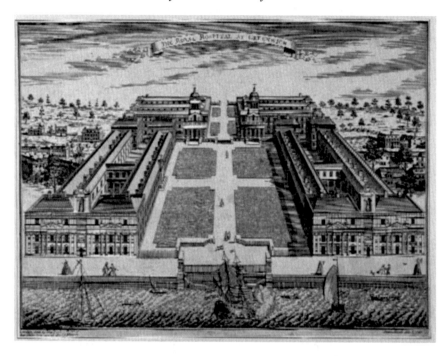

in the Queen Mary and King William buildings as they were constructed.
He did, of course, appreciate that detached buildings are safer than
contiguous ranges in case of fire, and generally easier to light and ventilate.
Isolated blocks could also be added gradually, as the money came in, and
money was usually a problem during Greenwich's construction. For all these
reasons they were used for the rebuilding of St Bartholomew's Hospital in
London, beginning in 1730, and in 1751 they were planned for the London
Hospital, which did not build them, and six years later for the naval hospital
at Plymouth, which did. At Plymouth, these blocks offered another
advantage. Unlike the veterans' and the civil hospitals, it regularly accepted
cases of 'infectious' and/or 'contagious' diseases, which could be isolated in
their own blocks.

Though they were readily available to see in engraved form, Wren's
detached ward buildings need not have inspired these later designs: they had

the self-evident advantages just mentioned. However, Greenwich would not have been ruled out as an architectural model simply because it was not a clinical hospital – or rather, was more than a clinical hospital. The distinction was explicitly dismissed by John Aikin (1747–1822), whose *Thoughts on Hospitals* (1771), was widely read until the early-nineteenth century. Aikin recommended Greenwich as a model for hospitals for the acutely ill, with the proviso that these patients would require a greater volume of circulating air and hence larger wards than for the aged and infirm.[20] He was clearly referring to the regular accommodation, and not to the separate Infirmary built between 1762 and 1768 to the designs of James Stuart (1713–88), but its planning was not dissimilar.[21] Among the laity, Greenwich and Chelsea prompted a mild and evergreen joke: because they seemed 'more fitted, by their grandeur and extent, for the residences of kings', while the palaces looked like pauper hospitals, foreigners were often confused.[22]

The naval hospitals

The Portsmouth garrison hospital, which measured one hundred and twenty by thirty-five feet overall, was an exceptional undertaking. Personally encouraged by Charles II, whose coat of arms it bore prominently, its construction was financed by the sale of £1,500, worth of timber from 'dotard & decayed trees' from the royal New Forest.[23] Though, at forty beds, its capacity was no greater than that of other regimental hospitals, they were more modest; and the hospitals following the Army's domestic and overseas manoeuvres occupied rented accommodation, or tents. It is to the Navy that we must look for new construction on any scale in this period.

The first of the purpose-built naval hospitals was at Port Mahon, Minorca, where in 1711 work began on a replacement for the sick-quarters set up a few years previously.[24] Minorca's hospital was, however, unique until the 1740s, when others were built on Jamaica and Gibraltar and begun on the Haslar peninsula.

As hospitals, these buildings had to be open to light and air, and as naval hospitals they had to secure their patients. The men were prone to 'run', or desert, or at least to wander off in search of a game and a drink, now defined as medical as well as disciplinary problems – they gambled away their clothes. Conflicting *desiderata* dictated a standard type, which was at first intended for Haslar too. Both the Jamaica and the Gibraltar hospitals consisted of the 'large Quadrangle[s], with a spacious piazza within' that the Admiralty specified for Haslar in mid-1745: that is, a great hollow rectangle whose wards' inner or 'piazza' sides were lined with arcades or colonnades.[25] These formed open but sheltered galleries, which served the staff for circulation and the men for healthful strolling, 'giv[ing] them Air', as the architect Nicholas Hawksmoor (1661–1736) explained Greenwich's equivalent colonnades.[26] The enclosure of the whole was to prevent running. The hospitals at Haslar and Plymouth retained the piazzas and the galleries, but abandoned physical enclosure.

Fever of one kind or another was the immediate stimulus for Britain's first programme of state hospital construction. It was endemic in the West Indies. The Jamaica hospital, which to discourage desertion was built beside a lagoon, was ordered moved and rebuilt in 1756: the site was disastrously conducive to outbreaks of 'intermittent' fever, malaria.[27] Equally terrifying was the 'continued' and 'malignant' fever, today identified as typhus, which swept through the British fleet between 1739 and 1741. The epidemic was understood to have started in the London prisons, and to be spreading with the mass impressment and mobilisation that attended the outbreak of hostilities with Spain. Though it did not admit its first patients until 1754, the hospital at Haslar was a 'monument to the disasters of 1740 and 1741', as Daniel Baugh has explained.[28]

Fever epidemics had long been observed among close populations: a favourite historical example, in the eighteenth century, was the deadly outbreak at the Oxford Assizes of 1577.[29] As explained in the final part of this essay, it was John Pringle who, beginning in the early-1750s, led the world to understand that the diseases still variously named for the environments which engendered them – the (army) camp, ship, hospital, and jail fevers – were one and the same. They comprised the continued, malignant, and/or 'putrid' fever today identified with louse-borne typhus (though loosely identified – contemporary reports accord with this mechanism of transmission, but the symptomatology is not always a perfect fit). The fever became more common over the course of the century in England, as armies and fleets were mobilised in greater numbers, towns grew, and residential institutions were built. It did not, however, become a regular problem in prisons or civil hospitals until the 1770s, when overcrowding became a regular problem; their architectural reform followed. Though the evidence is circumstantial, it seems as if the naval hospital planners, working in the wake of the epidemic of 1739–41, and of course aware that these hospitals must (unlike their civil counterparts) admit men already suffering from the fever, seem to have been particularly alert to the danger it presented, especially after Pringle's books began appearing.

The Royal Naval Hospital at Haslar was also a monument to far-reaching changes in naval–medical organisation that began around 1740. The new hospital's management, including its provisioning, was to rectify the long-acknowledged defects of the 'contract' system, now joined by another: hired hospitals and sick-quarters were clearly incapable of coping with a severe epidemic. As a building, the hospital was clearly preferable to those other royal hospitals, those on ships.[30] Hospital ships were excellent at reducing desertion, and could, when necessary, isolate cases of communicable disease, but because they were ships they were damp and malodorous, at a time when moisture and smells were believed to be powerful contributory, and even direct, causes of scurvy and the fever.[31]

When, in June 1745, the Admiralty informed the Commissioners for Sick and Wounded Seamen of the acquisition of the Haslar site, it handed over to them the hospital's 'Inner Parts', instructing them 'to consider attentively to the disposition, Situation, & Dimension of the Wards for sick Men, the Convenience of Light and Air; To avoid narrowness, as also crowding the Beds too close together'.[32] The three naval Boards were feeling their way around this new problem of building hospitals – which were, moreover, enormous by civilian standards – and the Admiralty asked the London merchant Theodore Jacobsen (d.1772) to look at the plan drawn up by the Navy Board's Surveyor Sir Jacob Ackworth. Amateur status was no disqualification for an architect then – Jacobsen had just designed the large new building for the Foundling Hospital, an orphanage, in London – and he might, the Admiralty hinted to the Commissioners, be more disinterested, as well as better qualified, than the widely-loathed Ackworth.[33] Not 'entirely approving' of Ackworth's plan, Jacobsen devised another, 'which he believes may be better for the Purpose'.[34]

The hospital at Haslar, begun in 1746, was handsomely illustrated in the *Gentleman's Magazine* five years later (Figure 9.4, overleaf). In the engraving we can see how the courtyard was lined, at ground-floor level, by arcading; and from it we can understand how each wing was formed by a pair of narrow ward ranges, rather like Greenwich's King Charles and Queen Anne buildings (seen in Figure 9.3). The picture does not, however, show Haslar as it was built. Sometime before early-1756 it was decided to substitute a wall with a gate for one of the wings, and in this way a quadrangular hospital approximating what was, after Gibraltar's and Jamaica's, becoming the standard naval type, took the form of a U.[35] The wing's omission saved money: what was immediately recognised as England's biggest brick construction would, when finished, even with three wings, cost around £100,000 – James Lind estimated in 1758 – two-and-a-half times the original prediction.[36] Other alterations are not so easily explained. Between 1756 and 1762, when the hospital was finished, it was decided to clear the narrow courts between the ward ranges in what were, now, the side wings. The buildings which Figure 9.4 shows in the centres of these wings were, in construction, replaced by pairs of free-standing blocks for storage, which face one another across the narrow inner courts. Two storeys high, they are a floor lower than the stacks of wards on either side and hence, according to the description published by the surgeon Johann Hunczovsky (1752–98) in

Figure 9.4

The Royal Hospital at Haslar as published in 1751.
Courtesy: Wellcome Library, London.

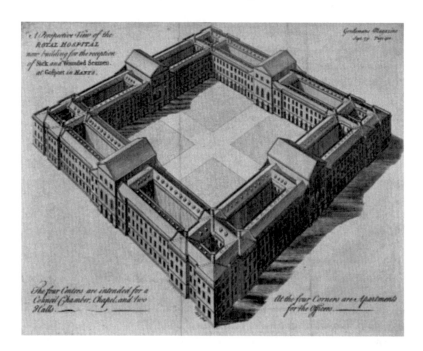

1783, did not interfere with air circulation.[37] After 1756, it was also decided to omit the kitchens, dining rooms, and stairs intended for the narrow courts (these are not shown in Figure 9.4), which meant that the wards could have more windows.

Between the storage and the ward blocks run terraces, resting on arcades; at ground level one could walk right through the side wings, under the terraces. Another Continental surgeon, Jacques Tenon (1724–1816) accordingly understood these wings, in 1787, as composed of pairs of isolated buildings – the end wards and the storage blocks – plus the wards attached to the central range (Figure 9.5).[38] The changes made to Haslar's plan during its construction, one way or another, all opened out, or perforated, the solid brick enclosure that was first envisaged. The result helped England's biggest hospital to enjoy, briefly, a reputation as its healthiest. Haslar was remarkable for the care with which it separated patients with different illnesses, and the clothing and bedding that they came into contact with, wrote Tenon, whose countryman Pierre-Jean Grosley had

Figure 9.5

Haslar, from John Howard's Account of the Principal Lazarettos... *(1789).*
Courtesy: Wellcome Library, London.

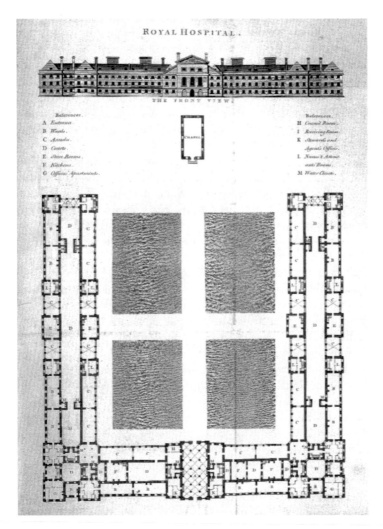

seventeen years earlier summarised architecture's contribution to these separations. The hospital had a 'variety of apartments for the reception of the different sorts of patients, built in solitary pavillions', which served both 'to prevent a communication... [and] to promote a circulation [*renouvellement*]

237

of air'.[39] Though the description is more obviously applicable to the Navy's next hospital on home soil, it is not inappropriate.

In July 1757, during the years of Haslar's construction, and changes to planned construction, the Admiralty minuted its approval of the plans put forward by the Navy Board for a hospital near Plymouth.[40] It admitted its first patients in early 1760, and the new Royal Hospital was finished just over two years later, about the same time as Haslars was. At Plymouth, fifteen detached buildings were arranged around a square and linked by a colonnade lining it (Figure 9.6).[41] The chapel faces the gate to the enclosure, both flanked by pairs of ward blocks. On each side are two more ward-blocks between lower, single-storey buildings for domestic offices. One also held wards for men suffering and recovering from smallpox, and another, cells for the insane, who would, like those at Haslar, be moved on to Bethlem in London.[42]

According to Tenon, Plymouth's surgical patients were separated from the medical, and the latter according to whether they suffered from fever, ship fever, dysentery, scurvy, phthisis, scabies, or venereal disease, as well as smallpox and insanity.[43] Actively 'contagious' patients, including victims of smallpox and the malignant fevers and fluxes, were assigned to the highest wards at both hospitals. This was because 'infected' and otherwise vitiated air rises, or so it was understood, and because these men might be emanating morbid *effluvia*, nothing and no one could lie safely above them.[44] (They were also, of course, dangerous in direct contact; hence the care for the clothing and the bed linen too.) Convalescents occupied ground-floor wards, adjacent to their *promenades*.

Hunczovsky and, in particular, Tenon described the naval hospitals' architecture in greater detail than any native – including John Howard – then did, because they were the emissaries of regents with a special interest in the subject. Hunczovsky inspected English hospitals at Joseph II of Austria's behest, and Tenon was there on behalf of Louis XVI and specifically the Paris Académie des Sciences' commission entrusted with the re-planning of the Hôtel-Dieu. National and professional pride dictated that the establishments put their best foot forward. Hunczovsky saw Haslar's convalescents playing a 'kind of ball game' to build up their strength, but in 1780, around the time of his visit, the Navy's Comptroller Charles Middleton (1726–1813) reported that its over-'numerous and ungovernible' patients instead refreshed themselves with liquor smuggled in by their friends and relations. Its officers enjoyed no 'Dignity or respect'.[45] By the same token, however, the foreign surgeons' descriptions of the buildings are particularly useful. From them we can appreciate the hopes that their local informants had for architecture and its capacity for effecting, less with walls

Figure 9.6

The Royal Hospital at Plymouth, from the French edition (1788) of
Howard's State of the Prisons. *Two ward-blocks at the front are omitted.*
Courtesy: Wellcome Library, London.

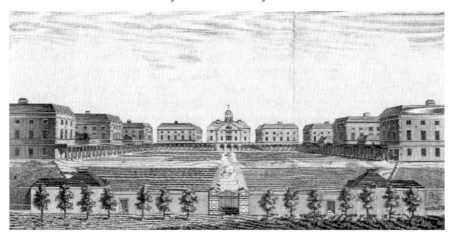

than with airy gaps, the necessary separations between different kinds of patients.

The hospital at Plymouth, was designed by Alexander Rovehead, or Rouchhead (d.1776), who was apparently from London.[46] His models do seem to have been metropolitan. Each floor of Plymouth's ward blocks consisted of two wards side-by-side, sharing a central chimney-stack, and in most cases, a front vestibule with its stairs, washtubs, and latrines. This planning resembles that of St Bartholomew's, the construction of whose fourth and final building (1757–69) coincided with Plymouth's, and it is even closer to that of the London Hospital. The London had rejected the detached ward blocks designed by Boulton Mainwaring (1702–78), but seems to have retained their internal arrangement for its new building, begun in 1752 and also still underway, whose plan was widely circulated.

Such resemblances were not pointed out at the time; the natural comparison was between the two naval hospitals. They look very different, but both formed great courts lined with galleries. Three storeys of doubled wards – end-to-end at Haslar, side-by-side at Plymouth – alternate with lower storage blocks, and the galleries between them were open on both sides, or were intended to be. At Plymouth, to cut the wind, a wall was built along the line made by the outer edges of the side pavilions, so the buildings were no longer entirely detached.[47] Even so, Plymouth was, its admirers thought, as fragmented and porous as any permanent, masonry hospital for

1,200 men could be. Its reputation was already fixed when, in 1788, Sir Joseph Banks (1743–1820) wrote that experience had shown that it was 'probably the best construction of its type in the kingdom'. Though with one qualification – Plymouth's wards should not have been doubled – the French students of the hospital type could find nothing better in the world.[48]

In 1799, the third edition of the *Observations on the Diseases Incident to Seamen*, by Gilbert Blane (1749–1834), subjected the naval hospitals' architecture to an unprecedented empirical comparison. It began with differences in their mortality rates during recent wars. Between 1793 and 1797, for example, Haslar's rate was one in 14.3, significantly higher than Plymouth's one in 24.7. Blane pointed out his controls: they were 'equally well supplied with accommodations, diet and attendance' and had the same kinds of patient, who each enjoyed equal volumes of space. The difference was presumably 'owing to the difference in point of air' and, even allowing for the local climates and soils, this point of air must rest on architecture:

> Haslar hospital consists of one great center building, and four pavilions running backwards from each corner of it. These are placed in pairs, standing parallel and very close to each other lengthwise, so as to intercept the free course of air. ...Plymouth hospital consists of twelve separate similar and equal buildings, ranged in a large square, with wide intervals between each. Of these twelve, however, ten only are occupied by the sick.

Blane's medical authority was John Pringle (1707–82), to whom we are indebted, he wrote, for placing the subject of pure air in such a 'strong and instructive point of view', that is, the hospital-planning point of view.[49] Pure air's centrality to health was a truism as old as writings about health – recall the Admiralty's instructions to the Commissioners for Sick and Wounded, in 1745, to consider the 'Convenience of Light and Air' at Haslar – but Blane was right. It was Pringle and his military followers, to whom we now turn, who had transformed the truism into a principle to be formulated through inductive reasoning. Their example prompted Blane's empiricism, a way of analysing hospital buildings that had arrived to stay. Paradoxically, their writings also have a distinctively fervent, even mystical flavour, and that would be equally lasting.

Redemption through ruin

In May 1750, more than fifty Londoners died of the gaol fever after attending an Old Bailey courtroom, victims of 'putrid streams from the bail dock', in which stood two prisoners from Newgate.[50] Pringle's *Observations on the Nature and Cure of Hospital and Jayl-fevers*, price one shilling, was printed thirteen days after the beginning of these, the 'Black Assizes'. In this pamphlet, the former Physician General to the forces in the Low Countries, and their hospitals, identified the outbreak with the fever he had observed among military populations. His *Observations on the Diseases of the Army in Camp and Garrison*, first published in 1752 and thereafter in many English, Italian, German, French, and American editions, expanded on the connection, remarking that the fever was, in effect, Britain's version of the 'true plague',[51] and explained the measures necessary for its, and other diseases' – especially dysentery's – prevention and containment.

When Pringle described how 'poisonous effluvia of sores, mortifications, dysenteric and other putrid excrements' accumulate when sick and wounded men are gathered, and how ventilation would dilute and dispel these *effluvia*, his pioneering study of military hygiene was not breaking new ground.[52] The mechanical 'ventilator' devised in 1741 by Stephen Hales (1677–1761), who also coined the word, had already been installed at a number of hospitals and jails for just this reason; and Pringle's own testimony played a big part in the invention's success. He, however, offered three corollaries of this observation about *effluvia*, which struck contemporary and later readers with considerable force. The first was the most general. When Florence Nightingale (1820–1910) famously wrote that the 'very first requirement of a hospital is that it should do the sick no harm', it was in a conscious, though unacknowledged, echo of Pringle's 'Among the great causes of sickness and death in an army, the Reader will little expect that I should mention... the hospitals'.[53] Secondly, the fuller the hospital, the bigger the danger. This maxim was generally applicable, and when generally applied had interesting implications for evaluating charitable 'success'. Beginning with John Aikin's *Thoughts on Hospitals* (1771), and the *Practical Remarks* (1776) by the American military surgeon John Jones (1729–91), it can be traced through subsequent attacks – some as political as they were medical – on the large London civil foundations until the early-nineteenth century, when James Tilton returned it to the military arena: the 'humane and benevolent design of large... hospital accommodation must necessarily be defeated in the execution... profusion and extravagance serve only to precipitate destruction and ruin'.[54]

Pringle also showed the irony in a third, even more specific problem of hospitals, and this was that patients and their nurses shut the ward windows once the physician's or surgeon's back was turned. The solution was at first simple, if radical. Unless Hales's ventilator ensured that the flow of air in military-hospital wards was proof against this fatal foolishness, the best expedient was to 'lay the sick, if numerous, in churches, barns, or ruinous houses only, where neither they nor their nurses can confine the air'.[55]

The *Observations'* fourth edition was published eight years later, in 1764. In it, the sick soldiers are still to be laid in the churches, barns, and ruinous houses, but now 'unless the wards be uncommonly well aired', not ventilated with the help of Hales's machine.[56] Later editions keep this wording, which is suggestively unspecific. Military physicians had backed off from the ventilator, which was expensive, hardly portable, and, man-powered as it was, required stricter discipline than they could muster.[57] Uncommonly good airing would have to be achieved by other means. Given that some jurisdictions – notably London and the Navy – could not manage with small hospitals, let alone ruinous houses, this seemed to rule out the makeshifts, and throw the onus on to management and design. Though a firm advocate of the benefits of 'land air', James Lind (1716–94), for example, Haslar's Physician since 1758, decided that ventilators were unnecessary if ward windows were opened as often as possible, especially since they were opposite one another.[58]

These wards got most, if not all of these opposed windows only in the late-1750s. Should we attribute the alterations made to Haslar's plan to Pringle's influence? Not in the (apparent) absence of documentation about the changes, but as two books newly published in 1764 show, his authority was becoming considerable.

The fourth edition of Pringle's *Observations* also stipulates for the first time that the sick were to be 'divided' from one another.[59] In his *Account* of the diseases of soldiers serving on the Continent, also published in 1764, Donald Monro (1727–1802) reinforced this stricture with exact figures. In churches and other lofty spaces, Monro wrote, one might allow thirty-six square feet per man, but forty-two to sixty-four square feet would be required in ordinary wards, depending on their height and the building's airiness and dryness.[60] Though volumetric specifications would soon be preferred, this was an important contribution to the methodology of institutional reform. However, *effluvia* could infect not just the men and their attendants, but buildings themselves, as Pringle had already suggested and Richard Brocklesby (1722–97) was then showing again in 1764, and no quantity of moving air would protect these sickening fabrics. With Brocklesby, Pringle's 'ruinous houses' began to take tangible form.

Brocklesby's *Observations... Tending to the Improvement of Military Hospitals* describes one of the 'close hovels, or miserable hospitals' he had been forced to use on the Isle of Wight in 1758: this level of corroborative detail, which Pringle also favoured, constituted another important contribution to reformist rhetoric. Four men put into the same corner died, poisoned one after the other. Only by scraping away at the floors and walls, and thereby 'substituting an intire new layer of the whole inside of the house', had Brocklesby managed to kill the infection. This was the bad hut; but he found the good one on another occasion, when, after cramming the sick into every house, barn, outhouse, and cottage that could be found, 'some Gentleman of the hospital' (was this Brocklesby himself?) 'proposed to erect a temporary shed with deal [softwood] boards, upon the open forest, and to have it thatched over with a coat of new straw'. The shed in the forest was big enough for 120 sick men and, though they were cold and wet there, remarkably fewer died of the same diseases, Brocklesby explained, than others under the same regimen did elsewhere, and convalescents recovered much sooner. Again, this time at Guildford, in 1760, when the putrid fever was rife, Brocklesby built a hut of wattle and thatch, big enough for forty. His 'mansions for the sick' could be quickly raised and destroyed as quickly again, if they became diseased; and by their very nature they could not be sealed against the air.[61]

The huts and ruined houses were always serendipitous. Pringle, Brocklesby, and Tilton did not (they implied) seek out such odd alternatives to hospitals, but were obliged to use them by the force of circumstance, after the windows were broken, and then discovered how well they worked.[62] Well into the next century, astonishment remained conventional in these narratives of health restored within, and, by apparent ugliness, transience, and ruin, even as the paradox was applied to effect. The sick soldiers in the Crimea 'lay looking up at the open sky', wrote Nightingale in 1858, 'thro' the chinks – & slits' of their wretched huts and tents, and there twice as many survived than in the truly wretched enclosure of the massive Scutari Hospital, in Constantinople.[63] The old ardour survived.

Pringle had written that he found existing books of no use at all,[64] but Brocklesby had two: one was Pringle's and the other was God's. Leviticus, Brocklesby explained, tells us what to do about the filth produced by 'infirmaries, or hospitals, in all countries', in which the 'seeds of infection once sown, continue, in some instances, to spread infectious diseases, and to contaminate the house', much as Israelites' 'tents, or hutts' were 'infected with the filthy leprosy' during their journey to the Land of Promise. It was the priests, the men of learning, who adhering to Mosaic precept had done the right thing: scraped the walls and if necessary pulled down the entire leprous house and carried the materials right out of the settlement.[65] In 1953, Owsei Temkin traced the eighteenth century's definitive 'secularisation' of ancient notions about ritual pollution: the 'laws of the Bible imposing the ritualistic stamp of clean and unclean were now explained as wise sanitary prescriptions by a shrewd law-giver'.[66] Today, we are less inclined, in general, to view the Enlightenment as a purely secularising phenomenon, and can acknowledge the messianic fervour with which the military physicians explained their hovels.

They found a wide readership because their audience shared a vested, Christian interest in humility. Moreover, in the two decades after 1750, a period of increasing civil and naval-hospital construction and apparently accelerating fevers, they offered an architectural 'type' in the strict, even theological, sense. The hut was not a model to be copied, at least not away from the encampments, but a prophetic or symbolic illustration of what hospitals could be. Christopher Wren would have appreciated the distinction, but he would have been even more pleased that great public buildings were still – as he put it – the 'Ornament of a Country'.[67]

Notes

1. J. Tilton, *Economical Observations on Military Hospitals; and the Prevention and Cure of Diseases Incident to an Army* (Wilmington: J. Wilson, 1813), 32–3.

2. *Ibid.*, 48–9.

3. H. Richardson (ed.), *English Hospitals 1660–1948: A Survey of their Architecture and Design* (Swindon: Royal Commission on the Historical Monuments of England, 1998), 87, from a chapter on the hospitals of the armed forces which provides a very useful overview on the basis of original research. See also the references (indexed) to hospitals in J. Douet and A. Saunders, *British Barracks 1600–1914: Their Architecture and Role in Society* (Norwich: The Stationery Office, 1998).

4. J. Evelyn, *Diary*, E.S. De Beer (ed.), 6 vols (Oxford: Clarendon Press, 1955), Vol. 2, 45. See also A.P.M. Langeveld, 'The Development of the Military Hospitals in the Netherlands' Army Medical Service', in Y. Kawakita, S. Sakai, and Y. Otsuka (eds), *History of Hospitals: The Evolution of Health Care Facilities*, Proceedings of the 11th International Symposium on the Comparative History of Medicine – East and West (Tokyo: Taniguchi Foundation, 1989), 89–126.

5. For the 'military revolution' and its historiography see J. Black, *European Warfare, 1660–1815* (New Haven and London: Yale University Press, 1994), 3–9. Black argues for dating it to circa 1660–1720, a reperiodisation which, though he does not discuss them, accords nicely with the construction of the first veterans' hospitals.

6. Notably by Le Jeune de Boulencourt's *Description Générale de l'Hôtel Royal des Invalides Etabli par Louis Le Grand... Avec les Plans, Profils et Elevations de Ses Faces, Coupes et Appartements* (Paris, 1683), discussed in C. Stevenson, *Medicine and Magnificence: British Hospital and Asylum Architecture, 1660–1815* (New Haven and London: Yale University Press, 2000), 68–9.

7. *Ibid.*, 69; R. Loeber, *A Biographical Dictionary of Architects in Ireland 1600–1720* (London: John Murray, 1981), 89.

8. M. Craig, *The Architecture of Ireland from the Earliest Times to 1880* (London and Dublin: B. T. Batsford and Eason, 1982), 153–5; E. McParland, *The Royal Hospital Kilmainham, Co. Dublin: A National Centre for Culture and the Arts in Ireland* (Dublin: Irish Architectural Archive, [1985]).

9. Quoted in G. Hutt (ed.), *Papers Illustrative of the Origin and Early History of the Royal Hospital at Chelsea, London* (London: Eyre & Spottiswoode, 1872), 14 (spelling modernised); from Charles's letter of October 1684 to William Sancroft, Archbishop of Canterbury and the King's former chaplain.

10. *Ibid.* M. Binney, 'The Royal Hospital, Chelsea', *Country Life* clxxvii (1982), 1474–7, 1582–5, on 1476, draws wider parallels with palaces as part of a useful account of Chelsea's architecture.

11. M. Whinney, *Wren* (London: Thames & Hudson, 1971), 147, who also describes Wren's six-ward-block plan for Greenwich as allowing the 'interiors the maximum of light and air' (188).

12. A. Wear, 'Making Sense of Health and the Environment in Early Modern England', in A. Wear (ed.), *Medicine in Society: Historical Essays* (Cambridge: Cambridge University Press, 1992), 119–47, on 141, 145–7.

13. F.N.L. Poynter (ed.), *The Journal of James Yonge (1647–1721), Plymouth Surgeon* (London: Longmans, 1963), 98, and see 200 for his introduction (by Robert Hooke) to Wren in 1686.

14. Nigel Barker found two contracts from 1681 relating to this hospital ('The Architecture of the English Board of Ordnance 1660–1750', 3 vols [unpublished PhD dissertation, University of Reading, 1985], Vol. 1, 288–91), the only one built by the Ordnance on home soil during his period. C.G.T. Dean, 'Charles II's Garrison Hospital, Portsmouth', *Papers and Proceedings of the Hampshire Field Club and Archaeological Society* 16 (1947), 280–3, describes what remained of it in 1947. Enclosed beds became suspect, as impediments to ventilation, in the 1760s (Edward Foster, *An Essay on Hospitals. Or, Succinct Directions for the Situation, Construction, and Administration of Country Hospitals* [Dublin: the author, 1768], 25) and twenty years later the Commissioners for Sick and Wounded Seamen recommended that they be abandoned at naval hospitals overseas, though in equivocal terms. No longer was the patient to be spared the 'dying looks of his companion': quoted Richardson (ed.), *op. cit.* (note 3), 82.

15. J. Bold, *Greenwich: An Architectural History of the Royal Hospital for Seamen and the Queen's House* (New Haven and London: Yale University Press, 2000), 98-108.

16. Stevenson, *op. cit.* (note 6), 74–5, 77 reproduces Wren's plan drawing for the twelve ward-block project and the perspective and plan engraved in 1699.

17. With the intriguing exception of the palace of Marly, built (1679–84) for Louis XIV as a private retreat in thirteen pavilions, and used later in the century to explain pavilion-hospital planning: *ibid.*, 190. He also departed from the Invalides model, otherwise still influential in England: John Bold, 'Comparable Institutions: The Royal Hospital for Seamen and the Hôtel des Invalides', *Essays in Architectural History Presented to John Newman. Architectural History* xliv (2001), 136-44.

18. In 1763: James Boswell, *The Life of Samuel Johnson*, 2 vols (London: Robert Rivière, [1906]), Vol. 1, 284.

19. Specifically, the largest, with the fourteen blocks: *The Sixth Volume of the Wren Society ...The Royal Hospital for Seamen at Greenwich 1694–1728*. A.T. Bolton and H.D. Hendry (eds) (Oxford: University Press for the Wren Society, 1929), 97; J.D. Thompson and G. Goldin, *The Hospital: A Social and Architectural History* (New Haven and London: Yale University Press, 1975), 149; T.A. Markus, *Buildings and Power: Freedom and Control in the Origin of Modern Building Types* (London and New York: Routledge, 1993), 117–18.

20. J. Aikin, *Thoughts on Hospitals* (London: Joseph Johnson, 1771), 20. The book, which was translated into French in 1777, perhaps prompted Jean-Noël Hallé's characterisation of Greenwich as one of three older hospitals 'dignes de servir d'exemple' of hospital construction (the other examples were French): 'Air. Hygiène' in F. Vicq d'Azyr (ed.), *Encyclopédie Méthodique... Médecine*, (Paris: Panckoucke, 1787), 492–590: 575. French visitors were however independently impressed by the healthiness of its architecture (enhanced by an impressive standard of housekeeping): [P.-J.] Grosley, *A Tour of London; Or, New Observations on England, and its Inhabitants*, trans. Thomas Nugent, 2 vols (London: Lockyer Davis, 1772), Vol. 2, 42; J. Tenon, *Journal d'Observations sur les Principaux Hôpitaux et sur Quelques Prisons d'Angleterre*, J. Carré (ed.) (Publications de la Faculté des Lettres et Sciences Humaines, n.s. 37. Clermont-Ferrand: Université Blaise-Pascal, 1992), 65–71.

21. For this building, which later housed the Dreadnought Seamen's Hospital and survives in altered form, see the National Monuments Record (Swindon) file no. 101280, and Bold, *op. cit.* (note 15), 206–20. Greenwich's exact role in the development of the modern hospital type remains uncertain, but it was bigger than was once assumed, at least by architectural historians, who used to adduce only Wren's unexecuted designs (see the references at note 19, above). Naval-medical historials did not assume this: see, for example, C. Lloyd and J.L.S. Coulter, *Medicine and the Navy, 1200–1900*, Vol. 3, *1714–1815* (Edinburgh and London: E. & S. Livingstone, 1961), 207, on Haslar's debt to Greenwich's architecture, an hypothesis also advanced in Richardson, *op. cit.* (note 3), 79.

22. [T. Faulkner], *An Historical and Descriptive Account of the Royal Hospital... at Chelsea* (London: T. Faulkner, 1805), 46.

23. Even so, the building had become a barracks by 1694: Dean, *op. cit.* (note 14), 283.

24. On this hospital, which survives in part, see J.G. Coad, *Historic Architecture of the Royal Navy: An Introduction* (London: Gollancz, 1983), 31, 143–5; and E. Buchanan, 'Naval Hospital Architecture in the Eighteenth Century'

(unpublished MA Dissertation, Courtauld Institute, London, 1996), 12–15;
thanks to the latter for allowing me to cite her dissertation here. It does not
form a closed quadrangle, but its siting on an island in the harbour answered
the problem of security.

25. National Maritime Museum (henceforth, NMM) ADM/E/11
    (Commissioners for Sick & Hurt Seamen. In Letters from the Admiralty,
    1744–5), not numbered, filed after (20.), 18 June 1745. Lloyd and Coulter,
    op. cit. (note 21), 101–4 and D. Baugh, *British Naval Administration in the
    Age of Walpole* (Princeton, NJ: Princeton University Press, 1965), 217–18
    describe the Jamaica hospital. For the Gibraltar hospital (which survives)
    completed in 1756, see C. Lawrance, *The History of the Old Naval Hospital
    Gibraltar 1741 to 1922* (Lymington: C. Lawrance, 1994) and Coad, *op. cit.*
    (note 24), 145–7.

26. N. Hawksmoor, *Remarks on the Founding and Carrying On the Buildings of
    the Royal Hospital At Greenwich* (London: N. Blandford, 1728), 16.

27. S. Gradish, *The Manning of the British Navy during the Seven Years' War*
    (London: Royal Historical Society, 1980), 186; P.K. Crimmin, 'The Sick and
    Hurt Board and the Health of Seamen, c.1700–1806', *Journal for Maritime
    Research* (December 1999), http://www.jmr.nmm.ac.uk/server/show/
    conJmrArticle.12.

28. Baugh, *op. cit.* (note 25), 51, and see 179–86, 216–22 for the epidemic's
    impact on manning and hospital construction.

29. R. Evans, *The Fabrication of Virtue: English Prison Architecture 1750–1840*
    (Cambridge: Cambridge University Press, 1982), 95, at the beginning of an
    excellent chapter on 'Gaol Fever'; see also M. DeLacy, *Prison Reform in
    Lancashire, 1700–1850: A Study in Local Administration* (Stanford: Stanford
    University Press, 1986).

30. On 7 February 1759, for example, the Sick and Hurt Board recommended
    to the Admiralty that the use of the *Blenheim* be discontinued (and that of
    another hospital ship at Plymouth, once the new hospital there was ready),
    as at the royal hospitals 'Patients may be as effectually secured as on board an
    Hospital Ship, and their Cure sooner Compleated' if the sentries 'do their
    Duty'; ships 'at best afford but very indifferent conveniences for the Sick'.
    The National Archives [hereafter NA] ADM 98/7 (Sick and Wounded
    Board's Out-Letters to the Admiralty from 10 October 1757 to 1759), 374.
    See Baugh, *op. cit.* (note 25), 50–1, 180–4 and Crimmin, *op. cit.* (note 27)
    for good introductions to medical contracting.

31. See, for example, K.J. Carpenter, *The History of Scurvy and Vitamin C*
    (Cambridge: Cambridge University Press, 1986), 57–61 on James Lind's
    belief, which he held until the early-1770s, that the moisture discouraging
    'insensible' perspiration was scurvy's principal cause; and C. Lawrence,
    'Disciplining Disease: Scurvy, the Navy, and Imperial Expansion

1750–1825', in D. P. Miller and P. H. Reill (eds), *Visions of Empire: Voyages, Botany, and Representations of Nature* (Cambridge: Cambridge University Press, 1996), 80–106, on 86, which quotes John Pringle: the 'corruption of the bilge water, is not only a main cause of sea scurvy, but often concurs in crowded ships, to raise a fever of the hospital or jayl kind'.

32. NMM ADM/E/11, not numbered, filed after (20.), 18 June 1745. Twelve years later, the Admiralty forwarded to the Commissioners, their interest in hospital planning now established, a proposal for an eighty-bed army hospital at Chatham. They approved of it, but suggested increasing the widths and heights of the wards, and that the building be enlarged to permit 'the Cradles being placed seperately', two feet apart, instead of coupled. NA, ADM 98/6 (Sick and Wounded Board's Out-Letters to the Admiralty from 30 October/1 November 1756–57 to 9 October 1757), 159–60 (26 January 1757).

33. That 'brute of a Shipwright': Baugh, *op. cit.* (note 25), 48, quoting a remark from 1747. Ackworth was blocking changes in ship design that the Admiralty wanted, and failing to improve efficiency at the dockyards: *ibid.*, 89, 251–2. The Admiralty Secretary explained to the Commissioners on 18 June 1745 that 'Their Lordships have directed Sr Jacob Ac[k]worth, who has been consulted in this Affair, and has Schemed a Plan for the Building, to meet you, when you shall apply to him, and Mr Jacobson, a Gentleman, who Voluntary was concerned in projecting the Plan for Building the Hospital for Foundlings, has likewise promised to give you his Company, whenever you shall send to him': NMM ADM/E/11, not numbered, filed after (20.). Admittedly, it was a very unusual 'Gentleman'-architect who designed big institutional buildings.

34. As the Commissioners reported to the Admiralty on 17 June 1745, after Ackworth and Jacobsen met on their premises that day: NMM ADM/F/6 (Admiralty. In Letters from the Sick & Hurt Board, May–August 1745), not numbered.

35. See the plan (Admiralty Library) annotated in early 1756, and reproduced by P.D.G. Pugh, 'The Planning of Haslar', *Journal of the Royal Naval Medical Service* 62 (1976), 103–20, on 115. The National Monuments Record (Swindon) file on the hospital, no. 100117, includes an excellent manuscript account (by Kathryn Morrison) of this complicated building in its present state.

36. Lloyd and Coulter, *op. cit.* (note 21), 216. Tenon, *op. cit.* (note 20), 179–80 called it England's biggest hospital, and J. Hunczovsky, in *Medicinisch-chirurgische Beobachtungen auf seinen Reisen durch England und Frankreich besonders über die Spitäler* (Vienna: Rudolph Graffer, 1783), 49, its biggest brick construction.

37. Hunczovsky, *op. cit.* (note 36), 50.

38. See the fast sketch that he made of the ground plan in 1787, reproduced in Tenon, *op. cit.* (note 20), facing 181.

39. Grosley, *op. cit.* (note 20), 2: 43, a precise translation from [P.-J. Grosley], *Londres. Ouvrage d'un François: Augmenté dans cette Édition des notes d'un Anglois*, 2nd edn, 3 vols (Neuchatel: Aux dépens de la Societé Typographique, 1770), 2: 386; Tenon, *op. cit.* (note 20), 183–4.

40. NA, ADM 3/65 (Admiralty Board minute book, 19 November 1756–16 January 1758), 7 July 1757.

41. Most of the buildings survive. See the National Monument Record's file no. 100373, which, besides a manuscript report (by Kathryn Morrison) on the hospital's current condition, includes particularly informative aerial photographs.

42. Tenon, *op. cit.* (note 20), 182 mentions Bethlem and in his *Memoirs on Paris Hospitals*, Dora B. Weiner (ed.) ([Canton, MA]: Science History Publications, 1996; a translation of his *Mémoires sur les hôpitaux de Paris*, 1788), 28, the smallpox wards. Another useful description of the hospital is that of Richard Creke (appointed its Governor in 1795), transcribed in Lloyd and Coulter, *op. cit.* (note 21), 267–9.

43. Tenon, *op. cit.* (note 20), 154–5: 'Les maladies sont classées par salles de fiévreux, de fièvre de vaisseau qui ressemble à celle d'hôpital, de dysenterie, de scorbut, de phtisiques, de petite vérole, de galeux, du mal vénérien, de blessés.'

44. Stevenson, *op. cit.* (note 6), 162, 182; Tenon, *op. cit.* (note 42), 28.

45. Wellcome Library MS 5992 (Observations by Charles Middleton on Reports of Conditions at Haslar Hospital, Gosport [1780]), ff. 4r, 6v. On this inspection see Lloyd and Coulter, *op. cit.* (note 21), 213; their account of the hospitals is useful on the continuing administrative problems. On the 'Art von Ballspiel', Hunczovsky, *op. cit.* (note 36), 51; I have not been able to discover when, exactly, he visited England.

46. H. Colvin, *A Biographical Dictionary of British Architects, 1600–1840*, 3rd ed. (New Haven and London: Yale University Press, 1995), s.v. 'Rouchhead, Alexander'.

47. As Tenon, *op. cit.* (note 20), 154, pointed out. He would have preferred complete detachment for ventilation's sake, but reported that the medical staff were happy with the new arrangement.

48. '[N]otre Hôpital Royal de Plymouth, qu'on a trouvé par experience être fort bon, et peut-être de la meilleure construction de tous ceux que nous avons dans le Royaume.' Banks was writing (2 October 1788) to the French physicist Jean-Baptiste Le Roy: British Library Add. MS 8097, fo. 111. I owe this reference to L.S. Greenbaum, 'Tempest in the Academy: Jean-Baptiste Le Roy, the Paris Academy of Sciences and the Project of a New Hôtel-Dieu', *Archives Internationales d'Histoire des Sciences*, xxiv (1974), 122–40, on

139. For Plymouth and the French see also Stevenson, *op. cit.* (note 6), 191–3.

49. G. Blane, *Observations on the Diseases Incident to Seamen*, 3rd edn (London: Murray & Highley, 1799), 175–6, 178n.

50. M. Ignatieff, *A Just Measure of Pain: The Penitentiary in the Industrial Revolution 1750–1850* (London: Macmillan, 1978), 44–5.

51. J. Pringle, *Observations on the Diseases of the Army, in Camp and Garrison: In three Parts: With an Appendix, Containing Some Papers of Experiments, Read at Several Meetings of the Royal Society* (London: A. Millar, D. Wilson, and T. Payne, 1752), 334.

52. Quoted in J.H. Woodward, *To Do the Sick no Harm: A Study of the British Voluntary Hospital System to 1875* (London: Routledge & Kegan Paul, 1974), 98.

53. F. Nightingale, *Notes on Hospitals*, 3rd edn (London: Longman, Green, 1863), iii; Pringle, *op. cit.* (note 51), vii. Tobias Smollett quoted this sentence in his (anonymous) review of the *Observations: Monthly Review* vii (July 1752), 52–6, on 53. For the durability of the formulation, see Stevenson, *op. cit.* (note 6), 158.

54. Aikin, *op. cit.* (note 20), 9, 11; J. Jones, *Plain Concise Practical Remarks, on the Treatment of Wounds and Fractures; To which is added, an Appendix, on Camp and Military Hospitals; Principally designed, for the use of young Military and Naval Surgeons, in North-America* (1776), repr. edn (New York: Arno Press & The New York Times: 1971), 101–5; Tilton, *op. cit.* (note 1), 15.

55. Pringle, *op. cit.* (note 51), 252.

56. J. Pringle, *Observations on the Diseases of the Army*, 4th edn (London: A. Millar, D. Wilson, T. Durham, and T. Payne, 1764), 293–4; Stevenson, *op. cit.* (note 6), 169–70.

57. The 'negligence, and laziness of the people in working them, and their diffidence of the utility of measures, which seem so simple and so trifling... made them fall very short of our expectations, whenever I attempted to enforce their use': R. Brocklesby, *Oeconomical and Medical Observations... Tending to the Improvement of Military Hospitals* (London: T. Becket & P.A. De Hondt, 1764), 57.

58. 'Es waren vormals zu Lüftung der Zimmer Ventilators bestimmt; Dr. Lind fand aber, daß dieselben bey weiten der Bestimmung nicht so ein Genüge thun, als die, so viel möglich, offen gehaltenen Fenster, zumal da sie einander angebracht sind': Hunczovsky, *op. cit.* (note 36), 52. According to Buchanan, *op. cit.* (note 24), 26, Lind had the sashes nailed open every spring.

59. Pringle, *op. cit.* (note 56), 293.

60. D. Monro, *An Account of the Diseases which were most frequent in the British Military Hospitals in Germany, from January 1761 to... March 1763: To which is added, An Essay on the Means of Preserving the Health of Soldiers, and*

Conducting Military Hospitals (London: A. Millar, D. Wilson, & T. Durham, 1764), 364.

61. Brocklesby, *op. cit.* (note 57), 62–6, 72–3, 77.

62. Tilton, *op. cit.* (note 1), 49 called his hut an experiment, but it was one forced by the hard winter. See Stevenson, *op. cit.* (note 6), 28–9, 163 for more extended discussions, from which I am borrowing here.

63. She was actually writing about a more prosaic question: do patients in satisfactorily-ventilated hospitals catch cold? M. Vicinus and B. Nergaard (eds), *Ever Yours, Florence Nightingale: Selected Letters* (Cambridge: Harvard University Press, 1990), 210.

64. Pringle, *op. cit.* (note 51), v.

65. Brocklesby, *op. cit.* (note 57), 59; compare Lev. 14:44–45.

66. O. Temkin, 'An Historical Analysis of the Concept of Infection' (1953), in *The Double Face of Janus and Other Essays in the History of Medicine* (Baltimore: Johns Hopkins University Press, 1977), 456–71: 468.

67. L.M. Soo (ed.), *Wren's 'Tracts' on Architecture and Other Writings* (Cambridge: Cambridge University Press, 1998), 153.

10

Internal Influences in the
Making of the English Military Hospital:
The Early-Eighteenth-Century Greenwich

Geoffrey L. Hudson

This chapter uses records at the Royal Greenwich Hospital for ex-sailors to analyse the nature of care, and to uncover how the chronically disabled patients themselves experienced the hospital. Greenwich became a 'reverse' institution, in that the ex-servicemen were closely regulated and treated like unruly visitors, while only officers and medics had free movement and influence. Although initially the inner workings of the Hospital owed much to almshouse and shipboard models, over time medical considerations became paramount. Physicians and surgeons became involved actively in governance and discipline, promoting environmental and dietary changes.

Whereas much has been written about the architecture of the Royal Greenwich Hospital, its inner life remains unexamined.[1] This chapter utilises the minutes of the Council that administered discipline at Greenwich to explore how its chronically disabled patients experienced the hospital.

The Greenwich Council met regularly and recorded the Hospital's internal regime in detail, including accusations brought against patients, nurses and officers, punishments meted out, as well as regulations made and amended as a result of the ongoing life of the institution. These records have never been examined systematically by historians. This chapter supplements them with other materials such as letters from the Admiralty about patient petitions.

Initially the inner life of the institution owed much to almshouse, monastic, and shipboard influences. Increasingly, however, medical considerations became influential, and a new type of institution for the chronically disabled took shape.

Relief of disabled servicemen, 1590–1700

Over four hundred years ago the English Parliament created Europe's first state system of benefits for rank-and-file disabled sailors and soldiers. A 1593 act created a county-based pension scheme that lasted, with changes, until 1679.[2] During the 1640s and 1650s Parliament ran a central fund that provided three hundred and fifty hospital places at the Savoy and Ely House, as well as 6,500 out-pensions to ex-servicemen, war widows, and orphans. With the Restoration, this central parliamentary provision ended. In the late seventeenth-century, the Royal Hospitals of Chelsea and Greenwich were created.

Historians who have considered the state's relief of disabled ex-servicemen in the early-modern period have tended to concentrate on the Royal Hospitals and give relatively scant attention to the county schemes. John Keevil, in *Medicine and the Navy*, dismisses the county system as 'no more than thinly disguised and inefficiently administered charity'.[3] Instead he concentrates on tracing developments 'which would in time lead to hospitals built exclusively for the sick and wounded of the fighting services'.[4] Thus the Savoy and Ely House hospitals created by Parliament in the mid-seventeenth century, 'afforded a striking contrast' to previous provision for the men which 'must have supplied many official arguments for the permanent retention of such state provision' and 'in their later use as homes for pensioners... were prototypes of the great hospitals at Chelsea and Greenwich founded at the end of the seventeenth century'.[5]

C.H. Firth in a chapter on the 'Provision for the sick and wounded and for old soldiers' maintained that the Long Parliament, in its creation of the two national military hospitals of the Savoy and Ely House, had thus 'recognised the moral obligation of the State to those who suffered in its service, and it was the *first* English government to do so'.[6] He argued that these hospitals were necessary in order to supplement the county pension scheme that, although revamped in the 1640s, was inadequate for the nation's needs. G. Hutt in *Papers Illustrative of the Origins and Early History of the Royal Hospital at Chelsea*, using the state papers to examine the county scheme at some length, comes to a similar conclusion to that of Firth. Parliament's national hospitals were an improvement on the county system and hence the Restoration brought detrimental change because these national hospitals were closed, the county pension scheme continuing in a new form from 1662 to 1679.[7] For both these scholars, with the creation of the army hospital at Chelsea in the 1680s, and the Greenwich hospital at the turn of the century, 'the example for the Long Parliament bore fruit'.[8]

C. Lloyd and J. Coulter, in the third volume of *Medicine and the Navy*, took Keevil's lead, arguing that the Greenwich hospital was a good thing for the disabled. Indeed, Lloyd and Coutler declare that 'there can be no doubt that one of the inscriptions on the hospital buildings rang true in the hearts of most of the old sailors: "Let them give thanks whom the Lord hath redeemed and delivered them out of the hands of the enemy".'[9] So too, Philip Newell in his book on Greenwich, declares that staff and patients were a 'happy family'.[10]

John Ehrman in *The Navy in the War of William II, 1689–1697* went so far as to state that Greenwich, designed as a hospital for the sick and wounded, 'as a home for pensioners and for the dependents of the disabled and the slain', was a 'magnificent monument' which by 1752 was 'to stand "the apotheosis of secular glory", as an unequalled monument to English sea power'.[11]

Historians of the English state's provision for disabled ex-servicemen have therefore provided us with a description of the state's beneficence in which it is assumed that the central government was more effective and efficient than local authorities and especially that the central government's hospitals provided an increasingly and relatively superior standard of provision for disabled ex-servicemen. I think that this interpretation can be called into question in a number of ways. Firstly, the county pension scheme provided for many more individuals than scholars have previously assumed. Enough treasurers' accounts survive around 1671 to permit a fairly reliable estimate of the numbers of county pensioners throughout England at this time. Given 123 pensioners per 100,000, and a population of 4,982,000 (5,331,000 with Wales), an estimate of the number of county pensioners in England, circa 1671, is 6,128 (6,557 in England and Wales).[12] It would be decades before the Royal Hospitals would be able to come close to this level of provision.

Although the county scheme had fiscal problems so too did the hospitals, especially in the early years. The governors of Chelsea reported in 1711, for example, that the out-pensioners had not received any pension monies for six months, and that they were:

[N]ow lying in the streets in and about the Cities of London and Westminster, and severall other parts of the Kingdom in a starving and perishing condition, severall of them not having wherewithall to cover their nakedness, and their wounds yet uncured all which tends very much to the discouragement of Her Majesty's Service... these Poore Creatures... having lost their limbs or been otherwise disabled in Her armies abroad.[13]

These facts beg the question as to whether the change to state military hospitals was simply dictated by the need to properly look after the men, and the example of the military hospitals of the Long Parliament, as historians argued. The needs of the military and intellectual fashion – the move to confinement – can be shown to have also been significant factors in the decision to create state national military hospitals. When these two factors are considered, they combine to fundamentally challenge the traditional view of unimpeachable progress because they involve an awareness of the changing use of power by the state over the bodies of the ex-servicemen.

Origins of Greenwich and Chelsea hospitals

From the outset, Greenwich and Chelsea were conceived as police operations. Proponents of such institutions such as John Evelyn (the first treasurer at Greenwich) and Stephen Fox (the first Paymaster-General of the Army) recommended their establishment on grounds of cost effectiveness.[14] In his proposal of March 1666 for a navy hospital at Chatham, Evelyn compared his scheme to the existing system of having the men relieved in public houses. He commented that with the creation of a hospital:

> [T]he almost indefinite number of Chirurgions & Officers [would be] exceedingly reduc'd: the Sick dieted, kept from drinke &, Intemperance; & consequently from most unavoydably relapseing: They are hindred from Wandring, slipping-away and dispersion: They are more fedulously attended; the Physitian better inspects the Chirurgions, who neither can, nor will be in all places, as now they are scattered in the nasty Corners of the townes.[15]

It would be expensive to admit those who did not need relief, or relieve men who were then allowed to misbehave in ways that would result in the necessity of further treatment. More to the point, however, proponents and planners also emphasised military considerations; the hospitals were to lead to a decrease in desertion and thus an increase in the numbers returning to active service.[16]

Roy Porter took exception to Foucault's claim that the mid-seventeenth century constituted a 'dramatic watershed in the process of institutionalisation' for the insane in any country, except perhaps for France. He also argued that England in particular is a country which 'does not easily square with the model of a 'great confinement'.[17] For the disabled ex-serviceman in England, however, Foucault's chronology has merit, as confinement began with the Parliamentary hospitals created in the 1640s. The English Civil War and Restoration complicate the story however.

Although Firth and Hutt argue that Chelsea and Greenwich were created as a result of the example of the Savoy and Ely House hospitals there is evidence to suggest that this is not the entire story; those in authority were also mindful of continental, and especially French, hospitals – as well as those of the rebels who ruled England in the mid-century. William Blathwayt, Secretary-at-War from August 1683, chose consciously to follow the administrative methods of the French army, including modelling the regulations that were employed at Chelsea, on those of the Hôtel des Invalides.[18] Blathwayt, writing to the minister to France, noted that:

> I am now reading a large description in folio of the Hotel des Invalides, which takes notice of several edicts and Regulations concerning the government and economy of that place which are said to be published and observed there, none of which are to be found in any of the volumes of Military Ordonnances, and if by your means they could be produced they would be of great use in the model of government for Chelsea Hospital his Majesty is now ordering to be prepared....[19]

When the Government was considering the construction of a navy hospital in the middle of the last decade of the century, the volume Blathwayt was examining – a 1683 description of the government of the Invalides – was translated and published in London – *Pattern of a Well-Constituted and Well-Governed Hospital...* – to serve as an example for those framing the regulations of the new hospital at Greenwich.[20]

Indeed, Blathwayt and others were being attentive to the political imperative to enhance royal authority over standing armed forces and as such were keen to follow the example of the confinement of ex-servicemen set by Louis XIV's France, with the opening of the Hôtel des Invalides in 1670. Louis himself stated that it was the one foundation he established that was most useful to the state.[21] The French had experience of the depredations ex-servicemen were capable of in mid-century – during and after the Fronde – and wished to discipline them. Indeed, the *Pattern* referred to the disabled pensioners as potential 'ravenous Wolves or wild Boars', to be kept within the hospital and only released with great care.[22]

In France and elsewhere, the creation of national military hospitals was deemed necessary as a result of changes concomitant with the creation of standing armies and navies, as well as the need to conserve troops given demands for more of them, and tactical changes which made it desirable that the state's fighters be experienced and trained. This process has been described for France by Colin Jones in his 'The Welfare of the French Foot-Soldier from Richelieu to Napoleon'. Jones also argued that the Hôtel des Invalides was erected as a hospital and retirement home for common foot-soldiers in the 1670s as a result of new ideas about social policy: it became fashionable to believe that it was in the state's interest to exclude 'alleged deviants from society within specialised institutions', such as the Invalides. Later, barracks were used to achieve the same purpose for those still in the lists.[23] These new institutions enabled the state to exercise greater discipline – 'greater bureaucratic control'. Not only did society need to be protected from the ex-servicemen's tendency towards crime but there was a desire to create 'a mode of bodily comportment' which included the regulation of sex.[24] For Jones 'military welfare policies were thus a kind of litmus test for social and political values, and also for the changing contours of the charitable imperative'.[25] He agrees with Isser Woloch that the ill or incapacitated ex-serviceman in the Ancien Regimé was at 'the frontier of social welfare'.[26] For the disabled in the military hospital this was especially so because:

> [H]ospitals shorn of their charitable carapace, administered by state bureaucrats rather than benevolent notables and run by paid orderlies rather than sisters of charity... were more directly accessible to trained medical staff.[27]

Jones is influenced by Foucault's interest in the great confinement of the mad, criminal, poor, and diseased in early modern France. In particular, Jones is drawn to Foucault's – now familiar – understanding of the new regime of power exercised by early modern states which manifested itself as bio-power: the body as an object to be controlled by various disciplinary technologies with the goal of improving it for the good of the state. These technologies included training of the body as well as enclosure and control of space.[28]

Although Jones is influenced by Foucault, he is careful to argue that Foucault tends to overestimate the repressive aspects of the institutions which used such technologies of power.[29] Instead, Jones points to research which shows that their civilian counterparts – the hôpitaux généraux, for example – often made a genuine contribution to the needs of the poor, who made use of them 'in particular at time of difficulty in the family life-cycle'.[30]

The records for the Savoy and Ely House, as well as those of Chelsea allow for only limited understanding of the inner life of those hospitals. For Parliament's hospitals, surviving materials include their regulations and various accounts, most of which are wage, laundry, and medicine bills. Firth, Keevil, and Gruber von Arni are able to reconstruct enough to allow only a glimpse of what confinement meant for the ex-servicemen.[31] For Chelsea, records of the inner life of the institution are more plentiful than the Savoy and Ely House, the hospital journals survive for example. The Chelsea journals, however, tend to focus on out-pensioners rather than in-pensioners, and there was no body, like the council at Greenwich, that administered discipline – and left a set of detailed minutes.

Overview of the operation of the Greenwich

Selection procedure included certificates from military superiors, including the surgeon. Invaliding boards reviewed the prospective applicants. The definition of pensionable disability continued – as in the county scheme – to focus on disability to work, with a vast majority being disabled in body, with a minority suffering from illness.[32]Greenwich, like Chelsea, was styled a royal charity, although it was financed by deductions from the pay of servicemen – 6d a month from 1696. Supplemental financing included unclaimed prize money, some parliamentary grants, and some estate income. This contrasts with the seventeenth century county scheme that had a statutory basis and was funded from the property tax.[33]

The Hospital's rules and orders, developed from August 1704, required twice-daily attendance at service, wearing of uniforms, and punishment for a variety of offences. The Council records include minutes of the meetings and a set of Council decisions – orders – that emerged from the experience of discipline.[34] The Council consisted of the Governor, Lieutenant-Governor, captains, lieutenants, chaplains, surgeon, and physician. Quorum was three and the lieutenant governor had to be present. It met about once a fortnight, sometimes more often, and dealt with in-house complaints and problems. The records are very full, especially for the first few years; details of testimony are notable. For example, one nurse who had listened in on a pensioner and nurse copulating reported what had been said between them in the act. It was duly noted in the minutes that the amorous nurse had exclaimed that he 'was the most charming man in the house.'[35]

Evidence was only exceptionally taken on oath.[36] There were penalties for lying to the Council, not appearing when summoned, and not providing information about infractions, 'crimes' against the hospital rules.[37] As numbers increased, informers were encouraged with cash rewards, and a number of petty offices were created – boatswains and boatswain mates – to enforce discipline, including complaining to the Council.[38] There is evidence that officers had latitude to inflict punishments without recourse to the Council. Practice contrary to the standing rules of the house was, however, forbidden.[39]

The Council records reveal the hospital's internal regime. This chapter will focus primarily on the crucial twenty-five-year period from 1704, when the first pensioners arrived. The range of accusations brought to the council include the following, in rough order of frequency: drunkenness; abusive language of various sorts including scolding; absence without leave, neglect of duty; not reporting crimes to the council; cursing; mutiny; threatening violence or assault; theft; sexual relations; nastiness (pee, shit, and spit); smoking; and bringing frivolous complaints.[40] Nurses were put in the stocks and deprived of food and wages. Irregular punishments included chaining. At times, pensioners were required to apologise on their knees in the Hall to individuals they had harmed.[41]

The type of punishment meted out to those judged guilty changed markedly over these years. Until 1714 the following were the main punishments: loss of food, being put on bread and water; losing allowance money; not being allowed out of the hospital for a period; being put in the house of confinement; standing in the elevated place in the Hall during meals; wearing a badge appropriate to one's crime; not being allowed out of the hospital; having to clean up the guard room for a period; being a scavenger – wearing the broom and shovel around one's neck during meals.[42]

Usually punishments were combined. It was common for men – and women – to be brought before Council on a number of occasions. One example, John Worley, has been immortalised by James Thornhill: Worley served as Thornhill's model for the figure of 'Winter' on the ceiling of Greenwich's painted hall. He was admitted on 2 February 1704/5 and died a pensioner on 9 June 1721.[43] Worley was cited before the Council on nine occasions between September 1706 and January 1713/14, for being absent without leave, drunk, quarrelsome, foul mouthed, abusive to his ward mates, and mutinous. On 2 March 1707/08 he declared that 'there was not any justice done' in the hospital. A few years later (17 January 1711/12) he came into his ward drunk, called a fellow pensioner 'a pitiful louzey Scotch dog' and declared that 'he was a better man than any offi[ice]r in the House'. For the latter misbehaviour he was sentenced to lose a day's meals, standing in the elevated hall for a week during meal time, refused permission to leave the hospital for a month, and ordered to wear a badge for 'swearing' for a week.[44]

In May 1714, the punishment of food deprivation was commuted to a monetary deduction.[45] As well as being deprived of their allowances, men were exposed in the Hall, and were made to wear a yellow frock and confined to the hospital. The purpose of the yellow frock was to enable those on guard duty to identify those who were not supposed to leave the hospital. In years to come those wearing the yellow were nicknamed canaries.[46]

In common with almshouse officers and county justices, the Council at Greenwich exercised discretion when sentencing in order to elicit improved behaviour: lighter sentences going to first-time offenders, those with good reputations, those making their humble submissions to the court. The Council also took age, poverty, and the accused's medical condition – disability – into consideration when sentencing. One Cresswell, pensioner, ordered a walking stick to be made with King George's head 'with a pair of horns' – thereby implying that the King was a cuckold. The Council decided to punish rather than expel him for the 'scandalous words… in consideration of his age & that (having lately broke his thigh) he is unable any ways to gett a living'[47] Those who were incorrigible were severely punished ultimately up to and including exclusion, with ten per cent being expelled or running away during the first fifty years of the hospital.[48]

Medicalisation

During the first few years at Greenwich the disciplinary regime owed much to almshouse, monastic, and shipboard models. The men were placed in cells, encouraged and required to pray and worship daily, dined communally, uniformed and ranked, with discipline and punishments influenced by life at sea.[49]

Increasingly, as medical considerations became influential, a new type of institution was being created. Whereas at first, the surgeon and doctor rarely attended council meetings, in time they attended regularly and influenced decisions. The man who set the pattern in this regard was the surgeon James Christie, who previously had been influential in the expansion of the numbers of hospital ships, the early transfer of infectious cases to land, and the move to having live animals on board. Christie had an explicit pride in the Navy medical services.[50] The result? The Council reduced sentences on the basis of the men's age and physical disabilities. The change in the whole nature of punishment, with the elimination of food deprivation, came about because of concerns about the effect of such punishments on the men's physical state. The physician secured an order opening the infirmary doors, with guards posted, so that there would be movement of air, an environmental health consideration. It was noted that 'the physician being of opinion that the locking up the infirmary doors at night is of ill consequenct [*sic*] to the sick by keeping them too close from air and especially in the summer season'.[51] There was also a concern about faeces and urine being tossed in and about the hospital, including tossing it out the windows, particularly directly above the infirmary wards that were on the ground floor.[52] Pensioners were told they would be rewarded for informing on the culprits. Rewards could be quite large: five shillings for information leading to a conviction in the mid 1720s.[53]

In the early-eighteenth century there was a growing relationship between drink, discipline and health. At first, alehouse servants were prohibited from selling alcohol in the hospital.[54] Then, infirmary patients were forbidden to leave the hospital, to prevent them from drinking and thus retarding their recovery.[55] Those visiting the sick were not allowed to bring alcohol. Later, bars were put on the infirmary windows to prevent the patients escaping to the alehouse.[56] The physician proposed depriving the infirmary patients of their allowance in order to stop them drinking, the money to be put towards better food. In the preamble to the proposal, the physician commented that drinking among the sick in the infirmary 'renders a great part of his endeavour fruitless'.[57] So too, a proposal to build a hospital alehouse with a monopoly, was prefaced by the comment that alcohol was destroying 'the good orders and discipline of the house' and ruined the men's health.

The drink/discipline/health nexus continued into the late-eighteenth century, with the hospital physician, Robert Robertson commenting that intemperance resulted in many deaths by way of drowning in ditches and other accidents but more importantly by the destruction of the interior of the body, as evidenced in his post-mortem examinations. Robertson complained that 'all the low arts imaginable are put in practice, to get liquor and sling the doctor, of which the natural consequences follow.'[58]

Ten years after the hospital first admitted pensioners the Council, on the advice of the physician and surgeon, opened a 'private' ward for those unable to take a turn at watch, attend chapel, and take their meals in the Hall. Many of these men 'by infirmity or weakness wet their Beds'. The private ward was on the ground floor ward and was considered part of the infirmary: it was under the control of the medics, who examined the nurses before they were permitted to serve in these wards. In addition, infirmary and private ward pensioners had to get permission from the medics to leave the hospital.[59] Men in the infirmary wore a red gown to distinguish them from the rest of the pensioners and thus aid in the prevention of their unauthorised departure.[60]

Eventually, the physician's authority was confirmed by order of the Directors of the Hospital. They ordered that the physician has the sole right to dispose of the pensioners in the infirmary and helpless/private wards and that the boatswain mates and nurses were to obey the physicians orders when they did not interfere with those of the commanding officer. In mid-century the medics pressed for a separate building for the infirmary, which was sanctioned and completed in 1771.[61]

One part of this process of medicalisation was the development of a medical monopoly. Seventeenth-century county pensioners were given money to help pay for their medical bills. Early on, hospital pensioners had leeway to pursue their own courses of treatment on the outside. Thomas Nichols, for example, was under the care of a Mrs Price of Deptford for his blindness in 1707.[62] This leeway to go outside the institution was, however, curtailed. Pensioners were punished if they resisted the course of treatment dictated by the hospital surgeon or physician, or sought alternative care outside the hospital. The buyer–seller relationship between patient and medical practitioner disappeared for disabled seamen while it remained predominant in society. One Roger Pannell, ordered to go to the surgeon to be bled in April of 1711 refused, saying 'he would not [go] for the surgeon had kill'd one man by letting his blood very lately'. The Council seriously considered expelling him, only to relent when Pannell apologised to the surgeon and the latter intervened on the pensioner's behalf.[63] In another example, Richard Mercer presented himself to the physician and surgeon in 1720 for treatment but was told he was not ill. He responded by going outside the hospital for treatment and medicines. He also went to the civil officers of the house and asked to be placed in a lower ward so that he could more easily enter and exit the institution. The civil officers agreed, only for the medics to protest in Council 'that the said Mercer has no distempers that may occasion his being admitted into the Infirmary'. The Council determined that Mercer had acted in contempt of the hospital officers 'by applying for Medicines abroad' and he was reprimanded.[64]

The medical monopoly included the imposition of novel treatments on pensioners with ruptures and other ailments by entrepreneurial medics – as discussed by Philip Mills in chapter 6. Greenwich, unlike the civilian hospitals of the Eighteenth century that catered particularly to the sick poor, was designed for the 'tedious incurable', thereby permitting military medics the opportunity to dissect, experiment on, and observe continuous subjects. This medical monopoly was such that Greenwich was to become, at the end of the eighteenth century, a significant site of research into geriatric medicine. The physician, Robert Robertson, examined thousands of men from the 1790s, dissecting, looking for reasons for death, and arguing for scientific observation as a method to aid in discovering interventionist medical procedures. It could be said that Robertson and later physicians at Chelsea such as Daniel McLachland, began the process of arguing in favour of transforming chronic conditions into acute curable diseases.[65] But that is another story. Study of the early life of the Greenwich Royal Hospital contributes to our knowledge of the development of hospitals and medicine in the eighteenth century. Until now, scholars have focused on the impact of private philanthropy and almost completely excluded these national military hospitals.[66] The inclusion of these hospitals alters the view that the development of hospitals in the eighteenth century was the product of civic philanthropy. With Greenwich and Chelsea, and later Haslar and Plymouth, the state is the creator and manager. Greenwich and Chelsea, as well as being more accessible for trained medical staff, presaged later developments in other hospitals. In these hospitals the control and influence of medics increased, which allowed the medicalisation of the institution and the objectification of the patient.

Confinement and negotiation

A persuasive case can be made that confinement was not a positive experience; that Greenwich was not a home for pensioners, but a monument for the Navy. The pensioners were not so much inhabitants as they were visitors, with only the officers, civilian staff, and medics given free movement and influence over the institution. The Council material confirms Christine Stevenson's application of the ideas of Bill Hillier and Julienne Hanson to this hospital and similar institutions: one who lives in a reversed, public building is not necessarily an inhabitant of that building.[67] The inhabitant is the one to have special access and control over the space, as did officers and medics at Greenwich.

Early on, pensioners were forced to remove the pictures they put on the walls, and the furniture they had brought in.[68] They were not permitted to show visitors around – only the porter could do that, and keep a portion of the gratuities.[69] When one visitor asked to see inside a pensioner's footlocker it was opened, despite the protests of the pensioner, who was subsequently punished.[70] After complaints by local ladies, pensioners were not permitted to walk in the park on Sundays.[71]

Sixty per cent of pensioners were married, thirty-five per cent with children. Pensioners' families were excluded from the wards and hall during meals.[72] Instead, wives and children were left to beg for leftovers at the gates.[73] When the town complained, the hospital ordered pensioners with families to either procure a certificate from another parish promising to provide for the family or 'see that they remove them elsewhere'.[74] For families, separation was evidently difficulty. On one occasion, a pensioner returned late to the hospital with the explanation that his wife had hidden his hospital clothes in order to prevent his return.[75]

The non-marrying rule was applied harshly. In one case, a superannuated nurse was discharged from her pension for marrying a pensioner.[76] Indeed, nurses and pensioners were prohibited from any 'private association' together, including kissing or drinking.[77]

Whereas, under the county scheme, pensioners had been free to work to supplement their pensions, this was curtailed. The Council forbade pensioners from engaging in any 'servile work' outside the hospital such as looking after horses and drawing drinks in alehouses. In so doing, the Council stated, the men spoiled the hospital's clothes and were regarded as 'a scandal and disgrace to the house'. The only exception to the rule permitted by the Council was that the pensioners remained free to wait on hospital officers.[78]

The seventeenth-century county pensioner was mobile and free, subject to little discipline: a vassal serving his master, a tenant at the feast if you will, treated as a member of the community of honour. His circumstances and behaviour were not looked into too closely. The Greenwich pensioner is confined, disciplined, treated as a cog in the machine of the modern standing armed forces; in perpetual service.

Colin Jones and others are right to point us in the direction of a close analysis of the way patients and pensioners negotiate the terms of their incarceration. Indeed, a close look at the Greenwich council records reveals that the men did negotiate their position in the institution, as had their predecessors within the context of the county scheme. That pensioners struggled against the harshness of the regime is clear from the *repeated* orders about matters such as remarriage, leaving the hospital on Sunday, and the porter being the only individual permitted to show the hospital to visitors for money.[79] The pensioners also used the Council to achieve some redress for themselves. Initially, officers and informers brought most allegations to the attention of the Council. This changed, with pensioners bringing their own concerns. The Council also took various complaints brought by infirmary patients against drunken, violent and/or thieving nurses, very seriously, and disciplined, transferred and/or expelled the latter.[80] A number of petty officers found themselves rejoining the ranks after being convicted of breach of orders on the complaint of an ordinary pensioner.[81]

Pensioners were adept at working the system in various ways, promising never to repeat certain behaviour, being submissive, then carrying on as before.[82] Some men collected pensions from the Chatham Chest at the same time as they were pensioners at Greenwich.[83] A number of pensioners also managed to get Council orders overturned by appealing to the Lords of the Admiralty.[84] Others applied to leave the hospital when employment opportunities presented themselves, and successfully returned to the hospital when age and service disabilities made further work impossible.[85]

Men mutinied. In the Council's first decade, for example, thirty-eight individuals were accused of mutiny, with fourteen expelled. Insubordination termed 'mutiny' included: denying authority of officers of the house (9 instances); threatening to go above the heads of house officers (5); not obeying officer(s) (14); complaining about food improperly — not taking it up first with the officers (12); disputing justice of punishment (1); speaking against Council in its presence (5); and in one case, stripping the hospital's clothes off before the hospital's Council.[86]

In one example a pensioner, struck by a Lieutenant Smyth for being out of line when marching to the chapel, complained loudly and the call went up for mutiny: 'one and all'. When the officer demanded who called for mutiny, one James Johnson:

> [S]tep'd up to him & flourishing his stick said he was the man & Damn him he [the officer] had struck a better man than himself & that they did not come here to be beat nor wou'd not & if the Men wou'd be ruled by him, they shou'd loose their lives before they wou'd suffer it.[87]

The man who was struck and Johnson were expelled. This was despite the fact that all but one of the other officers present at the time refused to help

Smyth, indicating their sympathy with the men. They left him to the mercy of the pensioners. Subsequently, the Council ordered that anyone refusing to assist any officer in 'quelling any mutiny, Riot, or disturbance' shall be adjudged mutinous themselves.[88]

N.A.M. Rodger in *The Wooden World* posits social cohesion and lack of class awareness in the Navy prior to the last two decades of the eighteenth century. Perhaps older men were more likely to feel division, given their long service.[89] Certainly, many did not seem to feel part of a happy family, as Newell views the hospital. Several pensioners complained about the lack of justice in the house, and expressed disrespect for the officers. A pensioner on guard, who was supposed to turn away the poor and vagrants from the hospital instead turned away all comers. He stated that he 'did not know one Gentleman from another'.[90] I don't think this is what Rodger meant by lack of class awareness!

Pensioners also combined with some success when they complained to the Council. An example is their ongoing concern over the quality and quantity of their food. Concerned about the cheese rations men went into town in order to get their portions of cheese weighed, coming back with certificates proving inadequate rations. Embarrassed, the Council ordered the purchase of a set of scales for this purpose that the pensioners could use within the institution.[91] The Council also allowed the pensioners to take turns in the kitchens watching the servants to ensure that the food was prepared and apportioned correctly. In the kitchen, at least, the pensioner as visitor had become the pensioner as inhabitant.

Conclusion

In conclusion, an examination of the inner life of Greenwich via its Council records alters the historiographical arguments and cultural traditions that celebrate Greenwich (and Chelsea) as both safe havens for the indigent and the incarnation of progress.

During its early years, almshouse, monastic, and shipboard models influenced the inner life of the institution, with medical considerations increasingly shaping a new type of institution that would be constructed at other locations: Haslar and Plymouth being examples. In time, Greenwich's inner life thus changed, with more emphasis on medical care for the men. This change then informed the architecture, with, for example, separate infirmaries built. For the patients this was a mixed blessing, with the men becoming subject to the introduction of a medical monopoly. At Haslar the Greenwich clerk was brought in at its inception to help form its administrative systems.[92] Haslar and Plymouth were run by hospital councils, chaired by physicians. In addition, the same architectural form was utilised as at Greenwich, with each side of Haslar consisting of a double row of buildings to allow for free movement of air.

To understand the shift from a county out-pension scheme in the seventeenth century to Greenwich and Chelsea – palaces for paupers – it is necessary to understand the shift in the nature of power relations. Greenwich and Chelsea promised greater and visible central control of ex-servicemen. In this political area as in others most county authorities were happy to transfer onto central funds – in time, a system of deficit financing ultimately borne by customs and excise duties – a burden previously borne on local rates – politically unpopular taxes on land. The development of hospitals is thus not only about civic philanthropy but also about the manifestation of the domestic face of the fiscal military state. In the wider European context this analysis accords with Colin Jones' examination of military medicine and the French hospital for disabled veterans. These institutions were police operations first and foremost, and it is no accident that medicalisation – and patient objectification – occurred early relative to other, civilian, hospitals.

The disabled pensioners never gave up negotiating improvements to the terms of their incarceration, despite the impediment of living in a national monument. Their stories are many and colourful. In the 1860s, a Parliamentary committee explicitly commented that the men preferred out-relief to 'imprisonment' in a hospital. The men were freed, given out-pensions, and the hospital turned into a naval college.[93]

Notes

1. J. Bold, *Greenwich: An Architectural History of the Royal Hospital for Seamen and the Queen's House* (New Haven and London: Yale University Press, 2000) and C. Stevenson, *Medicine and Magnificence: British Hospital and Asylum Architecture, 1660–1815* (New Haven and London: Yale University Press, 2000)

2. G. Hudson, 'Disabled Veterans and the State in Early Modern England' in D. Gerber (ed.), *Disabled Veterans in History* (Ann Arbor: University of Michigan, 2000), 117–44; and G. Hudson, 'Ex-Servicemen, War Widows and the English County Pension Scheme, 1593–1679' (unpublished DPhil thesis, University of Oxford, 1995).

3. J.J. Keevil, *Medicine and the Navy 1200–1900, Vol. I, 1200–1649* (Edinburgh: Livingstone, 1957), 52, 54. So too, John Childs, in his two books about the armies of Charles II and James II, dismissed the Elizabethan county pension scheme and the system of retaining old and disabled soldiers in the army as being two systems which combined to provide 'erratic' provision for soldiers. Only the lucky got a pension or a place. He concluded that 'a combination of these evils resulted in the foundation of the

Chelsea military hospital'. J. Childs, *The Army of Charles II* (London: Routledge, 1976), 53–6; *idem, The Army, James II, and the Glorious Revolution* (Manchester: Manchester University Press, 1980), 35–6.

4. Keevil, *ibid.* 193, 197.

5. J.J. Keevil, *Medicine and the Navy 1200–1900, Vol. II, 1649–1714* (Edinburgh: Livingstone, 1958), 24, 75.

6. C.H. Firth, *Cromwell's Army* (London: Methuen, 1962 edn), 270; my emphasis.

7. G. Hutt, *Papers Illustrative of the Origins and Early History of the Royal Hospital at Chelsea* (London, 1872), 41.

8. Firth, *op. cit.* (note 6), 270.

9. J.L.S. Coulter and C. Lloyd, *Medicine and the Navy 1200–1900, Vol. 3, 1714–1815* (Edinburgh: Livingstone, 1961), 206.

10. P. Newell, *Greenwich Hospital: A Royal Foundation, 1692–1983* (London: The Trustees of Greenwich Hospital, 1984), 35.

11. J. Ehrman, *The Navy in the War of William III, 1689–1697* (Cambridge: Cambridge University Press, 1953), 444. Ehrman was citing D. Matthew, *The Naval Heritage* (London: Collins, 1945), 62.

12. Corporation of London Record Office, 35B, military – and naval – maimed soldiers and sailors annual list of pensioners 1671/2–1678/9; Greater London Record Office, MJ/SBB/263, fs. 38–45; Gloucester Record Office, QSO, Order Book 1, 1672–1681, n.f. Hilary 1672/3; Somerset Record Office, Q/SO 6, f. 336; Shropshire Record Office, Quarter Sessions 177; Devon Record Office, Q/S, 1/11, n.f.; Wiltshire Record Office, A1/160/3, n.f.; Cheshire Record Office, QJF 100/2, f. 32, 100/3, f. 45; West Riding of Yorkshire Record Office, QS10/5, fs. 97–100. For the population of Cheshire see G. Walker, 'Crime, Gender and Social Order in Early Modern Cheshire' (unpublished PhD thesis, University of Liverpool, 1994), 110–11, n10.; for the population of London and Middlesex see R. Finley and B. Shearer, 'Population Growth and Suburban Expansion' in A.L. Beier and R. Findlay (eds), *The Making of the Metropolis: London, 1500-1700* (London: Longman, 1986), 37–59; for the West Riding, J.D. Purdy, 'The Hearth Tax Returns for Yorkshire' (unpublished MPhil thesis, University of Leeds, 1976), 316–17 cited in R. Bennet, 'Enforcing the Law in Revolutionary England—Yorkshire *c.*1640–*c.*1660 (unpublished PhD thesis, King's College London, 1988), 23. For the populations of the other jurisdictions see A. Whiteman (ed.), *The Compton Census of 1671: A Critical Edition* (London: British Academy, 1986), cx, cxi, lxxv. I accepted Whiteman's recommendation of forty per cent as it allows for the under-enumeration of communicants.

13. The National Archives [hereafter NA], Treas. 1/139, cited in R.E. Scouller, *The Armies of Queen Anne,* (Oxford: Oxford University Press, 1966), 334.

14. Hutt, *op. cit.* (note 7), 13.

15. Bod. Rawl. A 195A, ff. 249-54. See also Keevil, *op. cit.* (note 5), 105–6, 127.

16. J. Ehrman, *op. cit.* (note 11), 444–5; Coulter and Lloyd, *op. cit.* (note 9), 119, 192.

17. R. Porter, 'Madness and its Institutions', in A. Wear (ed.), *Medicine in Society* (Cambridge: Cambridge University Press, 1992), 277–301, 282–3.

18. Childs, *Charles II, op. cit.* (note 3), 103; *idem, James II, op. cit.* (note 3), 84; J.H. Plumb, *The Growth of Political Stability in England 1675–1725* (London: Macmillan, 1967), 24-5; G.A. Jacobsen, *William Blathwayt* (New Haven: Yale University Press, 1932), 223–4.

19. *HMC*, Downshire Mss, Trumbull Papers, Vol. I, pt I, 140, 163 cited in Jacobsen, *op. cit.* (note 18), 224.

20. *A Pattern of a Well-Constituted and Well-Governed Hospital: Or, a Brief Description of the Building, and Full Relation of the Establishment, Constitution, Discipline, Oeconomy and Administration of the Government of the Royal Hospital of the Invalids Near Paris. Partly Translated from a Large Book Printed Some Years ago in French; And Partly Extracted out of Some Other Manuscript Relations Never Before Published* (London, 1695).

21. B. Jestaz, *L'Hôtel et l'Eglise des Invalides* (Paris: Picard, 1990), 27.

22. *Pattern, op. cit.* (note 20), 169

23. C. Jones, *The Charitable Imperative: Hospitals and Nursing in Ancien Régime and Revolutionary France* (London: Routledge, 1989), 218.

24. *Ibid.*, 219–20.

25. *Ibid.*, 19.

26. *Ibid.*, 19; I. Woloch, *The French Veteran from the Revolution to the Restoration* (Chapel Hill: University of North Carolina Press, 1980), xvi, 316.

27. Jones, *op. cit.* (note 23), 38.

28. M. Foucault, *Discipline and Punish: The Birth of the Prison* (New York: Vintage, 1979), 139, 184–5. See also *idem, Madness and Civilization* (New York: Vintage, 1965); *idem, The Order of Things: An Archaeology of the Human Sciences* (New York: Vintage, 1970); *idem, The History of Sexuality, Vol. I* (New York: Vintage, 1979); M. Foucault and C. Gorden (eds), *Power/Knowledge: Selected Interviews and Other writings* (New York: Pantheon, 1980), 'The Politics of Health in the Eighteenth Century', 106–82; M. Hewitt, 'Bio-Politics and Social Policy: Foucault's Account of Welfare' in M. Featherstone, M. Hepworth and B.S. Turner (eds), *The Body: Social Process and Cultural Theory* (London: Sage, 1991), 225–55; G. Gutting, 'Foucault and the History of Madness', in G. Gutting (ed.), *The Cambridge Companion to Foucault* (Cambridge: Cambridge University Press, 1994), 47–70; J. Rouse, 'Power/Knowledge', *Cambridge Companion*, 92–114.

29. Jones, *op. cit.* (note 23), 8.

30. *Ibid.*, 9. For a discussion of 'Hospital History: New Sources and Methods' see G.B. Risse, R. Porter and A. Wear (eds), *Problems and Methods in the History of Medicine* (London: Croom, 1987), 175–203. See also R. Porter, 'The Patient's View: Doing Medical History from Below', *Theory and Society*, 14, 2 (March 1985), 175–98; L. Granshaw, 'Introduction' in L. Granshaw and R. Porter (eds), *The Hospital in History* (London: Routledge, 1989), 1–18 ; M. Fissell, *Patients, Power, and the Poor in Eighteenth-Century Bristol* (Cambridge: Cambridge University Press), Ch. 8, 'The Patient's Perspective', 148–70..

31. NA, SP 28/140, 141 A; Firth, *op. cit.* (note 6), 264–5; E. Gruber von Arni, *Justice to the Maimed Soldier* (Aldershot: Ashgate, 2001); Keevil, *op. cit.* (note 5), section I.

32. NA, ADM 73/36–39, 51–3 (pensioner entry books); For an example of an admiralty order concerning a disabled man, the requirement for a medical examination and the test of disability to work see NA, ADM 2/1133, 200 (14 February 1716/17).

33. Hutt, *op. cit.* (note 7), 104; P. Newell, *op. cit.* (note 10), 31, 62–3, 67, 69–70, 78, 79, 113, 116–18, 122, 124, 128, 150, 204; NA, ADM 65, 66, 68; Hudson, 'Ex-servicemen', *op. cit.* (note 2), Ch. 1.

34. NA, ADM, 67, 80/69.

35. NA, ADM 67/119, 70, 1 August 1707.

36. Example of the rare use of an oath: NA, ADM 67/120, 170, 16 March 1714/15.

37. NA, ADM, 80/69, 30, 24 April 1711.

38. NA, ADM 80/69, 45-49 25 May 1715); 59, 5 September 1716.

39. NA, ADM, 80/69, 22, 20 December 1708.

40. Sample: PR0, ADM 67/119, August 1705–August 1707, and ADM, 67/120 August 1713–August 1715.

41. Examples: Nurses in stocks, NA, ADM 67/119, 29, 2 December 1706, 38 27 January 1706/7; chaining, ADM, 67/120, 49 4 May 1711; begging forgiveness on knees, ADM, 67/119, 65 12 July 1707.

42. NA, ADM 67/119, 120.

43. NA, ADM 73/36.

44. NA, ADM, 67/119, 24, 25 September 1706; 46, 21 March 1706/07; 101, 2 March 1707/8; 122, 17 September 1708; 67/120, 30, 27 October 1710; 34, 19 December 1710; 79, 18 January 1711/12; 123, 2 February 1712/13; 142, 21 January 1713/14.

45. NA, ADM 80/69, 43, 20 May 1715

46. NA, ADM 80/69, 41, 13 April 1715; 45, 23 May1715; Newell, *op. cit.* (note 10), 82.

47. NA, ADM 67/121, 344, 16 March 1719.

48. NA, ADM 73/36 (entry book, which noted those expelled and those run on the books).

49. For an excellent discussion of the architectural influences of the monastery and almshouse at Greenwich see C. Stevenson, *Medicine and Magnificence: British Hospital and Asylum Architecture, 1660–1815* (New Haven and London: Yale University Press, 2000), 50.

50. J. Keevil, *op. cit.* (note 5), 246–7, 255–6. Other medical officers at Greenwich Hospital at this time including the physicians Drs S. Cade (appointed 1695), W. Maundy (1713), W. Oliver (1714) and R. Morton (1716). Surgeons were J. Christie (1704) and I. Rider (1714).

51. NA, ADM 80/69, 57, 23 May 1716.

52. NA, ADM 80/69, 55, 25 January 1715/16; 59, 5 September 1716.

53. NA, ADM 67/122, 154, 13 May 1724.

54. NA, ADM 80/69, 11, 11 December 1706.

55. NA, ADM 80/69, 24–5, 15 November 1709.

56. NA, ADM 67/121, 140, 22 February 1716/17.

57. NA, ADM 67/121, 153, 18 April 1717.

58. R. Robertson, *Observations on Diseases Incident to Seamen: Whether Employed on, Or Retired from Actual Service, Infirmities or Old Age*, Vol. IV (London: T. Cadell and W. Davies, 1870), 778.

59. NA, ADM 80/69, 37-38, 23 February 1714/15; 67/122, 275, 6 March 1726/27.

60. NA, ADM 67/122, 279, 28 April 1727.

61. NA, ADM 67/22 A, 27 November 1729 & 15 July 1730 (Director's minutes).

62. NA, ADM 67/119, 107, 16 April 1707

63. NA, ADM 67/120, 45, 4 April 1711.

64. NA, ADM 67/121, 357, 1 June 1720.

65. S. Katz, *Disciplining Old Age: The Formation of Gerontological Knowledge* (Charlottesville and London: University of Virginia Press, 1996), 87.

66. See, for example, G.B. Risse, 'Medicine in the Age of Enlightenment', 149–96, esp. 178–9, and L. Granshaw, 'The Rise of the Modern Hospital in Britain', 197–218, esp. 199, 202–4 in A. Wear (ed.), *Medicine in Society: Historical Essays* (Cambridge: Cambridge University Press, 1992). See also L. Granshaw and R. Porter, *The Hospital in History* (London: Routledge, 1989).

67. C. Stevenson, *Medicine and Magnificence* (New Haven: Yale University Press, 2000), 43; B. Hillier and J. Hanson, *The Social Logic of Space* (Cambridge: Cambridge University Press, 1984).

68. NA, ADM 80/69, 20, 5 December 1707.

69. NA, ADM 80/69, 23–4, 28 July 1709.

70. NA, ADM 67/119, 93, 3 January 1707/08.

71. NA, ADM 67/121, 78, 18 April 1716.

72. NA, ADM 80/69, 58, 25 July 1716.

73. NA, ADM 80/69, 49, 4 June 1715.

74. NA, ADM 80/69, 71–2, 30 May 1718.

75. NA, ADM 67/121, 101, 8 August 1716.

76. NA, ADM 67/120, 31, 8 November 1710.

77. NA, ADM 80/69, 18–19, 23 June 1707.

78. NA, ADM, 80/69, 51, 14 September 1715.

79. Examples: remarriage, NA, ADM 80/69, 43, 20 May 1715; 80/69, 72, 30 May 1718; leaving the hospital on Sundays, NA, ADM 80/69, 60, 17 October 1716, 78, 3 June 1719; Porter the only person permitted to show the hospital, ADM, 80/69, 76–7, 8 April 1719.

80. Example: NA, ADM 67/119, 8, 21 October 1705.

81. NA, ADM 67/119, 120. Example: 67/119, 65–6, 5 July 1707.

82. Example: NA, ADM 67/122, 183, 29 January 1724/25.

83. NA, ADM 2/1133, 99, 30 June 1711; 127, November 1712.

84. NA, ADM 67/122, 142, 31 January 1723/24.

85. Examples: NA, ADM 67/122, 261, 14 December 1726; 2/1133, 314, 11 April 1727.

86. NA, ADM 67/119 & 120. The Council at Greenwich was especially severe in punishing mutiny when pensioners threatened to petition the Admiralty or insulted members of the Council. N.A.M. Rodger maintains that mutiny was 'part of a system of social relations which provided an effective working compromise between demands of necessity and humanity, a means of reconciling the Navy's need of obedience and efficiency with the individuals grievances.' Words as well as actions, from individuals *and* groups, could be mutinous. N.A.M. Rodger, *The Wooden World: An Anatomy of the Georgian Navy* (Glasgow: William Collins, 1986), 243–4.

87. NA, ADM, 67/120, 60, 29 August 1711; 2/1133, 102, 12 September 1711.

88. NA, ADM 80/69, 67, 20 July 1717.

89. Rodger, *op. cit.* (note 86), 237.

90. NA, ADM 67/120, 49, 4 May 1711.

91. NA, ADM 80/69, 65, 20 February 1716.

92. Lloyd and Coulter, *op. cit.* (note 9), 215–16.

93. NA, ADM 67/15.

Notes on Contributors

James D. Alsop is professor in the History Department at McMaster University (Canada). His research has been focused upon social, administrative, and medical topics for early-modern England and the Atlantic world. He has been the recipient of Wellcome Trust and Associated Medical Services grants on various medical history topics and is currently involved in several research projects, including the treatment of malaria in seventeenth-century England and public health in the New South.

Patricia Kathleen Crimmin was formerly a senior lecturer in history at Royal Holloway College (University of London). Since retirement, she has been Caird Senior Research Fellow at the National Maritime Museum, Vice-President of the Navy Records Society, and an honorary research associate at the University of Greenwich's Maritime Institute. In addition, she has been a member of the Council of the Society for Nautical Research. Crimmin has published on various aspects of naval history in the eighteenth century. In recent years she has worked on subjects related to the health of seamen in that period including the care and treatment of British held prisoners-of-war (1793–1815), and on the fifteen volumes of Nelson manuscripts in the Wellcome Library for the History and Understanding of Medicine.

Eric Gruber von Arni is a freelance historian specialising in the history of military hospitals and military nursing. He has published *Justice to the Maimed Soldier: Nursing, Medical Care and Welfare for Sick and Wounded Soldiers and their Families during the English Civil Wars and Interregnum, 1642–1660* (Aldershot: Ashgate, 2001), co-authored (with G. Searle) *Sub-Cruce Candida: One Hundred Years of Army Nursing* (Aldershot: QARANC Association, 2002), and (with C.S. Scott and A. Turton), *Edgehill: The Battle Reintrepeted* (Barnsley: Pen & Sword, 2004). His most recent book is *Hospital Care and the British Standing Army, 1660–1714* (Aldershot: Ashgate, 2006). He is the official historian of Queen Alexandra's Royal Army Nursing Corps, a Trustee of the Army Medical Services Museum, and also an honorary research fellow at the

Centre for the History of Medicine at the School of Medicine at the University of Birmingham.

Mark Harrison is Professor of the History of Medicine, and Director of the Wellcome Unit for the History of Medicine, at the University of Oxford. Harrison has published widely on the history of disease and medicine, especially in relation to the history of war and imperialism from the seventeenth to the twentieth centuries. He is currently working on a history of medicine and British imperial expansion, *c.*1700–1850. He was awarded the 2004 Templer Medal for his book *Medicine and Victory: British Military Medicine in World War Two* (Oxford: Oxford University Press, 2004).

Geoffrey L. Hudson is Assistant Professor of the History of Medicine in the Northern Ontario School of Medicine (Lakehead and Laurentian Universities, Canada). His research interests are in the areas of the social history of medicine, as well as war and society. He is currently completing a study of war and disability in early-modern Britain.

Paul E. Kopperman is a professor of history at Oregon State University. Several of his published articles are on social and medical aspects of the eighteenth-century British Army including a recent article entitled 'The Medical Aspect of the Braddock and Forbes Expeditions', *Pennsylvania History,* 71 (2004), 257–83. He is the author of two books: *Braddock at the Monongahela* (London: Feffer and Simons, 1977) and *Sir Robert Heath, 1575–1649: Window on an Age* (Woodbridge: Boydell Press, 1989); a third work, *Theory and Practice in Eighteenth Century British Medicine, with Particular Reference to 'Regimental Practice', by John Buchanan, MD,* is awaiting publication.

Margarette Lincoln is Director of Research and Planning at the National Maritime Museum, Greenwich, and Visiting Fellow at Goldsmiths College, University of London. She has published widely in eighteenth-century studies, including *Representing the Navy: British Sea Power 1750–1815* (Aldershot: Ashgate, 2002). She edited the catalogue for the Museum's special exhibition, 'Nelson and Napoleon' in 2005. Her book *Naval Wives and Mistresses, 1750–1815,* which explores the domestic role of these women and their social position within the context of Britain's growing imperial power, will be published in 2007.

Philip R. Mills graduated from the University of York with a BA in History in 1997, before completing an MSc in the History of Science, Technology and Medicine the following year at Imperial College, London. Subsequently, he spent over two years full time researching a doctoral thesis on British military medicine in the eighteenth century at The Wellcome Trust Centre for the History of Medicine at UCL, before leaving to start a new career. He currently works as an analyst developer for a major investment bank in London.

Christine Stevenson is a senior lecturer at the Courtauld Institute of Art, University of London. Stevenson began teaching at the Institute in 2002, after ten years as a lecturer at the University of Reading, and previously, as an academic editor at the then Wellcome Institute for the History of Medicine, and Macmillan Publishers. She is the author of *Medicine and Magnificence: British Hospital and Asylum Architecture, 1660–1815* (New Haven: Yale University Press, 2000). Stevenson is now writing a book about the politics of architecture in Restoration London.

Index